LIPPINCOTT'S REVIEW SERIES

Mental Health and Psychiatric Nursing

FOURTH EDITION

Ann Isaacs, RN, MS, APRN-BC
Professor
Luzerne County Community College
Nanticoke, Pa.

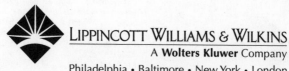
LIPPINCOTT WILLIAMS & WILKINS
A **Wolters Kluwer** Company
Philadelphia • Baltimore • New York • London
Buenos Aires • Hong Kong • Sydney • Tokyo

Staff

Executive Publisher
Judith A. Schilling McCann, RN, MSN

Senior Acquisitions Editor
Elizabeth Nieginski

Editorial Director
David Moreau

Clinical Director
Joan M. Robinson, RN, MSN

Senior Art Director
Arlene Putterman

Art Directors
Elaine Kasmer, Mary Ludwicki

Electronic Project Manager
John Macalino

Editorial Project Manager
Coleen M.F. Stern

Clinical Project Manager
Beverly Ann Tscheschlog, RN, BS

Editor
Diane M. Labus

Copy Editors
Kim Bilotta (supervisor), Karen C. Comerford,
Amanda Bradford Cortright, Pamela Wingrod

Designer
Lynn Foulk

Digital Composition Services
Diane Paluba (manager), Joyce Rossi Biletz

Manufacturing
Patricia K. Dorshaw (director), Beth J. Welsh

Editorial Assistants
Megan Aldinger, Karen J. Kirk, Linda Ruhf

Indexer
Karen C. Comerford

LRSMHPN010505 – 020706

Library of Congress Cataloging-in-Publication Data

Mental health and psychiatric nursing. — 4th ed.
p. ; cm. — (Lippincott's review series)
Rev. ed. of: Mental health and psychiatric nursing /
Ann Isaacs. 3rd ed. c2001.
Includes bibliographical references and index.
1. Psychiatric nursing — Examinations, questions, etc. I.
Isaacs, Ann. Mental health and psychiatric nursing. II.
Lippincott Williams & Wilkins. III. Series. [DNLM: 1.
Mental Disorders — nursing — Examination Questions. 2.
Psychiatric Nursing — Examination Questions.]
RC440.L57 2006
616.89'0231 — dc22
ISBN 1-58255-454-4 (alk. paper)   2005002597

Introduction

Lippincott's Review Series is designed to help you in your study of the key subject areas in nursing. The series consists of eight books, one in each core nursing subject area:

> *Critical Care Nursing*
> *Fluids and Electrolytes*
> *Maternal-Newborn Nursing*
> *Medical-Surgical Nursing*
> *Mental Health and Psychiatric Nursing*
> *Pathophysiology*
> *Pediatric Nursing*
> *Pharmacology*

Lippincott's Review Series was planned and developed in response to your requests for comprehensive outline review books that address each major subject area and also contain a self-test mechanism. Each book is a complete source for review and self-assessment of a single core subject — all eight together provide an excellent comprehensive review of entry-level nursing.

Each book is all-inclusive of the content addressed in major textbooks. The content outline review uses a consistent nursing process format throughout and addresses nursing care for well and ill clients. Also included are necessary teaching and other concepts, such as growth and development, nutrition, pharmacology, body structures and functions, and pathophysiology. Special features include:

• **Nursing process overview sections** ✪ review each step of the nursing process for the system or group of disorders in discussion. These reviews improve your ability to apply principles to practice by highlighting common assessment findings, diagnoses, goals, interventions, and outcomes.

• **Nursing alerts** ✋ are fundamental guidelines you can follow to ensure safe and effective care.

• **Drug charts** ⊘ provide quick reference for medications that are commonly used in treating the disorders discussed within a given chapter. The drug classification, indications, and selected nursing interventions are provided.

• **Key questions** boxes ⓠ present assessment questions crucial to patient evaluation.

• **Client and family teaching** boxes detail health teaching information, which may be applied in the clinical setting.

• **Chapter study questions** help you chart your progress through each chapter. Answer keys are provided with rationales for correct and incorrect responses.

• **Comprehensive examination** mimics the *National Council Licensure Examination* (NCLEX) and allows you to assess your strengths and weaknesses. An answer key is provided with rationales for correct and incorrect responses.

• **Alternate-format questions**, designed after the NCLEX's new-style questions, challenge you to grasp the complete clinical picture.

• **Accompanying CD-ROM** provides 210 additional NCLEX-style questions so you can practice computer adaptive test-taking skills. Answers are provided with rationales for correct and incorrect responses.

You can use the books in this series in several different ways. Overall, you can use them as subject reviews to augment general study throughout your basic nursing program and as a review to prepare for the NCLEX-RN. How you use each book depends on your individual needs and preferences, and on whether you review each chapter systematically or concentrate only on those chapters with subject areas you find particularly challenging. You may instead choose to use the comprehensive examination as a self-assessment opportunity to evaluate your knowledge base before you review the content outline. Likewise, you can use the study questions for pre- or post-testing after study, followed by the comprehensive examination as a means of evaluating your knowledge of an entire subject area.

Regardless of how you use the books, one of the strengths of the series is the self-assessment opportunity it offers, in addition to guidance in studying and reviewing content. The chapter study questions and comprehensive examination questions have been carefully developed to cover all topics in the outline review. Unlike the NCLEX, which tests the cumulative knowledge needed for safe practice by an entry-level nurse, these practice tests systematically evaluate the knowledge base that serves as the building block for the entire nursing educational process. In this way, you can prepare for the NCLEX throughout your course of study. Good study habits throughout your educational program are not only the best way to ensure success, but will also prove the most beneficial way to prepare for the licensing examination.

Keep in mind, these books are not intended to replace formal learning. They cannot substitute for textbook reading, discussion with instructors, or class attendance. Every effort has been made to provide accurate and current information, but class attendance and interaction with an instructor will provide invaluable information not found in books. Used correctly, these books will help you increase understanding, improve comprehension, evaluate strengths and weaknesses in areas of knowledge, increase productive study time, and, as a result, help you improve your grades.

Dedication and acknowledgments

To my husband, Bob; son, Jeff; daughter-in-law, Jaime; son, Dennis; and grandson, Taylor —
thank you for your love and support.

To all my LCCC students, past, present, and future —
thank you for your interest and questions.

I would like to thank Beverly Ann Tscheschlog, Clinical Editor, and the staff at Lippincott Williams & Wilkins for their careful editing and helpful suggestions.

I would also like to thank the following individuals, who reviewed the CD-ROM material: Linda Carman Copel, PhD, RN, CS, DAPA, Associate Professor at Villanova (Pa.) University College of Nursing, and Connie S. Heflin, RN, MSN, Professor of Nursing at West Kentucky Community and Technical College, Paducah, Ky.

Contents

1 Introduction to Mental Health and Psychiatric Nursing

I. EVOLUTION OF MENTAL HEALTH TREATMENT

A. Pre-1960

1. Treatment was provided in large mental hospitals (state or private) usually located away from well-populated areas.
2. Length of stay was typically prolonged; few mechanisms for follow-up care after discharge existed.
3. Clients commonly became dependent and institutionalized; they were not active participants in their health care and treatment.
4. Family members were not part of the treatment team.

B. 1960 to 1970

1. The Civil Rights movement of the 1960s served as a catalyst for focusing on the rights of the mentally ill.
2. The Community Mental Health Centers Act (1963) dramatically affected delivery of mental health services.
3. Focus and funding for treatment shifted from large mental hospitals to newly established community mental health centers that provided the following services:
   a. **Emergency care:** immediate assessment and initiation of appropriate treatment
   b. **24-hour inpatient care:** hospital-based care for symptom stabilization (short-term care)
   c. **Partial hospitalization:** treatment programs for individuals requiring daily support but not 24-hour hospital care; allowed clients to participate in various therapies (group or individual therapy, social skills training) for 6 to 8 hours per day
   d. **Outpatient care:** assessment, psychotherapeutic support, and medication management; clients seen for 1 to 2 hours per week
   e. **Consultation and education:** outreach programs for community groups on mental health topics (training for police on handling rape trauma, training for employers to assist employees with alcohol problems)

C. 1970 to 1980

1. Treatment shifted from long-term hospital care to shorter inpatient stays, followed by community-based treatment after discharge.
2. Client populations decreased in large mental hospitals, forcing many hospitals to close.
3. Community mental health centers were often unable to provide services for the resulting greater numbers of clients.
4. Homelessness became a problem for people with persistent chronic mental illness who lacked family resources and adequate social support.

D. 1980 to 1990

1. The high cost of health care and the need for cost containment became national issues, leading to the establishment of **managed care systems,** which oversee the relationship among payers, providers, and consumers of health care.

    a. These systems monitor distribution of services, provider care, and treatment outcomes.

    b. The goal of managed care is to decrease cost while promoting quality of service.

    c. Under these systems, managers and insurers of health care monitor and often dictate the relationship between providers and consumers of health care.

  2. Types of managed care systems include:

    a. **Health maintenance organizations (HMOs),** which offer a preset fee for clients in a particular population in exchange for delivery of health care services (by a provider) during a given time period

    b. **Independent practice organizations,** in which groups of health care providers contract with HMOs

    c. **Preferred provider organizations (PPOs),** in which an HMO approves provider groups to provide services to its client population

E. 1990 to 2000

  1. Significant changes in the delivery of mental health treatment occurred.

  2. Managed care incorporated several new structures and services:

    a. **Case management:** involves assignment of a case manager to coordinate services for individual clients and collaborate with a multidisciplinary team

    b. **Critical pathways** and **care maps:** serve as clinical management tools to designate the organization, sequence, and timing of interventions provided by a treatment team for an identified client disorder

    c. **Population-based community care:** focuses on primary preventive services and not just illness-based care; includes identification of high-risk groups and education for lifestyle changes to prevent illness

  3. Alternative settings were designed to provide treatment and tertiary prevention (reducing the severity of the mental health problem and helping the client to maintain the highest functioning capacity) in the least restrictive environment, including:

    a. Mental health centers and community crisis centers

    b. Short-term inpatient psychiatric units located in community hospitals

    c. Partial hospitalization and day-care programs

    d. Residential treatment programs in halfway houses, board-and-care homes, and foster homes

    e. Mobile crisis units and homeless shelters

    f. Clubhouse programs offering transitional services to promote independent community living

    g. Prisons

    h. Nursing homes

  4. The Americans with Disabilities Act (1990) helped ensure that people with disabilities, including mental illnesses, can fully participate in the economic and social mainstream of society.

  5. Growth of the consumer movement led to national changes.

   a. The National Alliance of the Mentally Ill helped remove the stigma of mental illness and provided local community support for mentally ill people and their families.

   b. Other national and local organizations lobbied to increase funding for the research and treatment of mental illness.

  6. During the "Decade of the Brain," medical advances and genetic research led to profound knowledge about the workings of the brain, reshaping our understanding of the causes and treatment of mental illness.

F. 2000 to present

  1. The **recovery and rehabilitation model,** which was founded on the beliefs of individual client empowerment and control, focuses on prevention or reduction of impairment in clients with severe, persistent mental illness.

  2. Assertive community treatment uses a team approach to provide comprehensive, community-based treatment and rehabilitation services for clients with severe, persistent mental illness.

  3. Evidence-based practice integrates clinical expertise with the best clinical research evidence and incorporates the use of clinical practice guidelines, critical pathways, and clinical algorithms.

  4. Increased awareness of cultural diversity has contributed to the use of **complementary and alternative medicine** health care practices in treating mental illnesses.

II. HISTORY OF PSYCHIATRIC NURSING

A. Key figures

  1. Florence Nightingale was the founder of modern nursing and author of the first nursing text, *Notes on Nursing,* published in 1859.

  2. Harriet Bailey wrote the first psychiatric nursing textbook, *Nursing in Mental Diseases,* published in 1920.

  3. Hildegarde Peplau wrote *Interpersonal Relations in Nursing,* a landmark book published in 1952 that described a framework for psychiatric nursing practice; her emphasis on nurse-patient relationships and theoretical constructs to explain patient problems provided the foundation for psychiatric nursing practice.

B. Nursing organizations

  1. The National League for Nursing (NLN), established in 1937, recommended the inclusion of mental health and psychiatric nursing in nursing school curricula.

  2. The American Nurses Association (ANA), founded in 1958, established the Conference Group on Psychiatric Nursing.

   a. The Conference Group worked to define the practice of psychiatric-mental health nursing.

   b. In 1973, the ANA was the first to publish standards of mental health and psychiatric nursing practice; revised standards were published in 1982, 1994, and 2000.

c. In 2000, the ANA and the Coalition of Psychiatric Nursing Organizations jointly revised and updated a description of two levels of psychiatric and mental health nurse practice, the **generalist** and the **specialist,** which were originally defined in 1994.

III. CURRENT PSYCHIATRIC AND MENTAL HEALTH NURSING PRACTICE

A. Psychiatric-mental health nurse generalist

1. Education required is a baccalaureate degree in nursing.
2. Certification involves a formal process regulated by the American Nurses Credentialing Center (ANCC) that validates clinical competence; designation following certification is *RN, C.*
3. A generalist works with individual clients, families, groups, and the community to assess mental health needs, develop diagnoses, and plan, implement, and evaluate nursing care.
4. Focus of care covers the spectrum of mental health and psychiatric concerns: health promotion and maintenance; intake screening and evaluation; case management; provision of a therapeutic environment (milieu therapy); teaching clients and assisting them with self-care activities; administering and monitoring psychobiological treatment regimens; crisis intervention and counseling; and outreach activities in the home and community.
5. Practice settings include hospitals, home health agencies, employee assistance programs, mental health clinics, HMOs, primary care centers, homeless clinics, senior centers, emergency and crisis centers, daycare centers, schools, and prisons.

B. Psychiatric-mental health nurse specialist

1. Education required is a master's degree in psychiatric–mental health nursing.
   a. A **psychiatric nurse practitioner** is an advanced-practice RN (APN or APRN) with a master's degree who provides primary care; individual state nursing practice acts govern the scope of practice, including the nurse's ability to prescribe drugs.
   b. A **clinical nurse specialist (CNS)** is a master's-prepared RN who provides direct care as a therapist or indirect care as a consultant, educator, or researcher.
2. Certification by the ANCC involves a formal process to validate clinical competence.
   a. Advanced practice mental health nurses may also become certified as clinical specialists.
   b. The designation *RN, CS*, applies to both psychiatric nurse practitioners and clinical nurse specialists.
3. The specialist performs all of the functions of a generalist as well as the following:
   a. Primary mental health care: includes prescribing psychoactive medications and ordering appropriate diagnostic tests according to state nursing regulations

    b. Analysis of the health needs of individuals and populations

    c. Development of programs that target at-risk groups as well as cultural and environmental factors that foster health and prevent mental illness

  4. Practice settings include those described for the generalist as well as solo and group practices; may include contracts with employee assistance programs, HMOs, PPOs, and other settings where specialized services are delivered.

IV. THERAPEUTIC RELATIONSHIPS

A. Definition

  1. A **therapeutic relationship** is a nurse-client interaction that is directed toward enhancing the client's well-being.

  2. The client may be an individual, a family, a group, or a community.

B. Elements of the therapeutic relationship

  1. A **contract** establishes the time, place, and purpose of meetings between the nurse and client as well as conditions for termination

  2. **Boundaries** establish the relationship as therapeutic (as opposed to a social relationship)

    a. The roles of participants are clearly defined.

    b. The nurse is defined as a professional helper.

    c. The client's needs and problems are the focus of the interaction.

  3. **Confidentiality** helps build trust and must be maintained by the nurse throughout the relationship.

    a. The nurse shares client information with professional staff only on a need-to-know basis.

    b. The nurse must obtain the client's written permission to share information with any others outside the treatment team.

TABLE 1-1
Empathic behaviors

In a therapeutic relationship, the nurse should use appropriate verbal and nonverbal behaviors to communicate empathy, the emotional and intellectual ability to identify and understand another person's feelings and perspective objectively.

Verbal behaviors	**Nonverbal behaviors**
■ Asking open-ended questions	■ Fully attending to the client
■ Focusing on the client's feelings	■ Using a warm vocal tone
■ Paraphrasing the client's comments to check perceptions	■ Maintaining a relaxed, unhurried manner
■ Seeking clarification	■ Leaning forward slightly in an open body posture
■ Communicating an understanding of the client's feelings and perceptions	■ Nodding head and smiling periodically
	■ Synchronizing movements with those of the client
	■ Maintaining eye contact (*Note:* In some cultures, direct eye contact is inappropriate; the nurse should be respectful of cultural differences.)

    4. Therapeutic behaviors and practices involve the demonstration of the following consistent practices by the nurse when interacting with the client:

      a. Self-awareness

      b. Genuinely warm, respectful behavior

      c. Empathy (See *Table 1-1, Empathic behaviors.*)

      d. Cultural sensitivity

      e. Collaborative goal setting

      f. Responsible, ethical practice

C. Phases of the therapeutic relationship

    1. Orientation, the initial phase, involves assessment and analysis.

      a. The nurse establishes trust with the client.

      b. The nurse assesses the client. (See *Table 1-2, Nursing assessment of the psychiatric client.*)

      c. A nursing diagnosis is formulated.

TABLE 1-2
Nursing assessment of the psychiatric client

During the orientation phase of a therapeutic relationship, the nurse gathers data to help assess the client's mental health status and formulate a plan of care. This table highlights information typically collected during a client assessment.

Area to assess	Specific data collected
Client identification data	Name, address, phone number, date of birth, marital status, education, employment, emergency contact person, primary care provider, type of housing (independent of assisted living)
Physical assessment, past medical history	Allergies, vital signs, weight, nutritional and dietary history, sexual orientation, reproductive history, head-to-toe or body systems assessment (as required by client status or agency protocol), major illnesses and surgeries, medications used
Past psychiatric history	First occurrence (date and duration), hospitalizations, treatments, community follow-up care, case manager or primary therapist
Substance use	Use of any drugs (name, route, length of time used, amount and frequency of use, history of withdrawal symptoms)
Current problem and stressors	Description of problem (using client's own words), including developmental or situational stressors related to current problem
Family and cultural data	Names and ages of family members or significant others, characteristics of relationships, family history of mental illness, cultural or spiritual factors (beliefs about health and illness, specific health practices, identification of cultural health practitioner or religious affiliation)
Mental status (based on standard mental examination or agency protocol)	General appearance, behavior, attention, and orientation; use of language and speech patterns; cognitive processes, memory, and general intellectual functioning; mood and affect; thought patterns and content; degree of insight

  d. The nurse prioritizes the client's problems.

  e. The nurse and client establish mutually agreed-on goals.

 2. The **working phase** involves planning outcomes and related interventions to help the client achieve goals.

  a. The nurse helps the client to express problems, thoughts, and feelings.

  b. The nurse collaborates with the client using a problem-solving approach to resolve problems.

  c. The nurse teaches and encourages the use of coping measures.

  d. The nurse encourages the client to practice adaptive behaviors and evaluates their effectiveness.

 3. **Termination** (evaluation) marks the ending of the nurse-client relationship.

  a. The nurse evaluates outcomes, reassessing the problems, goals, and interventions, if necessary.

  b. The nurse and client express feelings about termination.

  c. The nurse observes the client for regressive behaviors.

  d. The nurse evaluates the entire nurse-client relationship.

V. THERAPEUTIC COMMUNICATION

A. Key concepts

 1. **Therapeutic communication** is composed of verbal and nonverbal techniques that the nurse uses to focus on the client's needs.

 2. Basic elements of a completed interaction include:

  a. Sender—originator of the message

  b. Message—information transmitted; may have both latent and manifest content

  c. Receiver—recipient of the message

  d. Feedback—receiver's response to the message, indicating understanding

 3. For successful communication, the nurse must be available to listen to the client.

B. Verbal communication techniques

 1. Asking neutral, **open-ended questions** encourages the client to express concerns. ("How are things going today?")

 2. Providing opening remarks or general statements based on assessment data gives the client an opportunity to begin sharing thoughts and feelings. ("I noticed that you seem anxious today.")

 3. **Restating,** repeating to the client the main content of the communication, reinforces that the nurse is listening to the client. ("You've told me about how the accident has affected every area of your life...")

 4. **Reflecting** directs feelings and questions back to the client to encourage elaboration. ("You're feeling really sad since you've been unable to go back to work.")

 5. **Focusing** allows the nurse to ask goal-directed questions to help the client focus on a specific area of concern. ("Let's talk about your difficulty with your father.")

6. Encouraging elaboration helps the client to describe more fully the concerns or problems being discussed. ("Tell me more about that.")
7. Seeking clarification helps the client put unclear thoughts or ideas into words. ("Do you mean that you become more anxious each time you leave your house?")
8. Sharing information that is relevant to the client's health care and well-being promotes trust and encourages the client to share thoughts and feelings. ("I have a card describing your medication that I'll review with you.")
9. Examining alternatives allows the client to explore options. ("Have you thought about requesting an extension on that deadline?")
10. Validating information assures the client that he was heard and understood. ("Did I understand you correctly when you said...?")
11. Summarizing key points of the discussion helps ensure accurate communication. ("We've talked about your mother's illness, your relationship with your husband, and your concerns about your children.")

C. Nonverbal aspects of communication

1. **Kinetics** involves body movements, such as gestures, facial expressions, and other mannerisms.
2. **Proxemics** refers to the physical distance between communicators; therapeutic communication generally takes place within the confines of personal space.
   a. Intimate space: up to 18 inches
   b. Personal space: 18 inches to 4 feet
   c. Social-consultative space: 9 to 12 feet
   d. Public space: more than 12 feet
3. **Touch** should be used deliberately, only after assessing the client's condition and likely response; it may be inappropriate in some situations and with some clients (such as suspicious and mistrustful clients, abuse victims, clients with tenuous ego boundaries, or clients whose culture prohibits or restricts touch).
4. **Silence,** often a powerful tool, allows periodic pauses to give nurse and client time to reflect.
5. **Paralanguage** refers to voice quality (tone, inflection) or how a message is delivered; the nurse should moderate voice quality according to the message being given to the client.

VI. CULTURAL CONSIDERATIONS IN PSYCHIATRIC NURSING

A. Key terms

1. **Culture** encompasses learned values, beliefs, and norms that are shared within a family, group, community, and nation.
2. **Enculturation** is the process of learning about one's culture.
3. **Ethnicity** is one's sense of belonging to a particular cultural group.
4. **Stereotyping** is the expectation that all persons from a particular group will behave, think, and respond in certain ways based on preconceived ideas.

5. **Cultural diversity** refers to a variety of cultural groupings, based not only on race and ethnicity, but also on age, gender, socioeconomic status, religion, mental illness, and physically challenged conditions.
6. **Culturally competent nursing** reflects sensitivity to diverse cultures; the nurse demonstrates awareness, knowledge, and respect of a client's particular cultural background.

B. Cultural issues

1. The United States is made up of more than 100 ethnic groups; population percentages (based on race and ethnicity) are as follows: 75.1% White, 12.9% Black/African American, 12.5% Hispanic, 3.6% Asian, and 0.9% American Indian/Alaskan Native.
2. Although there is no conclusive evidence that mental illness rates vary with race or other intrinsic human characteristics, researchers have identified some distinctions:
   a. African Americans are more likely than Whites to be diagnosed with schizophrenia rather than with affective disorders (caregiver bias may be a factor in this).
   b. Socioeconomic status is a significant factor in mental illness; poverty profoundly affects child and adolescent development.
3. Ethnicity seems to play a role in the efficacy of psychoactive medications; these differences result from biological and nonbiological factors.
   a. Differences in enzyme activity and metabolism affect the efficacy of psychotropic medications.
   b. Nutrition and diet may influence the effectiveness of psychotropic medications.
4. Currently, no single psychotherapy has been studied or cross-validated with relation to ethnic groups.
5. Values and beliefs about health, illness, mental disorders, and acceptable treatments may differ among cultural groups.
   a. Some cultural groups believe mental illness is caused by supernatural factors.
   b. Cultural perception may determine what is considered normal and abnormal.
   c. Some cultural groups use the services of a spiritual healer who usually has a mind-body-spirit approach to care.

C. Culturally competent nursing

1. The following variables should be considered when performing a cultural assessment:
   a. The client's understanding and interpretation of verbal and nonverbal communication
   b. The nurse's proximity to the client (especially personal space)
   c. The client's social organization (cultural group, defined family group, and characteristics of relationships)
   d. The client's concept of time (orientation to present and future)
   e. Environmental factors (includes special cultural health practices, beliefs about health and illness)

f. Biological variations among different groups (for example, the increased incidence of hypertension among African Americans may influence the type of psychotropic medication prescribed)

2. Nurses need to rely on their sensitivity and knowledge combined with cultural assessment, communication, and other mental health nursing skills to care for a culturally diverse population of clients.

3. Nurses should take appropriate steps to preserve cultural differences while helping clients to change only those patterns that are not helpful (for example, the nurse may consult the client's spiritual healer when developing a plan of care).

4. Nurses should modify their communication approaches, as needed, to accommodate the client's culture and practices.

   a. It may be necessary to avoid direct eye contact with a client whose culture deems it inappropriate.

   b. Use of validation can be a helpful communication tool, especially when the client speaks a foreign language; in some cases, an interpreter may be needed.

VII. LEGAL ISSUES IN PSYCHIATRIC NURSING

A. Development of mental health laws

1. Federal and state legislation, along with significant case law, provides the basis for psychiatric practice.

2. All states legislate their own laws to govern the treatment of mentally ill persons.

3. Several federal laws have been passed to protect the basic rights of mentally ill and physically challenged U.S. citizens.

4. In 1976, the Supreme Court of California found that a therapist must warn others when a mentally ill client poses a serious danger or threat to them; the "duty to warn," has since been adopted as law in many states.

B. State commitment laws

1. Each state has its own laws to determine types of admission for psychiatric treatment.

2. Clients are either admitted voluntarily or committed involuntarily.

   a. With **voluntary admission,** the client willingly enters and consents to treatment.

   – Clients retain all of their civil rights and may discontinue treatment whenever they choose (some states require the client to sign a 72-hour notice of intent to leave).

   – If the treatment team disagrees with a client's decision to discontinue treatment, the client signs a form acknowledging that he has been discharged against medical advice, or the treatment team may decide to seek involuntary commitment of the client.

   b. With **involuntary inpatient commitment,** the client is institutionalized against his will.

   – State laws define which persons can be committed and generally include those who pose a threat to self or others, those who lack the capacity for

meeting basic needs, and those who are seriously mentally ill but fail to seek treatment.
- State guidelines specify time limits for various types of involuntary commitment, including evaluation and emergency care, observation and treatment of a mental disorder, and extended or indeterminate care.
- Clients who are committed for extended care are entitled to legal representation and a court hearing before being committed and at specified times during their care.

   c. **Involuntary outpatient treatment** involves treatment mandated by a court order.
- This option has been used as deinstitutionalization has progressed.
- Clients typically include substance-impaired individuals, homeless mentally ill persons, and sex offenders.

   d. **Important note:** Involuntary commitment does not mean that an individual is incompetent; the client retains the right to consent to and refuse treatment.

C. Federal legislation

1. All clients admitted for psychiatric treatment retain their civil rights; however, in an emergency involuntary commitment, state law covers deprivation of liberty.
2. The **Patient's Bill of Rights,** which was originally published in 1973 by the American Hospital Association (AHA) and adopted into law by the Mental Health Systems Act in 1980, includes the following rights (among others not specified here):
   a. The right to appropriate treatment in the least restrictive setting
   b. The right to participate in the planning of treatment
   c. The right to refuse treatment except in an emergency or as permitted by law
3. The **Americans with Disabilities Act**, which was passed in 1990, ensures that those with a mental illness can fully participate in the economic and social mainstream.
4. The **Social Security Act**, passed in 1993, provides clients with the right to an individual treatment plan of care, the right to participate in a plan of care, and the right to refuse treatment.
5. The **Health Insurance Portability and Accountability Act (HIPPA)**, signed into law in 1996, mandates standards for the privacy of individually identifiable health information for all health plans and health care providers.
   a. The law protects any health information that is kept, filed, used, or shared in oral, electronic, or written form.
   b. It includes mental health records, such as psychotherapy and drug and alcohol treatment

D. Key legal concepts

1. Client information is considered privileged and must be treated with **confidentiality**.
2. A client's **informed consent** ensures that he received adequate information about his care and treatment prior to his consenting to treatment.
3. All clients (including those committed involuntarily) have the **right to refuse treatment**; however, in an emergency, a client can be given medication or con-

fined by seclusion or restraints (institutional guidelines are important in these situations).

4. The court determines client **incompetence** (or the inability to legally make decisions regarding one's health care, finances, and property) when self-management is so impaired that the client is at risk for grave harm.
    a. The client will have legal representation during this period.
    b. If the client is found to be incompetent, a legal guardian is appointed by the court to make decisions for him.

5. **Seclusion** and **restraint** are methods of preventing a client from harming himself or others during a violent outburst; both methods are regulated by specific legal and ethical guidelines.
    a. Federal agencies, professional associations, and health care facilities are all involved in a concerted effort to eliminate and/or reduce the use of these restrictive measures (a statement by the American Psychiatric Nurses Association can be accessed through the Web site http://apna.org).
    b. The guiding principle of managing client acting-out behavior is the use of **least restrictive measures,** in which the nurse attempts to calm the client before advancing to interventions that require seclusion or restraint.
        – Effective initial measures include limit setting, verbal interventions (including forming a therapeutic relationship with the client), and offering medication.
        – When initial measures fail or are inappropriate, the client may be involuntarily confined (secluded) in a room or area to prevent him from physically leaving.
        – In some cases, the client may require restraint; this refers to any method (such as manually holding a client or applying a device or piece of equipment that is attached or adjacent to the client's body) to restrict freedom of movement or normal access to his body.

VIII. ETHICAL ISSUES IN PSYCHIATRIC NURSING

A. Guiding principles
1. Both nursing and psychiatric nursing are governed by ethical and legal principles.
2. Historical and contemporary issues involving morals and ethics, spiritual and cultural beliefs, social justice and preservation of human rights, and concern for society's sick, injured, and vulnerable influence these principles.

B. Acts and ethical codes
1. Each state has issued a **nurse practice act,** which defines nursing and describes boundaries and standards of nursing practices.
2. The **ANA Code of Ethics for Nurses with Interpretive Statements,** published in 2001, provides ethical guidelines for nursing practice.

3. The **ANA Scope and Standards of Psychiatric-Mental Health Clinical Practice,** published in 2000, provides direction for professional nursing practice and reflects the standards and values of psychiatric nursing.
4. Madeline Leininger's **Transcultural Care Principles, Human Rights, and Ethical Considerations,** published in 1991, has been used as a model and source of inspiration for nursing education, research, and practice.

C. Ethical principles applicable to nursing

1. **Autonomy** is the client's freedom to make choices about his life.
2. **Beneficence** means acting in ways that benefit the client.
3. **Nonmaleficence** means acting in a manner to avoid causing harm to a client.
4. **Veracity** is the practice of telling the truth.
5. **Confidentiality** means nondisclosure of information with which one is entrusted.
6. **Justice** means acting in a fair, equitable, and appropriate manner.
7. **Fidelity** is faithfulness and the practice of keeping promises.

D. Ethical issues in psychiatric nursing

1. Nursing uses a holistic body-mind-spirit view of individuals.
   a. Nurses are ethically bound to honor a client's spiritual beliefs and to incorporate them, whenever possible, into the client's plan of care.
   b. **Spirituality** is defined as an animating force, life principle, or essence of being that permeates life and is expressed in multifaceted connections with self, other, nature, and God or Life Force.
2. Due to widespread acceptance of **complementary and alternative medicine (CAM)**, spurred by the consumer movement and the public's desire to maintain greater control over health care, nurses are ethically bound to consider a client's treatment choice when planning care.
   a. Examples of CAM include acupuncture, herbal medicine, homeopathy, naturopathy, meditation, relaxation, tai chi, and massage therapy.
   b. Nurses should become familiar with alternative choices and may obtain information about the safety and efficacy of treatments from the National Center of Complementary and Alternative Medicine (NCCAM), which hosts a Web site (www.nccam.nih.gov) exploring current topics, research, and trends.
   c. In some cases, psychiatric nurses may have difficulty accepting a client's choice of CAM.
3. Although nurses may not share the same culture or values as their clients, they have a duty to employ culturally sensitive techniques in all interactions and treatments.
4. Nurses must respect their client's autonomy while attempting to practice beneficence.
   a. In many cases, the nurse will feel conflicted in wanting to help the client but knowing that she must honor the client's wishes.
   b. This may be particularly difficult when a seriously mentally ill client refuses to take a medication or undergo a treatment that the nurse knows will help.
5. Nurses sometimes feel a sense of failure and frustration regarding decisions involving limited health care resources.

a. Under a managed care system, nurses are considered providers of care and must follow the dictates of HMOs and PPOs.

b. In some cases, this results in a client's early discharge from treatment before maximum beneficial effects occur.

6. Controversial client choices, such as abortion and active euthanasia, are often troubling to nurses; in such cases, nurses are forced to reconcile their own conflicts over values and beliefs that differ with the client's beliefs.

7. Many nurses may have strong feelings regarding the use of seclusion and restraint, which may differ from institutional, professional, and legal guidelines.

Study questions

1. A nurse employed in a managed care system collaborates with the treatment team to monitor a client's progress from psychiatric inpatient care to a community-assisted living program. Which role is the nurse assuming?
1. Advanced practice nurse
2. Case manager
3. Nurse manager
4. Staff nurse

2. When the nurse establishes a therapeutic relationship with a client, which of the following is the primary focus for the client's care?
1. The medical diagnosis
2. The client's needs and problems
3. The nursing diagnosis
4. The client's social interaction skills

3. Which of the following is the overall purpose of therapeutic communication?
1. To analyze client problems
2. To elicit client cooperation
3. To facilitate a helping relationship
4. To provide emotional support

4. The nurse is fully attentive to her client, seeks clarification of unclear statements, and periodically tells the client about her perception of the client's feelings. Which of the following is the nurse demonstrating?
1. Congruence
2. Empathy
3. Reflection
4. Summarization

5. Which legal-ethical principle would the nurse use when interacting with a psychotic client who refuses psychotropic medication?
1. Autonomy
2. Confidentiality
3. Empathy
4. Fidelity

6. While teaching a client about psychotropic medication, the nurse obtains data indicating the client's understanding of what was taught. On which part of the communication process is the nurse focusing?
1. Feedback
2. Message
3. Receiver
4. Sender

7. When the nurse interacts with a client from a different cultural background, which technique would provide sensitive care?
1. Confronting issues of noncompliance
2. Use of therapeutic silence

3. Use of therapeutic touch
4. Validation of communication

8. Shortly after his voluntary admission to a psychiatric inpatient unit, a client tells the nurse, "I don't know if I should be here. What will my family think?" Using reflection, which response by the nurse is most appropriate?
1. "Your family can visit you here, and they will see that this is a helpful place."
2. "You think your family will be upset because you have a psychiatric problem?"
3. "There is still a stigma associated with mental illness. Hopefully your family won't feel this way."
4. "You are wondering if you made the best decision, and you are concerned about your family's reaction."

9. A nurse is assigned to a client who has a domineering and demanding attitude, similar to the nurse's own mother. The nurse seeks out a colleague to share feelings about this situation. The nurse's action indicates:
1. Appropriate self-awareness
2. An inability to cope effectively
3. Lack of knowledge about the client's problems
4. A need to change client assignment

10. After an initial nurse-client interaction, the client asks for the nurse's home phone number, indicating a desire to date the nurse. Which response is most appropriate?
1. "I may consider dating you once you are fully recovered."
2. "I'm sorry, but I already have a special relationship."
3. "It's against hospital policy for me to date clients."
4. "This is a professional relationship, and we need to stay clear on that."

11. A client who was hospitalized involuntarily wants to call an attorney about a personal matter involving a lawsuit. Which of the following nursing actions would be most appropriate?
1. Allow the phone call without seeking further information.
2. Ask the client questions about the pending lawsuit.
3. Call the attorney, and explain that the client is in the hospital.
4. Tell the client that the lawsuit would be best settled after discharge from the hospital.

12. The advanced practice RN (APRN) who provides primary psychiatric care, including writing prescriptions, is legally authorized to practice under which of the following?
1. ANA Standards of Psychiatric Practice
2. Certification by the ANCC
3. Graduation from accredited master's program
4. State Nurse Practice Act

13. A client has become increasingly unable to maintain self-care, with worsening symptoms of a chronic mental illness and refusal to accept psychiatric treatment. The community psychiatric nurse explains to the client's family that a legal procedure can be initiated to empower another person to give consent for treatment. Which of the following would a court hearing legally establish about this client?
1. Autonomy
2. Competence
3. Sanity
4. Client rights

14. The nurse and client are entering the termination phase of the nurse-client relationship. Which of the following nurse behaviors are appropriate at this phase? Select all that apply.
  1. Evaluate outcomes of intervention.
  2. Facilitate the client's expression of problems.
  3. Facilitate expression of feelings regarding the nurse-client relationship.
  4. Establish mutually agreed-on goals.
  5. Note any regressive behaviors initiated by client.
  6. Use a problem-solving approach with client issues.

15. A community psychiatric nurse visits a client's home after a referral from a case manager who is concerned about the client's increased delusions. A spiritual healer from the family's cultural group is present in the home and indicates the desire to work with the client and family. Which action would be most appropriate?
  1. Explain that the healer's efforts would be incompatible with psychiatric care.
  2. Proceed with data collection only after requesting a private interview with the client.
  3. Plan to collaborate with the healer to provide care to the client and family.
  4. Refuse to continue with the client and family, and contact the case manager immediately.

16. The nurse interacts with the psychiatric client using empathy. Which of the following demonstrates empathic behaviors? Select all that apply.
  1. Determining which medications are used by the client
  2. Focusing on the client feelings
  3. Maintaining a relaxed, unhurried manner
  4. Paraphrasing the client's comments to check perception
  5. Performing a body systems assessment
  6. Synchronizing movements with those of the client

Answer key

1. The answer is **2**.
In a managed care system, the case manager is responsible for monitoring and ensuring continuity of care in collaboration with the treatment team. Although they provide different levels of care, both the staff nurse and the advanced practice nurse provide primary care. The nurse manager supervises other nursing personnel.

2. The answer is **2**.
The primary focus of a therapeutic relationship is to help the client work on his needs and problems. Although the medical diagnosis and nursing diagnosis are important in identifying and understanding the client's disorder, they are not part of the therapeutic relationship. Improving social interaction skills may be one of the nursing interventions, but it is not the purpose of the relationship.

3. The answer is **3**.
The purpose of therapeutic communication is to foster a helping relationship, so that the client can more effectively cope with problems. The other tasks described are part of the helping relationship but are not the overall purpose.

4. The answer is 2.

These behaviors illustrate the nurse's empathy. The other options are examples of therapeutic communication techniques.

5. The answer is 1.

Autonomy is the client's legal right to make decisions affecting himself. This right applies regardless of whether the client has a mental illness, unless he is declared incompetent. Confidentiality is an important aspect of the nurse-client relationship in which the nurse maintains the privacy of client information and shares it with only those on a need-to-know basis. Empathy is the ability to understand another person's feelings and perspective, an important part of the therapeutic relationship. Fidelity is the ethical principle of keeping promises.

6. The answer is 1.

The communication sequence is complete when the receiver of the message provides feedback regarding the content of the message. The remaining options reflect other important parts of the communication process.

7. The answer is 4.

Frequent validation is key to preventing cultural misunderstandings when the nurse and client have different backgrounds. Confronting the client's noncompliance is inappropriate because the nurse's interpretation of this situation may be quite different from the client's perspective. Therapeutic silence is important; however, validating communication will ensure culturally sensitive care. Touch may be inappropriate in some cultures; when used, the nurse must be extremely cautious and evaluate the client's anticipated response before using it.

8. The answer is 4.

Reflection involves rewording the client's statement to indicate the nurse's understanding of the client's experience.

9. The answer is 1.

Analyzing and sharing perceptions about herself in relation to her client demonstrates self-awareness and helps the nurse to work through counter-transference feelings, which could hinder the therapeutic process. Seeking colleague consultation regarding a difficult interaction does not indicate poor coping or a lack of knowledge about the client's problem. If consulting the colleague fails to improve her ability to interact therapeutically with this client, a change of assignment may be indicated.

10. The answer is 4.

At the beginning of a nurse-client relationship, it is important for the nurse to clarify parameters of the relationship and establish clear boundaries.

11. The answer is 1.

A client who is committed involuntarily retains all of his civil rights, including the right to consult an attorney and the right to sue. The nurse should not ask the client about the lawsuit because this is intrusive behavior on the nurse's part. Calling the attorney and telling him that the patient is in the hospital violates the client's rights, as does telling the client that the lawsuit would best be settled after discharge from the hospital.

12. The answer is 4.

State Nurse Practice Acts provide legal parameters and boundaries for the practice of nursing. ANA Standards provide ethical guidelines for practice. Certification is a credentialing issue but does not provide legal authorization. An adequate knowledge base is acquired through education but does not establish legal authority.

13. The answer is **2.**

Competence is a legal issue indicating an *ability* to make decisions for oneself. When a client experiences severe impairments in this area, the court may declare the client incompetent and then appoint a legal guardian who can make decisions regarding the client's care and treatment. Autonomy is the legal *right* of each individual to make decisions affecting himself. When a client becomes so impaired that self-care is not possible, the court may intervene and declare the client incompetent. A client with a mental illness has a right to make decisions about his care unless the court declares that the client is incompetent. A court proceeding is unnecessary to establish client's legal rights; they are guaranteed by the U.S. Constitution.

14. The answer is **1, 3, 6.**

During the termination phase, the nurse evaluates outcomes, encourages the client to express feelings about the relationship, and expresses her own feelings about what has transpired. The nurse must also remain alert to any regressive behaviors, which can occur during termination. These behaviors express the client's fear of ending the relationship and may be an unconscious mechanism for getting the nurse to continue with the process. Establishing goals is part of the initial phase. Facilitating the client's feelings and using a problem-solving approach are commonly part of the working phase of the relationship.

15. The answer is **3.**

The nurse providing culturally sensitive care will respect a client's beliefs and collaborate with the client, family, and spiritual healer. The other options are actions that do not indicate understanding and respect for diversity, and therefore they are inappropriate.

16. The answer is **2, 3, 4, 6.**

Focusing on the client's feelings, maintaining a relaxed manner, paraphrasing the client's comments to better understand his perception, and synchronizing movements with those of the client are examples of verbal or nonverbal empathic behaviors. Determining the client's medications and performing an assessment are part of the assessment phase of the nursing process.

2 Conceptual Frameworks for Psychiatric Care

I. FRAMEWORKS FOR NURSING

A. Key concepts

1. **Conceptual frameworks** are methods of organizing knowledge that provide a basis for understanding human behavior and the relationship of biological factors, developmental processes, and environmental influences.
2. Conceptual frameworks help nurses to organize information according to the nursing process.
   a. They guide data collection.
   b. They provide explanations for assessed behaviors.
   c. They help with developing plans of care.
   d. They provide rationales for selecting interventions.
   e. They determine evaluation criteria for outcome measurement.
3. Conceptual frameworks help guide research by providing assumptions to be tested.

B. Commonly used conceptual frameworks

1. The **psychobiology framework** focuses on biological processes and their relation to human behavior.
2. The **developmental framework**, which is based on the works of such theorists as Freud, Sullivan, Erikson, and Piaget, explains behavior according to how individuals develop and mature.
3. The **behavioral framework** focuses on an individual's functioning in terms of identified behaviors.
4. The **cognitive framework** focuses on how thought patterns produce certain behaviors.
5. The **humanistic framework** focuses on an individual's current behaviors and problems in relation to shared human experiences.

II. PSYCHOBIOLOGY FRAMEWORK

A. Key concepts

1. **Psychobiology** is the scientific study of the relationships among the structure and function of the brain, biochemical and hormonal processes, genetics, environmental experiences, and human behavior.
2. Biological research and technological advances guide psychobiology.
   a. The 1990s, known as the "Decade of the Brain," saw an explosion of knowledge about brain functioning.
   b. Genetic research has established a relationship between genetics and mental illnesses.
   – Genetic makeup can affect vulnerability to mental illness.
   – To date, no cause-and-effect relationship has been identified.
   c. Psychopharmacologic research has led to the development of many new drugs that affect the brain's neurotransmitters, neurotransmitter receptor sites, and metabolic and electrical processes.

d. Brain imaging techniques (computed tomography, positron emission tomography, single-photon emission computed tomography, magnetic resonance imaging) are used to study individuals with mental illness.

B. Neuroanatomy and behavior

1. The **cerebrum,** the most superior part of the brain, is composed of two cerebral hemispheres; each hemisphere is divided into four lobes.

   a. The **frontal lobe** is responsible for higher-order thinking, abstract reasoning, decision-making, speech, and voluntary muscle movement; dysfunction is associated with illogical or psychotic thinking, uninhibited behaviors, and incoherent speech.

   b. The **parietal lobe** is responsible for sensory function and body position information; dysfunction is associated with impaired spatial ability and body image, as well as self-care deficits.

   c. The **occipital lobe** is responsible for visual function; dysfunction is associated with visual illusions and hallucinations.

   d. The **temporal lobe** is responsible for judgment, memory, smell, sensory interpretation, and understanding sound; dysfunction is associated with aggressive and violent behaviors, olfactory and auditory hallucinations, and language abnormalities.

2. The **diencephalon,** which is embedded in the cerebrum, is superior to the brain stem and composed of several structures.

   a. The **thalamus** receives and relays sensory information and plays a role in memory and mood regulation.

   b. The **hypothalamus,** the main visceral control center of the body, is vitally important to body homeostasis; it regulates the autonomic nervous system, body temperature, food intake, water balance, biological rhythms and drives, and hormonal output of the anterior pituitary gland.

   c. The **limbic system** comprises the limbic lobe and the numerous structures functioning with it, including the frontal cortex, hypothalamus, amygdala, hippocampus, brain stem, and autonomic nervous system; called the *emotional brain*, the limbic system regulates emotional responses.

C. Neurotransmitters and receptor sites

1. **Neurotransmitters** are chemical messengers that carry an inhibitory or stimulating message from one neuron to another across the space between them **(synapse)**.

2. Many psychiatric disorders are associated with abnormal interactions between neurotransmitter systems.

3. There are many neurotransmitters, and research is ongoing to identify their effects on behaviors.

   a. **Serotonin** (also called 5-hydroxytryptamine or 5-HT) mediates multiple areas of brain-behavior functioning.

   – Serotonin affects cognition and memory; emotional responses of anxiety and panic, violence, and aggression; sexual function; and sleep-wake cycles.

   – Many antidepressants increase levels of serotonin at synapses.

b. **Dopamine** (also referred to as DA) has multiple functions depending on which specific dopaminergic brain receptor pathway is involved.
- Dopamine affects pleasurable sensations (including euphoria resulting from drugs of abuse); delusions and hallucinations (related to excessive dopamine); and the control of complex motor functions.
- Many antipsychotic medications block dopamine from binding to receptor sites and therefore decrease psychotic symptoms.
- The motor side effects of antipsychotics are related to dopamine's effect on complex motor movements in the extrapyramidal system of the central nervous system.

c. **Norepinephrine** is a catecholamine neurotransmitter of the sympathetic nervous system, which mediates emergency response; changes in norepinephrine levels are associated with depressive disorders, including bipolar disorder.

d. **Gamma-aminobutyric acid (GABA)** is an inhibitory neurotransmitter.
- When neurons are stimulated (such as in anxiety), GABA decreases neuronal stimulation.
- Antianxiety medications stimulate GABA activity and therefore promote relaxation.

e. **Acetylcholine** is a major neurotransmitter of the parasympathetic nervous system, which controls muscle activity, memory, and coordination.
- Dopamine and acetylcholine have a reciprocal relationship in the modulation of motor activity and movements and possibly psychotic thinking.
- Decreasing this neurotransmitter produces the anticholinergic side effects common to many psychotropic drugs.
- Changes in acetylcholine levels have been associated with the memory deficits in Alzheimer's disease.

f. **Histamine** is a chemical messenger that mediates allergic and inflammatory reactions; its role in mental illness is not well understood.

g. Other neurotransmitters being researched include glycine, aspartate, somatostatin, neurotensin, substance P, cholecystokines, vasopressin, endorphins, and enkephalins.

4. Receptor sites are channels or openings on presynaptic and postsynaptic cell membranes.
   a. Each neurotransmitter can latch onto more than one kind of receptor.
   b. Receptor sites vary in affinity for different neurotransmitters.
   c. Receptor subtypes are often located in different brain areas and, therefore, can mediate different behavioral effects.

D. Genetics

1. Research on the role of genes in many mental illnesses is ongoing.
2. According to current thinking, certain genetic patterns may interact with other neurological, biochemical, and environmental factors, contributing to increased vulnerability to certain mental illness.
3. Genetic vulnerability has been established for mood disorders, schizophrenia, substance disorders, and Alzheimer's disease.

E. Hormonal influences

1. The hypothalamic-pituitary-adrenal (HPA) axis has been found to be hyperactive in individuals with depressive disorders.
2. An underactive thyroid gland is linked to depression.
3. The **stress response** is a neuroendocrine response that causes significant hormonal releases, which affects multiple body systems and can lead to psychological and physiologic symptoms. (See page 43.)

F. Biology and environment

1. Researchers are currently studying how an individual's environment affects brain development and functioning.
2. Early life experiences (such as physical or psychological abuse) can alter brain structure and affect production of hormones and neurotransmitters, which can produce symptoms of mental illness later in life.
3. Severe abuse early in life (such as physical or sexual abuse in infancy and early childhood) can permanently increase gene expression for corticotropin-releasing factor (CRF) and increase the risk of depression in adulthood.
4. The **Kindling model** proposes that repeated environmental stimuli lead to progressively greater neural responsiveness, which changes brain excitability and therefore behavioral responses over time (for example, an early life experience can contribute to an initial experience of mental illness, which may increase brain sensitivity and thus predispose the client to later episodes of mental illness, given continued life stressors).

G. Treatments

1. Psychiatric diagnoses are established according to *DSM-IV TR* criteria and laboratory and diagnostic studies (such as brain imaging).
2. Use of psychotropic medications is a well-established approach in the treatment of mental illness.
3. Electroconvulsive therapy and light therapy are also used based on their effect on the brain's electrical and chemical functioning.
4. Psychobiological treatments are often used in conjunction with psychotherapy for maximum effectiveness.

H. Application to nursing

1. Psychiatric nurses integrate knowledge of psychobiology and psychopharmacology into practice.
2. The American Nurses Association (ANA) has established guidelines for basic nursing practice related to the use of psychobiology in restoring client health.
3. The nurse assesses physiologic, emotional, and behavioral aspects of client functioning.
4. For nurses working in primary prevention, developments in genetic research can enhance the nurse's understanding of at-risk families.
5. Understanding psychobiology helps the nurse teach clients and families about the biology of mental illness, symptom recognition, medication management, and relapse prevention.

6. Nurses educated at master's level (APRN) may have primary responsibility for care of the client with mental illness (including prescriptive authority).

III. DEVELOPMENTAL FRAMEWORK

A. Developmental theories

1. Several important developmental theories have emerged to explain how an individual learns about himself in relation to his surroundings and others.

2. Development begins at birth and continues through various stages of an individual's life.

B. Freudian (psychodynamic) theory

1. **Psychodynamic theory,** based on the work of Sigmund Freud (1856-1939), focuses on intrapsychic processes and psychosexual development.

2. This theory identifies three levels of awareness.

  a. **Conscious** refers to experiences (memories, feelings, thoughts, and wishes) within an individual's awareness.

  b. **Preconscious** describes experiences that may be recalled to conscious awareness.

  c. **Unconscious** refers to experiences not available to conscious awareness.

3. Freudian theory also describes personality structure.

  a. **Id,** the most primitive component, is responsible for instincts and impulses, operating by the pleasure principle and primary-process thought (thinking that is characteristic of infancy, as well as "dream" thinking).

  b. **Ego,** the reality-based "I" component, validates and tests reality; it operates by secondary-process thought (reality-based thinking), balancing impulses from the id and demands from the superego.

  c. **Superego** is the component of moral principle, or the conscience; it consists of culturally acquired values, beliefs, and standards of behavior.

4. **Psychodynamics** are assumptions made by Freud and psychoanalysis in general that human behavior—especially emotional problems—occurs because of unconscious conflicts and basic instincts.

  a. **Psychic energy (cathexis)** is a force required for mental functioning, and it arises from drives (instincts).

  b. **Instincts (drives)** are inborn psychological representations or wishes and include self-preservation and preservation of species; Freud postulated that humans have both a life and a death instinct.

  c. **Anxiety** is a response to unconscious conflict or a threat to ego.

  d. **Defense mechanisms** are mental mechanisms (largely unconscious) that operate to protect the ego. (See *Table 2-1, Common defense mechanisms*, page 26.)

5. Freud's theory of psychosexual development includes various stages (oral, anal, phallic, latent, and genital), spanning infancy through adolescence. (See *Table 2-2, Comparing developmental theories*, page 27.)

6. Mental illness may be explained in a Freudian context as follows:

TABLE 2-1
Common defense mechanisms

Defense mechanism	Definition	Clinical example
Repression	Exclusion of unpleasant or unwanted experiences, emotions, or ideas from conscious awareness	The victim of an automobile accident does not remember anything about the accident.
Projection	Attributing one's own feelings or wishes (which are unacceptable to oneself) to another person	A frightened client lashes out at the nurse, saying the nurse is a timid, fearful person and should not be in the role of nurse.
Reaction formation	Adoption of behavior or feelings that are exactly opposite one's true emotions	A client is angry about the care he is receiving but behaves in a very ingratiating manner.
Displacement	Transferring emotions associated with a particular person or event to another person, object, or situation that is less threatening	A client who is angry with a doctor becomes verbally abusive to the nurses.
Identification	Adopting the thinking or behavioral patterns of another	A teenager hospitalized for diabetes wants to become a nurse as a result of her experience.
Denial	Refusal to believe or accept an unpleasant reality	A client who drinks alcohol daily and cannot stop fails to acknowledge that he has a problem.
Isolation	Separation of emotions from precipitating event or situation	A rape victim talks about her rape experience without showing any emotion.
Intellectualization	Use of thinking to avoid experiencing unpleasant emotions	A father talks with his child about what love should be like but fails to demonstrate love toward the child.
Rationalization	Attempts to justify one's behavior by presenting reasons that sound logical	A client being treated for a drug addiction claims she is unable to stop taking drugs because of her bad marriage.
Sublimation	Substituting constructive and socially acceptable behavior for strong impulses that are unacceptable in their original form	A mother who lost a child in a drunk-driving accident joins an organization that works to educate the public about the dangers of drunk driving.

    a. All behavior has meaning, although meaning may be unconscious.

    b. Symptoms of mental illness are caused by unconscious internal conflicts arising from unresolved issues in early childhood; situations occurring in adulthood that are similar to the conflicts of childhood will precipitate symptoms.

TABLE 2-2
Comparing developmental theories

Freud's (psychodynamic) theory	Erikson's (psychosocial) theory	Sullivan's (interpersonal) theory	Piaget's (cognitive) theory
Infancy (birth to 18 months): *Oral stage;* the infant learns to deal with anxiety by gratification of oral needs.	**Infancy:** *Trust versus mistrust;* the infant learns to trust others.	**Infancy:** The infant learns to trust others.	**Sensorimotor stage** (birth to 18 months): The infant learns about self and the environment through senses and motor activities.
Toddler (18 months to 3 years): *Anal stage;* the toddler learns muscle control and social control.	**Toddler:** *Autonomy versus shame and doubt;* the toddler learns self-control and beginning of independence.	**Childhood** (18 months to 6 years): The child accepts the influence of others.	**Preconceptual stage** (2 to 4 years): The child develops language and symbolic play.
Preschool (3 to 6 years): *Phallic stage;* the child establishes sexual identity.	**Preschool:** *Initiative versus guilt;* the child learns assertiveness and the ability to affect interpersonal environment.	**Juvenile** (6 to 9 years): The child forms peer relationships.	**Intuitive stage** (4 to 7 years): The child learns to classify and group things; period marked by egocentric thinking.
School age (6 to 12 years): *Latency stage;* the child establishes same-sex relationships.	**School age:** *Industry versus inferiority;* the child learns self-confidence through cooperation and competition.	**Preadolescence** (9 to 12 years): The child forms friendships with same-sex peers.	**Concrete operations stage** (6 to 12 years): The child learns to reason in a systematic way.
Adolescence (12 to 18 years): *Genital stage;* the adolescent establishes relationships with the opposite sex and finds gratifying work.	**Adolescence** (12 to 18 years): *Identity versus role diffusion;* the child develops a sense of self.	**Early adolescence** (12 to 14 yeas): The child is becoming more independent and begins to establish relationships with the opposite sex.	**Formal operations stage** (12 to 18 years and older): The child develops abstract thinking and conceptual thought.
	Young adult (18 to 25 years): *Intimacy versus isolation;* the young adult develops intimate relationships.	**Late adolescence** (14 to 21 years): The young adult develops enduring relationships with members of the opposite sex.	
	Middle adult (25 to 55 years): *Generativity versus stagnation;* the adult guides others and contributes to society.		
	Older adult (55 years to death): *Integrity versus despair;* the adult feels satisfied with his life.		

– For example, an adult who has unresolved conflicts related to toilet training may be vulnerable to situations in adulthood that call for giving of one-

self or sharing one's possessions.
  – These situations create anxiety that is largely unconscious.
  c. Defenses are fixed at an early development stage.
7. Treatment is insight-oriented and focuses on interpersonal conflicts, anxiety, defenses, and sexual and aggressive drives.
  a. Unresolved conflicts are brought to a conscious level by various techniques (free association, dream analysis, transference analysis).
  b. Psychoanalytic treatment is often long-term and expensive.
8. Nurses working within a Freudian framework use psychodynamic theory to understand client behavior and to gain a developmental perspective of behavior.
  a. It is important to assess the client's anxiety levels and use of defense mechanisms.
  b. The nurse should be aware of transference and countertransference in managing a therapeutic relationship.
    – **Transference** refers to client feelings toward a therapist arising from unconscious experiences with early significant others (such as parents).
    – **Countertransference** refers to a therapist's feelings that arise from early experiences.

C. Sullivan's (interpersonal) theory
1. **Interpersonal theory,** developed by Harry Stack Sullivan (1892-1949), focuses on interactions between an individual and his environment.
2. According to this theory, personality is shaped through interaction with significant others; the child internalizes approval or disapproval from the parents, and therefore the self is shaped by the parental view of the child.
3. **Self-system** is a way of conceptualizing the three components of personality.
  a. **"Good-me"** develops in response to behaviors receiving approval by parents or significant others.
  b. **"Bad-me"** develops in response to behaviors receiving disapproval by parents or significant others and leads to anxiety states.
  c. **"Not-me"** develops in response to behaviors generating extreme anxiety in parents or significant others; these behaviors are denied as being part of oneself.
4. Anxiety is an interpersonal phenomenon that occurs when one experiences conflict or problems in a significant relationship.
5. The basic needs of an individual include satisfaction (biological needs) and security (emotional and social needs).
6. Sullivan's theory incorporates developmental changes that are tracked from infancy through late adolescence. (See *Table 2-2, Comparing developmental theories*, page 27.)
7. Mental illness is explained in terms of interpersonal conflicts.
  a. Symptoms are related to conflictual or problematic interpersonal relationships (such as anxiety or depression in the spouse of an alcoholic).
  b. Causes of mental illness are related to past relationships, inappropriate communication, and the current relationship crisis.
8. Treatment focuses on anxiety and its cause.

a. The therapist is a participant-observer in relationship with the client; the role of the therapist is more active than passive when compared with psychoanalytic therapy.

b. The client is encouraged to verbalize feelings and to work on modifying problematic relationships.

9. Hildegarde Peplau (1909-1999), renowned nurse theorist, developed an interpersonal theory of nursing.

a. The nurse and client participate in and contribute to the relationship. The relationship itself can be therapeutic.

b. The nurse uses the nurse-client relationship as a corrective interpersonal experience for the client.

c. Nursing interventions commonly focus on current interpersonal concerns (as opposed to past problems or early relationship issues) and problem solving related to interpersonal issues.

d. Anxiety intervention is an important nursing function. (See pages 55 and 56.)

D. Erikson's (psychosocial) theory

1. **Psychosocial theory,** developed by Erik Erikson (1902-1994), proposes eight developmental phases spanning infancy through older adulthood. (See *Table 2-2, Comparing developmental theories,* page 27.)
2. According to this theory, ego development results from social interaction.
3. Developmental tasks are sequential and depend on prior successful mastery; an individual who fails to master a developmental task at the appropriate age can return later in life to work on mastery.
4. Views of mental illness and treatment are similar to those of Freud's theory.
5. Nurses use psychosocial development throughout the nursing process.

a. The nurse assesses a client's psychosocial development according to expected norms for specific age.

b. The nurse can use knowledge of developmental tasks in selecting appropriate interventions for the client.

c. The nurse fosters healthy behaviors and encourages hope that relearning is possible (for example, the nurse would establish trust with the client and encourage him to act autonomously or otherwise adopt the positive behaviors associated with each of the eight life stages).

E. Piaget's (cognitive) theory

1. **Cognitive theory,** developed by Jean Piaget (1896-1980), focuses on the innate development of thinking ability from infancy to adulthood. (See *Table 2-2, Comparing developmental theories*, page 27.)
2. According to Piaget, individuals are born with the tendency to organize and to adapt to their environment.
3. Although cognitive theory does not specifically address mental illness and treatment, it has various nursing applications.

a. Understanding the way an individual thinks enables the nurse to communicate in an age-appropriate manner.

    b. Nursing interventions can be adapted to the individual's cognitive level (for example, the nurse can use dolls or toy medical equipment to try to explain surgery to a preschooler who is about to undergo surgery).

    c. The nurse can select teaching strategies according to the client's age-appropriate cognitive processes.

IV. BEHAVIORAL FRAMEWORK

A. Key concepts

1. A **behavioral framework** is used to describe a person's functioning in terms of identified behaviors.

   a. People learn to be who they are by environmental shaping.

   b. Behavior can be observed, described, and recorded.

   c. Behavior is subject to reward or punishment.

   d. Changing one's environment can modify behavior.

2. Maladaptive behaviors are learned through classical and operant conditioning; they continue because they are rewarding to the individual.

3. Maladaptive behaviors can be changed, without developing insight into underlying causes, by altering the environment.

B. Classical conditioning (Pavlov's theory)

1. **Classical conditioning** was developed by Ivan Pavlov (1849-1936).

2. He established that learning or conditioning can occur when a stimulus (a bell) is paired with an unconditioned response (a dog's salivating in response to the sight of food); in other words, the dog learns to salivate at the sound of the bell and no longer needs the sight of food to elicit the response.

   a. A **conditioned response** is the pairing of a stimulus with a response (the bell eventually elicits salivation in the dog).

   b. **Acquisition** refers to gaining a learned response (once a response is learned, it continues).

   c. **Extinction** is the loss of a learned response.

C. Operant conditioning (Skinner's theory)

1. Developed by B.F. Skinner (1904-1990), **operant conditioning** involves the use of reinforced consequences to change behavior.

2. **Positive reinforcement** is a reward given to help continue the behavior.

3. **Negative reinforcement** removes undesirable consequences to help continue the behavior.

4. **Positive punishment** involves the use of aversive consequences to decrease a particular behavior.

5. **Negative punishment** involves withdrawing the reward to decrease a particular behavior.

D. Behavioral treatments

1. **Behavioral modification** involves the use of various learned techniques to change maladaptive behavior; it is commonly used with clients who have anxiety disorders, substance abuse problems, or other specific behavioral problems.

2. **Modeling** refers to new behaviors that are learned by imitating the behavior of another person.
3. **Operant conditioning** involves the use of tokens (rewards) for desirable behaviors *(token economy)*.
4. **Systematic desensitization** involves gradually confronting a stimulus that evokes intense anxiety; it is especially helpful for treating phobias.
    a. The therapist initially teaches the client how to relax, and then begins with a stimulus that causes mild anxiety.
    b. The client learns to invoke the relaxation response when confronted with the stimulus.
    c. The process continues until an intensely anxiety-provoking stimulus no longer causes the client to feel anxious.
5. **Aversive therapy** operates on the principle that unpleasant consequences result from undesirable behavior; it may be used to treat paraphilias (electric shocks may be paired with the patient's impulse to humiliate or hurt a nonconsenting sexual partner).
6. **Biofeedback** involves training techniques used to control physiologic responses (such as the stress response and its physiologic manifestations, including tachycardia and vasoconstriction of blood vessels leading to hypertension).
7. **Relaxation techniques** are training techniques used to counteract anxiety symptoms.
8. **Assertiveness training** incorporates techniques to overcome passivity or aggression in interpersonal situations.

E. Application to nursing
1. In the behavioral framework, the nurse assesses both adaptive and maladaptive behaviors.
2. The nurse and client collaborate to identify behaviors that require change.
3. As a member of the treatment team, the nurse uses various behavioral modification techniques to help the client.

V. COGNITIVE FRAMEWORK

A. Key concepts
1. The **cognitive framework** focuses on distorted or negative thought patterns that lead to maladaptive or symptomatic feelings and behaviors.
    a. Distorted thinking leads to and perpetuates maladaptive behaviors.
    b. Certain common thought patterns can be identified as misperceptions. (See *Table 2-3, Common misperceptions of thought patterns*, page 32.)
2. Patterns of thinking are learned, become automatic, and significantly affect a person's feelings and behaviors.
3. The amount of perceived control over a situation affects how an individual responds to stressors and problems.
    a. **Internal locus of control** refers to an individual's belief in his own ability to affect the outcome of life situations; although many external circumstances

TABLE 2-3
Common misperceptions of thought patterns

Misperception	Definition	Clinical example
Arbitrary inference	Holding beliefs in absence of supporting evidence	"I don't care what things you do to help me. I know you dislike me."
Selective abstraction	Concentrating on a single detail while ignoring others	"Look at how fat my thighs are." (Said by person who is underweight.)
Overgeneralization	Making global assumptions based on an isolated incident	"People who are in authority are like my boss—unfair and critical."
Magnification	Greatly exaggerating a situation	"I don't understand this one paragraph— I'll never be able to read this book."
Minimization	Making light of a situation or problem	"Getting arrested is no big deal. My family will understand."
Dichotomous thinking	"All or nothing" patterns of thought	"If you don't agree with me on this issue, then you're not my friend."

    of life cannot be changed, the individual can change his response to the situation.

    b. **External locus of control** refers to an individual's belief that others control his life and he is unable to improve his own functioning or well-being; he may also believe that other people or circumstances have to change for his own life to improve.

    c. The cognitive therapist may challenge the belief of a client who clings to an external locus of control.

B. Treatments

    1. Cognitive therapy encompasses various treatment methods in which the therapist and client work closely to identify maladaptive thought patterns and develop alternative ways of thinking and behaving.

      a. The therapist helps the client to become aware of negative thinking and recognize the effect of negative thinking on feelings and behaviors.

      b. The client is encouraged to practice alternative thought patterns that lead to healthier behaviors.

    2. In **rational-emotive therapy**, developed by Albert Ellis (1913-), the therapist actively disputes a client's irrational beliefs.

    3. In **Gestalt therapy,** based on the collaborative efforts of Fritz Perls (1893-1970) and Paul Goodman (1911-1972), the therapist promotes the client's self-awareness and increased self-responsibility for meeting needs.

    4. In **Beck's cognitive therapy,** developed by Aaron Beck (1921-), the therapist teaches the client to identify and correct dysfunctional thoughts about the self, the world, and the future.

5. Cognitive techniques may be used by the therapist to teach the client new thinking skills.

   a. **Cognitive restructuring** teaches the client to change maladaptive beliefs through positive self-statements and refuting irrational beliefs.

   b. **Thought stopping** teaches the client to consciously say, "stop" to maladaptive thoughts.

C. Application to nursing

1. The nurse assesses the client's thought patterns and identifies misperceptions. (See *Table 2-3, Common misperceptions of thought patterns.*)
2. The nurse encourages the client to assume responsibility for his behaviors and fosters awareness of the effect of negative thinking on feelings about self-image.
3. The nurse uses cognitive techniques in intervention strategies.

VI. HUMANISTIC FRAMEWORK

A. Key concepts

1. A **humanistic framework** focuses on the "here and now"—current behaviors, issues, and problems—as well as spiritual values and meanings.
2. Human nature is viewed as positive and growth-oriented, and existence involves search for meaning and authenticity.
3. Abraham Maslow's (1908-1970) theory of **human motivation** describes human needs that are organized according to levels **(hierarchy of needs),** in which individuals move on to higher needs as lower, more basic needs are met.

   a. **Physiologic needs** include the basic needs required to sustain life (air, food, water).

   b. **Safety and security** is the need to establish security, stability, and consistency out of the chaos of life.

   c. **Love and belonging** refers to an individual's desire for acceptance and belonging to others.

   d. **Self-esteem** and **esteem for others** are the needs for self-mastery and recognition by others.

   e. **Self-actualization,** the highest need, describes self-awareness and the desire to become the best that one can become.

4. The failure to develop one's full potential leads to poor coping.
5. Lack of self-awareness and unmet needs interfere with feelings of security (self-esteem) as well as with relationships.
6. Fundamental human anxiety is the fear of death, which leads to existential anxiety (concern about the meaning of one's life).

B. Treatments

1. **Client-centered therapy,** developed by Carl Rogers (1902-1987), is based on the belief that mental illness results from an individual's failure to develop fully as a human being.

   a. Psychotherapy fosters the process of learning to be fully one's own self.

    b. The therapist is genuine and without facade when relating to the client; she is an active participant in the therapeutic relationship and expresses her own feelings and emotions directly and honestly.

    c. The client's behavior changes toward positive self-functioning when the therapist conveys acceptance, respect, and genuine empathy for the client.

  2. Existential therapy is a form of talk therapy that focuses on life issues of freedom, helplessness, loss, isolation, aloneness, anxiety, and death; through psychotherapy, the client discovers his own meaning of existence.

C. Application to nursing

  1. Humanism establishes a theoretical framework for the caring component of nursing.

  2. The nurse-client relationship is based on positive regard, respect, and empathy.

  3. The nurse must analyze herself when working with the psychiatric client.

  4. The nurse assesses the client's spiritual aspects, including beliefs and values about spirituality or religion, the meaning of one's life, and the meaning of suffering and painful experiences; relationship with a higher being; connection with people, society, and nature; and the importance placed on such values as truth, beauty, love, tolerance, patience, and forgiveness.

  5. Through reflective listening and empathic responses, the nurse helps the client gain self-understanding.

  6. The nurse advocates the client's freedom to choose alternative behaviors in congruence with beliefs about the meaning and value of one's life.

Study questions

1. The nurse is teaching a schizophrenic client and his family about treatment for the chemical imbalance associated with his disease. Which neurotransmitter would the nurse identify as being the target for antipsychotic medications?
1. Acetylcholine
2. Dopamine
3. Norepinephrine
4. Serotonin

2. The nurse is reviewing the laboratory findings of a client being treated for depression. Which hormone level should she focus on?
1. Testosterone
2. Insulin
3. Parathyroid hormone
4. Thyroid hormone

3. A client diagnosed with cancer does not talk about or acknowledge her diagnosis. Which of the following defense mechanisms is this client using?
1. Denial
2. Identification
3. Projection
4. Rationalization

4. In planning care for a client, the nurse identifies certain privileges (telephone use, participation in recreational activities) to be used as rewards for desirable behavior. These privileges serve as:
1. an extinctive response.
2. an operant conditioning.
3. a behavioral technique.
4. positive reinforcers.

5. The nurse listens carefully to a client talk about choices and responsibilities in life, then encourages him to clarify his values in terms of choices to be made. The client begins to discuss the meaning of life in accordance with his spiritual values. Which conceptual framework is the nurse using?
   1. Behavioral framework
   2. Humanistic framework
   3. Psychodynamic framework
   4. Psychobiologic framework

6. During an assessment, the client tells the nurse, "I don't know what to do. My marriage is terrible, and I just got fired from my job." Which of the following is a client-centered response?
   1. "Your thoughts are negative right now, and this keeps you from making decisions."
   2. "Things in your life are not working well now, and you feel unsure about what to do."
   3. "Have you considered marriage counseling? Many people have benefitted from this."
   4. "Other people have difficulties too. Have you thought about joining a support group?"

7. Based on Erikson's theory, assessment of an adolescent client for age-appropriate development task work is conducted by asking questions about:
   1. ability to complete tasks.
   2. development of an intimate relationship.
   3. level of trust in others.
   4. self-identity.

8. According to Piaget's theory, which of the following is the typical age in which children would be able to participate in a group discussion about the concept of self-esteem?
   1. Age 6 to 7
   2. Age 4 to 5
   3. Age 8 to 10
   4. Age 12 to 14

9. A primary nurse encourages her client to record ongoing thoughts in a daily diary. The nurse then reviews the diary with the client to identify thought patterns that contribute to feelings of depression and anxiety. Which of the following conceptual frameworks is the nurse using?
   1. Behavioral framework
   2. Cognitive framework
   3. Interpersonal framework
   4. Psychodynamic framework

10. A client's possessions were stolen while he was sleeping at a homeless shelter, and now he has neither shoes that fit nor a winter coat. The client is well known to the community nurse and has been treated for persistent mental illness. He tells the nurse that the theft is proof of an FBI plot against him. Which nursing intervention is the nurse's priority?
    1. Discuss the client's feelings about loss.
    2. Encourage the client to interact with other residents.
    3. Obtain appropriate clothing for the client.
    4. Refer the client for outpatient treatment.

11. A man who was released from prison for selling narcotics has been rehabilitated and now works for a youth drug prevention agency. His current behavior reflects which defense mechanism?
    1. Denial
    2. Displacement

3. Identification
4. Sublimation

12. A client tells the nurse that because she failed an important test in school, she will never have an opportunity for a good job. Using cognitive theory, the nurse would identify the client's misperception as:
1. dichotomous thinking.
2. minimization.
3. overgeneralization.
4. reaction formation.

13. The nurse applies Maslow's theory of human needs when establishing priority of care for the psychiatric client. From the following list, order the needs from the most basic to the highest according to Maslow's hierarchy.
1. Safety and security
2. Self-esteem and esteem for others

3. Love and belonging
4. Physiologic needs
5. Self-actualization

14. The nurse uses cognitive theory when working with a client who believes that because her boyfriend broke up with her, she is unattractive, worthless, and will never marry. Which of the following interventions are examples of the use of cognitive theory? Select all that apply.
1. Encourage the client to analyze early parental relationships.
2. Encourage the client to practice positive thinking.
3. Help the client to analyze the underlying meaning of her behavior.
4. Help the client to identify negative thoughts.
5. Help the client to understand the effect of thoughts on feelings and behaviors.

Answer key

1. The answer is 2.
The neurotransmitter dopamine is associated with schizophrenia. In general, antipsychotic medications will block receptor sites for this chemical. The remaining options are all neurotransmitters, but they are not the targets for antipsychotic medications.

2. The answer is 4.
Research has shown that decreased functioning of the thyroid gland is associated with depression. The other hormones have not been associated with depression.

3. The answer is 1.
Failure to acknowledge the reality of the diagnosis is an example of the defense mechanism of denial. The other defense mechanisms do not apply to this situation.

4. The answer is 4.
In behavioral theory, the use of rewards for desirable behaviors will reinforce those behaviors. The stated examples are positive reinforcers. Extinction refers to stopping undesirable behavior by withholding reinforcers. Operant conditioning is the process used in behavioral change, not the particular reward system. The use of rewards is a behavioral technique; however, this response is not specific enough to answer the question.

5. The answer is 2.
Humanistic framework focuses on individual choice and responsibility. Using this framework, the nurse provides client-centered care.

6. The answer is 2.

Client-centered responses are based on active listening techniques. In this example, the nurse reflects what the client said. Client-centered responses help the client attain greater self-understanding. Option 1 is incorrect because the nurse is focusing on the client's cognitive processes. Options 3 and 4 are incorrect because the nurse is ignoring the client's feelings by suggesting that the client discuss them with someone else.

7. The answer is 4.

The developmental task of the adolescent is *identity versus role diffusion*. The nurse is assessing the client's sense of identity by asking how he views himself. The remaining options would be used to assess other developmental tasks or stages of development.

8. The answer is 4.

According to Piaget, children develop the ability to think in a conceptual manner from age 12 to adulthood. The other options are incorrect because children in these age groups are developmentally unable to use abstract thinking.

9. The answer is 2.

The cognitive approach is based on the idea that thoughts influence behavior and feelings. In this example, the client must first identify recurrent thought processes that are related to depression and anxiety. The behavioral approach focuses on identifying and changing particular behaviors by changing the environmental reinforcers that allow symptoms to persist. The interpersonal framework focuses on the client's relationships with significant others and the effects of these relationships on the client's behavior and symptoms. The psychodynamic framework focuses on the role of unconscious processes and the way in which these processes influence the client's behavior or symptoms.

10. The answer is 3.

The client's basic needs are not being met because essential items of clothing have been taken. The nurse establishes priorities for intervention based on Maslow's hierarchy of human needs. Options 1 and 4 would be more appropriate following resolution of the current problem (when the client again has appropriate clothing). Option 2 is inappropriate at this time because the client is experiencing delusional thoughts about others.

11. The answer is 4.

Sublimation is the defense mechanism whereby an individual substitutes constructive, socially acceptable behavior for strong impulses that are unacceptable. The other defense mechanisms do not apply to this situation.

12. The answer is 3.

The client is making a global assumption that a good job cannot be attained because of an isolated incident (failing an important test). This is a common misperception as identified by cognitive theory. Dichotomous thinking and minimization are also misperceptions identified by cognitive theory, but they do not apply to this example. Reaction formation is a defense mechanism.

13. The answer is 41325.

The physiologic needs are the first priority followed by the need for a safe and secure environment. The feeling of being loved and belonging to a social group is the next need in the hierarchy. In order to feel self-esteem and to esteem others, humans must have experienced the next need, which is love and belonging. The highest human need is self-actualization.

14. The answer is 3, 4, 5.

These interventions are based on cognitive theory, which emphasizes relationships among thinking, feeling, and behavior. Options 1 and 3 are interventions based on Freud's psychoanalytic theory.

3 Stress, Anxiety, and Anxiety-Related Disorders

I. OVERVIEW OF STRESS AND ANXIETY

A. Key concepts

1. **Stress** is a stimulus or situation that produces distress and creates physical and psychological demands on an individual, requiring coping and adapting.

   a. **General adaptation syndrome,** a theory developed by Hans Selye (1907-1982), describes stress as wear and tear on the body occurring regardless of whether the stressor is positive or negative; the body's response is predictable without regard to the particular stressor or cause.

TABLE 3-1

The "fight or flight" response

During the initial response to stress (alarm reaction), the body prepares for "fight or flight," producing the adaptations listed below.

Body part or system	Adaptation to stress
Hypothalamus	▪ Sympathetic nervous system is stimulated.
Sympathetic nervous system	▪ Adrenal medulla is stimulated.
Adrenal medulla	▪ Epinephrine and norepinephrine are released.
Eyes	▪ Pupils dilate.
Lacrimal glands	▪ Tear secretion increases.
Respiratory system	▪ Bronchioles and pulmonary blood vessels dilate; respiratory rate increases.
Cardiovascular system	▪ Force of cardiac contraction increases. ▪ Cardiac output increases. ▪ Heart rate increases. ▪ Blood pressure increases.
Gastrointestinal system	▪ Gastric motility (stomach and intestines) decreases. ▪ Secretions decrease. ▪ Sphincters contract.
Liver	▪ Glycogenolysis (glucose breakdown) and gluconeogenesis (glucose manufactured from other body substances) increase. ▪ Glycogen synthesis decreases.
Urinary tract	▪ Ureter motility increases. ▪ Bladder muscle contracts. ▪ Bladder sphincter relaxes.
Sweat glands	▪ Secretion increases.
Fat cells	▪ Lipolysis is initiated.

FIGURE 3-1

Understanding the sustained-stress response

When a continuing "fight or flight" response becomes a sustained-stress response, the whole body is affected. The hypothalamus stimulates the pituitary gland, which in turn directs the release of various hormones, including adrenocorticotropin, which stimulates the adrenal cortex: vasopressin, growth hormone, thyrotropin, and gonadotropins.

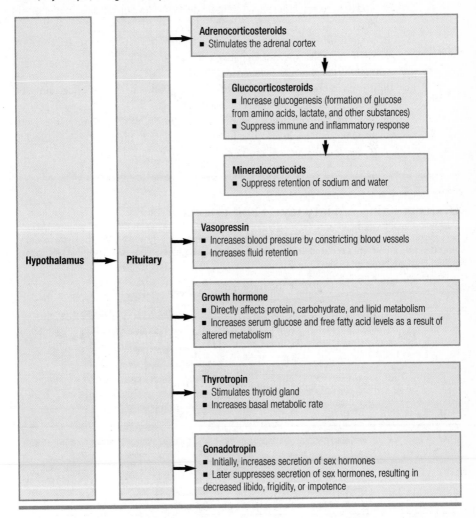

- An **alarm reaction** (also known as the **"fight or flight" response**) occurs when the sympathetic nervous system and endocrine system react to stress. (See *Table 3-1, The "fight or flight" response,* and *Figure 3-1, Understanding the sustained-stress response.*)
- The **stages of resistance** are adaptive responses that attempt to limit the damage of stress.

      – The **stage of exhaustion** occurs when physiologic and psychological resources are depleted and the immune system becomes depressed.

    b. Positive or negative transitions and changes can be sources of stress.

    c. In 1967, Thomas Holmes and Richard Rahe developed a numerical scale ranking stressful life events and the amount of distress they cause; according to their research, the greater the number of stressful life events over a given period of time, the more likely the individual is to develop physical or mental illness.

    d. In the *DSM-IV TR*, psychosocial stressors are rated in terms of severity on Axis IV of the multiaxial system of diagnosing mental illness.

  2. Anxiety is the subjective response to stress.

    a. It is characterized by feelings of apprehension, uneasiness, uncertainty, or dread, resulting from a real or perceived threat.

    b. Anxiety occurs in degrees of increasing intensity, ranging from mild anxiety to panic, which can affect an individual's ability to function. (See *Figure 3-2, Understanding anxiety levels and effects.*)

FIGURE 3-2

Understanding anxiety levels and effects

Depending on the degree of severity, anxiety produces various effects ranging from heightened alertness to complete inability to focus. Generally, the more severe the anxiety, the greater the dysfunction, as evidenced in the client's reduced ability to focus and deal with stress. Nursing interventions for each anxiety level are provided below.

ABILITY TO DEAL WITH STRESS AND TO LEARN IS REDUCED

| Mild | Moderate | Severe | Panic |

PERCEPTUAL FIELD AND ABILITY TO FOCUS ARE REDUCED

Anxiety levels	Effects	Nursing interventions
Mild	Increased alertness; enhanced learning	Use cognitive strategies, stress-management education, and problem-solving approach
Moderate	Ability to focus on central concerns; difficulty staying attentive and being able to learn	Use relaxation techniques; assist in using problem-solving approaches; teach coping strategies; and encourage verbalization of feelings
Severe	Inability to focus or solve problems; sympathetic nervous system activated	Encourage physical activity to stimulate large muscle groups and to release energy from "fight or flight" response (structured tasks and exercise are helpful)
Panic	Complete inability to focus; disintegrated ability to cope; physiologic symptoms from "fight or flight" response	Decrease environmental stimuli; stay with the client; using a quiet voice, assist him with relaxation breathing

DISPLAY 3-1
Coping strategies for stress reduction

- Seek out a supportive person.
- Strive for self-discipline and perseverance.
- Vent strong emotions.
- Think through options and use problem-solving techniques.
- Perform physical activities and exercise to release energy.

- Use relaxation techniques, such as:
  - listening to music
  - taking a warm shower or bath
  - meditating
  - performing imagery or visualization exercises
  - using progressive muscle-relaxation techniques.

3. Stress and anxiety can motivate and challenge a person as well as cause distress.
4. An individual's response to stress and anxiety depends on, but is not limited to, the following factors:
   a. Age, developmental maturity, or both
   b. Physical and mental health status
   c. Genetic predisposition (increased sensitivity to stress)
   d. Perceived meaning (stress can be viewed as harmful, threatening, or challenging)
   e. Cultural and spiritual values
   f. Social and environmental supports
   g. Learned coping responses. (See *Display 3-1, Coping strategies for stress reduction.*)

B. Psychobiological aspects of stress and anxiety

1. Neurobiologic changes involved in the alarm phase of the "fight or flight" response (stimulation of the hypothalamic-pituitary axis) produce cardiovascular, neuromuscular, gastrointestinal, and respiratory system effects (See *Table 3-1, The "fight or flight" response*, page 40); the client may experience tachycardia, headache, diarrhea, nausea, or tachypnea.
2. Neurotransmitter alterations in the brain, especially in the limbic system, have been implicated in stress, anxiety, and some anxiety-related disorders.
   a. **Gamma-aminobutyric acid (GABA)** is an inhibitory neurotransmitter associated with the relaxation response; because medications used to treat anxiety enhance GABA, researchers believe that a relative deficiency or imbalance in GABA is directly related to anxiety.
   b. **Serotonin** is a complex neurotransmitter associated with many aspects of brain functioning; deficits or imbalance of serotonin in the amygdala are thought to be significant in anxiety and anxiety-related disorders.
   c. **Norepinephrine** is an excitatory neurotransmitter responsible for cardiovascular changes in stress and anxiety; the noradrenergic dysregulation theory identifies norepinephrine systems as either overactive or underactive in areas of the brain associated with anxiety.
3. Biological differences in some individuals can lead to an overly active stress response (such as overproduction of hormones and neurotransmitters involved in the stress response), as hypothesized by **Jerome Kagan** in 1996.

4. Genetic studies have validated increased susceptibility to certain anxiety-related disorders in families.

C. Psychological variables that affect stress

1. Four psychological variables affect the physiological mechanisms of the stress response:
   a. **Control:** the belief that one has some control over stressors can lessen the intensity of the stress response.
   b. **Predictability:** stressors that can be predicted lessen the impact of the stress response (as compared with the response to unpredictable stressors).
   c. **Perception:** an individual's view of the world and perception of the current stressor either increases or decreases the intensity of the stress response.
   d. **Coping responses:** the availability and effectiveness of defense or coping mechanisms may increase or decrease the stress response.
2. Therapists and nurses consider these variables when developing a client's plan of care.

D. Psychosocial theories of stress and anxiety

1. According to the **psychodynamic theory,** the unconscious conflicts resulting from repressed wishes and drives cause guilt and shame, which lead to anxiety; anxiety threatens the ego, and protective defense mechanisms are used to respond to this threat.
2. With the **interpersonal theory,** early interpersonal relationships directly affect development of self-concept and self-esteem; individuals with poor self-concept and decreased self-esteem are more susceptible to anxiety and anxiety-related disorders.
3. **Behavioral theory** suggests that anxiety is a conditioned response to internal and external stressors.
4. **Cognitive theory** purports that the subjective feeling of anxiety is directly related to an individual's thoughts about himself, his future, and the world; faulty cognitive patterns can lead to misperceptions about the meaning of events (and therefore cause anxiety).
5. According to the **humanistic theory,** anxiety is related to the loss of meaning in one's life.

NURSING PROCESS OVERVIEW

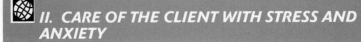

II. CARE OF THE CLIENT WITH STRESS AND ANXIETY

A. Assessment

1. Review the client's history for precipitating stressors.
2. Note the physiologic symptoms of the client's anxiety. (See *Table 3-1, The "fight or flight" response,* page 40.)
3. Determine the client's degree of anxiety, on a scale from mild to panic level. (See *Figure 3-2, Understanding anxiety levels and effects,* page 42.) Ask the client

to rate her experience of anxiety on a scale of 1 to 10 (10 being the highest level of anxiety).

4. Determine the client's cognitive responses, including her belief about the degree of control she has, her perception of stressors, and her ability to concentrate and make decisions.

5. Observe for behaviors typically noted in anxiety states, including irritability and anger, restlessness and pacing, crying and sighing, and complaints of tension and nervousness.

6. Determine the effect of the client's distress on her family, including the level of family involvement, the quality of family relationships, and the amount of support the family provides to the client.

7. Determine the client's use of coping strategies. (See *Display 3-1, Coping strategies for stress reduction*, page 43.)

B. Nursing diagnoses

1. Analyze the internal and external stressors affecting the client as well as the effectiveness of the client's coping strategies and defense mechanisms. (See *Table 2-1, Common defense mechanisms*, page 26).

2. Establish individualized nursing diagnoses for the client (and the client's family, as needed):
   a. Disturbed sleep pattern
   b. Impaired adjustment
   c. Readiness for enhanced coping
   d. Readiness for enhanced family coping
   e. Risk for self-directed or other-directed violence

C. Planning and outcome identification

1. Work with the client and her family, as needed, to set realistic goals.

2. Establish desired outcome criteria—measures that can be used to evaluate the client's improvement as a result of nursing interventions and her independent change in thinking, feeling, or behaving.
   a. Acknowledge the presence of anxiety and stress.
   b. Identify the stressors causing the anxiety.
   c. Use established coping strategies or learn new ones to reduce anxiety and stress.
   d. Modify thoughts and behaviors to enhance coping.

D. Implementation

1. The nurse helps the client to identify precipitating stressors and teaches her to monitor physical and psychological responses to stress. (See *Client and family teaching 3-1, Guidelines for clients with anxiety disorders*, page 46.)

2. For a client with mild or moderate anxiety, see *Figure 3-2, Understanding anxiety levels and effects*, page 42.

3. For a client with severe or panic-level anxiety, take the following measures:
   a. Stay with the client and provide support.
   b. Keep demands on the client to a minimum.
   c. Limit environmental stimuli (turn off loud music, avoid crowded areas).

CLIENT AND FAMILY TEACHING 3-1
Guidelines for clients with anxiety disorders

Provide information about the client's specific disorder and treatment:
- Anxiety-related disorders have both physical (brain chemical) and psychological causes (experience of stressful life events).
- The client with an anxiety disorder does not have control over symptoms. Part of the treatment is to learn how to control the anxiety.

Include information about how the family can be helpful:
- Remaining calm when the anxious client is upset, fearful, and panicky is helpful. You cannot control the client's response — only your own.

- Treatment may take time, and providing encouragement for small changes in positive directions is helpful.
- Encouraging the client to refrain from such substances as caffeine, nicotine, and alcohol can help reduce anxious feelings.
- Maintain your own normal lifestyle and functioning; giving up things you normally do in order to decrease the client's anxiety will create resentment.
- Learn about any medications used in the client's treatment.

---

     d. Encourage physical activity (such as walking) to release energy.

     e. Administer prescribed anxiolytic medications in a timely manner.

     f. Help the client to perform relaxation-breathing techniques.

  4. Provide additional measures as needed.

     a. Encourage the client to limit caffeine and nicotine intake.

     b. Promote sleep with comfort measures (warm bath, music, back rub).

     c. Protect the client from impulsive acts using one-to-one supervision.

     d. Help the client to express her feelings through active listening and empathic responses.

     e. Provide the client with information regarding community support systems, such as crisis hotline numbers, referral to a mental health center, self-help groups, and stress management clinics and programs.

     f. Teach the client and her family about prescribed medications, including the reason for use, dosage and timing, measures to counteract minor side effects, side effects that require notification of a health care provider, and what to do if a dosage is missed.

E. Outcome evaluation

  1. The nurse evaluates the client to determine whether established outcome criteria have been met as a result of nursing interventions.

  2. Possible outcomes include the following:

     a. The client recognizes and verbalizes her feelings of anxiety.

     b. The client identifies the stressors causing anxiety.

     c. The client reports a reduction in anxiety, an increased ability to cope, or both.

     d. The client modifies her behaviors to enhance coping.

     e. The client demonstrates improvement on standardized anxiety assessment scales.

III. ANXIETY-RELATED DISORDERS

A. Key concepts

1. The most common of all psychiatric disorders, **anxiety disorders** cause an individual to feel frightened, distressed, and uneasy without a specific cause (the specific stressor[s] may be out of the client's conscious awareness, and therefore the client attributes uneasy feelings to "bad nerves").
2. More than 23 million people in the United States are affected by anxiety disorders yearly (about 1 out of every 4 persons); those with anxiety disorder typically experience the physiologic, cognitive, and behavioral symptoms of anxiety.
3. The *DSM-IV TR* specifies the following types of anxiety disorders:
   a. Generalized anxiety disorder
   b. Panic disorders
   c. Obsessive-compulsive disorder
   d. Phobic disorder
   e. Post-traumatic stress disorder

B. Generalized anxiety disorder (GAD)

1. The essential feature of GAD is excessive anxiety and worry occurring more days than not for at least 6 months; other characteristics include restlessness, feeling "keyed-up" or "on edge," easy fatigue, difficulty concentrating, irritability and muscle tension, and sleep disturbances.
2. The exact etiology is unknown; however, associated factors have been suggested.
   a. **Biologic vulnerability:** This disorder is thought to be associated with neurotransmitter abnormalities (GABA, serotonin, or norepinephrine dysregulation) within the limbic system.
   b. **Gender:** Women are affected twice as often as men.
   c. **Other psychiatric disorders:** GAD has a high co-morbidity rate with other psychiatric disorders, including major depression and panic disorder.
   d. **Psychosocial factors:** GAD is associated with low self-esteem, decreased tolerance for stress, and the tendency to believe in an external locus of control.
3. Treatment generally takes place in community settings, including the primary care physician's office.
   a. **Antianxiety medications,** especially benzodiazepines, are used on a short-term basis (long-term use is not recommended because these drugs cause tolerance and dependence); nonbenzodiazapine antianxiety medications, such as buspirone (BuSpar) and various antidepressants, are also used. (See *Drug chart 3-1, Selected medications for treating anxiety disorders*, page 48.)
   b. **Cognitive-behavioral therapy,** including relaxation training and biofeedback, is recommended. Other cognitive techniques (questioning evidence, examining alternatives, reframing) may be used.

DRUG CHART 3-1
Selected medications for treating anxiety disorders

Classification	Drug	Rationale for use
Benzodiazepines	alprazolam (Xanax) chlordiazepoxide (Librium) clonazepam (Klonopin) lorazepam (Ativan)	Increase levels of gamma-aminobutyric acid, which decreases stimulation of limbic system, thereby decreasing anxiety; used for short-term treatment of generalized anxiety disorder (GAD), panic disorder, and social phobia.
Azapirones	buspirone (BuSpar)	Acts on serotonin receptors, causing presynaptic neurons to release less serotonin; decreased serotonin is thought to lead to decreased anxiety; used for GAD, panic disorder, and social phobia.
Tricyclic antidepressants	clomipramine (Anafranil) imipramine (Tofranil)	Block reuptake of neurotransmitters (serotonin and norepinephrine), thus allowing increased levels at synapse; deficits of serotonin in amygdala thought to be significant in anxiety disorders; used for GAD, panic disorder, social phobia, and obsessive-compulsive disorder (OCD).
Selective serotonin reuptake inhibitors	fluoxetine (Prozac) fluvoxamine (Luvox) paroxetine (Paxil) sertraline (Zoloft)	Selectively block serotonin reuptake at synapse, thereby increasing serotonin levels; used for GAD, panic disorder (Paxil, Zoloft, Effexor), and OCD.
Other antidepressants	venlafaxine (Effexor)	Affects serotonin reuptake and norepinephrine and dopamine levels; used for GAD.
Monoamine oxidase inhibitors	phenelzine (Nardil)	Inhibits action of enzyme oxidase (monamine oxidase), which breaks down serotonin, thereby increasing serotonin levels; used for panic disorders and agoraphobia.
Beta blockers	atenolol (Tenormin) propranolol (Inderal)	Induce peripheral beta-adrenergic blockade, therefore reducing physiologic effects of anxiety; used for social phobia and post-traumatic stress disorder.

C. Panic disorder

1. Panic disorder is characterized by panic attacks that recur at unpredictable times with intense apprehension, fear, and terror. (See *Display 3-2, Characteristics of panic attacks.*)

2. Panic disorder may occur with or without **agoraphobia** (anxiety about being in places or situations from which escape might be difficult or embarrassing, or in which help may not be available in the event of having panic-like symptoms).

   a. **Panic disorder without agoraphobia** is characterized by recurrent, unexpected panic attacks followed by at least 1 month of persistent concern about

DISPLAY 3-2
Characteristics of panic attacks

The hallmark of panic disorder, panic attacks produce various physiologic and psychological symptoms, as listed below.

- Physiologic symptoms of "fight or flight" response:
  - racing heart
  - chest pains
  - dizziness and nausea
  - difficulty breathing
  - choking sensations
  - numbness and tingling sensations
  - trembling and diaphoresis

- Feeling that one is having a heart attack
- Feeling that one is "going crazy"
- Fear of loss of control
- Decreased perceptual ability
- Decreased cognitive abilities

having another attack, worry about the possible implications or consequences of the attack, or a significant behavioral change related to the attack.

  b. **Panic disorder with agoraphobia** is defined as recurrent, unexpected panic attacks along with agoraphobia.

3. Although the exact etiology is unknown, associated factors include the following:

  a. **Biologic vulnerability:** Panic disorder may result from irregularities in the synthesis and release of norepinephrine, receptor hypersensitivity to serotonin or GABA, or both.

  b. **Lactate sensitivity:** Sodium lactate produces the physical symptoms associated with panic disorder in 4 out of 5 people with panic disorder; this same sensitivity is often found in family members of those with the disorder.

  c. **Suffocation alarm theory:** The rapid, heavy breathing (hyperventilation) that occurs during panic attacks may result from a false signal from the brain indicating a shortage of oxygen or an increase in carbon dioxide, thus triggering the panic attack.

  d. **Mitral valve prolapse:** Women with mitral valve prolapse have increased incidence of panic disorder; both disorders appear to have a genetic basis.

  e. **Family history:** Individuals with a family history of panic disorders are 4 to 7 times more likely to develop this disorder.

  f. **Psychosocial factors:** Stressful life events and faulty thinking pair together in such a way that normal bodily reactions are interpreted as catastrophic.

4. Treatment of the initial panic attack usually occurs in the emergency department because the individual may think she is having a heart attack; other medical conditions must be ruled out before diagnosis of panic disorder is made.

  a. **Antianxiety medications,** such as benzodiazepines and buspirone, and **antidepressants** are commonly used to treat panic disorder; although **monoamine oxidase inhibitors** can be used, they require dietary restrictions. (See pages 275 and 276.)

    - Benzodiazepines must be used cautiously because they are highly addictive.

    – The antidepressants paroxetine (Paxil), sertraline (Zoloft), and venlafaxine (Effexor) are considered effective in treating panic disorder and were approved by the FDA for this purpose. (See *Drug chart 3-1, Selected medications for treating anxiety disorders*, page 48.)

    b. **Cognitive-behavioral therapy** targets the panic-generating thought process and behaviors that originate and maintain anxiety-laden symptoms; specific techniques include client education and awareness, cognitive restructuring, and controlled relaxation breathing.

D. Obsessive-compulsive disorder (OCD)

    1. The essential features of OCD are recurrent **obsessions** (persistent ideas) or **compulsions** (uncontrollable urges to perform an act repetitively) that are severe enough to be time-consuming, cause marked distress, or lead to significant impairment in functioning (see *Display 3-3, Characteristics of obsessive-compulsive disorder*); the disorder often begins in childhood and adolescence.

    2. The exact etiology is not established, but associated factors include the following:

      a. **Biologic vulnerability:** OCD is associated with increased serotonin responsiveness, as validated by the success of antidepressant medications (both tricyclic antidepressants and the selective serotonin reuptake inhibitors [SSRIs]) in treating OCD.

      b. **Striatum dysfunction theory:** The striatum is the part of the brain that controls voluntary movement; repetitive motor acts (walking, chewing) stimulate release of serotonin, which in turn elevates mood; individuals with OCD may be performing repetitive rituals to "self-medicate" for their serotonin deficiency.

      c. **Genetic vulnerability:** The risk of OCD increases for an individual with a family history of the disorder.

    3. Once established, OCD tends to recur, and many clients experience increased symptoms associated with stressful events.

    4. Treatments include appropriate medication and cognitive-behavioral therapy.

      a. **Antidepressants,** especially tricyclic antidepressants, have been used for many years; currently, the **SSRIs** fluvoxamine (Luvox), fluoxetine (Prozac), sertraline (Zoloft), and paroxetine (Paxil) are recommended. (See *Drug chart 3-1, Selected medications for treating anxiety disorders*, page 48.)

DISPLAY 3-3
Characteristics of obsessive-compulsive disorder

In obsessive-compulsive disorder, the obsessions and compulsions commonly occur together.

- The most common *obsessions* are repeated thoughts about contamination, repeated doubts, a need to have things in particular order, aggressive or horrific impulses, and sexual imagery.
- Most common *compulsions* involve washing and cleaning, counting, checking, requesting or demanding assurances, repeating actions, and ordering.

- The individual is aware of the unrealistic, intrusive, and inappropriate nature of obsessions and compulsions (described as ego-dystonic symptoms).
- Attempt to resist obsessive thought or compulsive behavior causes the individual to experience increased anxiety.
- Indulgence in obsessive thoughts and performance of compulsive behaviors causes temporary anxiety relief (termed *primary gain*).

    b. **Cognitive-behavioral therapy** includes behavioral techniques, such as flooding and response prevention (putting the client in situations that usually trigger OCD behaviors and then preventing the OCD response); cognitive techniques are also used, in which cognitive distortions are identified and then restructured through psychoeducation.

E. Phobic disorder

    1. A phobic disorder is an irrational fear of a specific object, activity, or event (see *Display 3-4, Characteristics of phobic disorder*); individuals may have panic attacks or severe anxiety when exposed to these situations or objects.

    2. The exact etiology is unknown; however, the disorder may be linked to the following factors:

        a. **Genetic susceptibility:** Twin studies suggest phobias have genetic factors.

        b. **Conditioned response:** Behavioral theory suggests that phobia results from a conditioned response in which an individual learns to associate a phobic object with uncomfortable feelings; avoidance behaviors serve to reduce anxiety and reinforce the phobia.

    3. Effective treatment involves the use of appropriate medication and cognitive-behavioral therapy.

        a. Commonly used medications include **antidepressants** (tricyclic antidepressants and SSRIs) and **benzodiazepines** (can be used alone or in combination with antidepressants and **beta blockers**).

          – Social phobia can be treated with beta blockers in combination with an antidepressant or a benzodiazepine.

          – Benzodiazepines must be used cautiously because they are addictive. (See *Drug chart 3-1, Selected medications for treating anxiety disorders*, page 48.)

        b. **Systematic desensitization** (in which the client learns the relaxation response, establishes a hierarchy of phobic situations, and then gradually is exposed to each situation while maintaining the relaxation response) is commonly used.

        c. **Cognitive restructuring techniques** are also helpful in changing the client's perception of phobic situations.

F. Post-traumatic stress disorder (PTSD)

    1. PTSD is characterized by recurrent thoughts and feelings associated with a severe, specific trauma (combat experiences, rape, serious accident, severe depri-

---

DISPLAY 3-4
Characteristics of phobic disorder

Phobic disorder is marked by irrational fear of an object, person, or situation accompanied by persistent avoidance of the object, person, or situation.

■ The individual recognizes the fear as irrational and inappropriate (ego-dystonic), but he feels powerless to control it.

■ *Simple phobia* is the fear of specific things (elevators, airplanes, heights, insects).

■ *Social phobia* is the fear of potentially embarrassing social situations (the fear of eating or speaking in public or of using public restrooms).

DISPLAY 3-5
Characteristics of post-traumatic stress disorder

This disorder, which is characterized by recurrent thoughts and feelings of a severe trauma, may be an acute or delayed response or a chronic condition.
- Symptoms include an exaggerated startle response, sleep disorders, guilt (survivor's guilt), nightmares and flashbacks, and anger with numbing of other emotions.
- Affected individuals often use drugs, alcohol, or both to self-medicate for relief of distressful symptoms.

---

vation or abuse). (See *Display 3-5, Characteristics of post-traumatic stress disorder*.)

2. The cause of PTSD is the severe trauma experienced by the individual, but other factors may contribute to vulnerability.

   a. **Direct relationship:** There is a direct relationship between severe trauma and the risk of PTSD; out of 100 veterans who have suffered severe trauma, 31 of them will develop PTSD at some point in their life.

   b. **Psychosocial factors:** Other factors (separation from parents during childhood, family history of anxiety disorders, and preexisting anxiety or depression) can increase vulnerability to PTSD following severe trauma.

3. The client with PTSD may be treated with medication and a combination of individual and group therapy.

   a. **Antianxiety medications,** specifically benzodiazepines, are used cautiously because of risk of abuse or dependency; **antidepressants** are used to treat coexisting depressive disorders; **beta blockers** can be used to reduce the physiologic effects of anxiety. (See *Drug chart 3-1, Selected medications for treating anxiety disorders*, page 48.)

   b. **Cognitive-behavioral therapy,** especially cognitive restructuring, may be used to help the client view himself as a survivor rather than a victim.

   c. **Support group therapy,** especially with individuals who have experienced similar traumas (combat veteran groups, rape trauma groups), is also used.

G. Dissociative disorders

1. An individual with a dissociative disorder has an altered conscious awareness that may include periods of forgetfulness, memory loss of past stressful events, feeling disconnected from daily events, or an emergence of distinctly different personalities. (See *Display 3-6, DSM-IV TR subtypes of dissociative disorder*.)

2. Dissociative disorders are generally associated with traumatic events.

   a. **Trauma:** An individual reacts to trauma by "splitting off," or dissociating himself, from the memory of the trauma.

   b. **Abuse:** Dissociative identity disorder is generally thought to result from severe, traumatic abuse in early childhood; it is associated with a high comorbidity rate with substance abuse and depressive disorders.

   c. **Sexual and physical abuse in early childhood:** Early abuse has been found to affect neurodevelopment, especially in the left hemisphere and the limbic

---

DISPLAY 3-6
DSM-IV TR subtypes of dissociative disorder

The *DSM-IV TR* identifies five separate disorders characterized by dissociation, or the feeling of being detached from usual experiences or in a dreamlike state.
- *Dissociative amnesia* is the sudden inability to recall important personal information.
- *Dissociative fugue* is the sudden, unexpected flight from home with an inability to recall events from one's past.

- *Depersonalization disorder* is feeling detached from, and as if one is an outside observer of, one's thoughts or body.
- *Dissociative identity disorder* is the presence of two or more distinct personalities, each with its own pattern of perceiving, relating to, and thinking about the environment.
- *Dissociative disorder not otherwise specified* is a disorder that does not fit criteria for any of the other dissociative disorders.

---

system; these alterations in normal brain development are associated with problems involving mood, memory, and aggressive behavior.

    d. **Gender:** Diagnosis of dissociative identity disorder is 3 to 9 times more common in women than in men.

3. Dissociative disorders tend to be difficult to diagnose, and clients typically have multiple psychiatric diagnoses; consequently, treatment is often lengthy.

    a. **Medications** may be used when specific symptoms, such as anxiety or depression, are problematic.

    b. **Psychotherapy,** especially psychodynamic therapy with hypnosis, is used to elicit a conscious awareness of traumatic events and to facilitate coping with them.

    c. **Support group therapy** is useful in providing a supportive and psychoeducational approach.

NURSING PROCESS OVERVIEW

IV. CARE OF THE CLIENT WITH AN ANXIETY-RELATED DISORDER

A. Assessment

1. Note the physiologic symptoms of anxiety. (See *Table 3-1, The "fight or flight" response*, page 40.)
2. Use key nursing assessment questions to elicit information about the client's specific anxiety-related disorder. (See *Key questions 3-1, Assessing clients with anxiety disorders*, page 54.)
3. Note any cognitive-behavioral responses by the client that are congruent with established *DSM-IV TR* diagnostic criteria for an anxiety disorder.
4. Use standardized assessment tools (Yale-Brown Obsessive-Compulsive Scale, Dissociative Experiences Scale) for gathering detailed information regarding the client's anxiety-related disorder.
5. Review the client's history for previous diagnosis or treatment of anxiety-related disorders.

> **KEY QUESTIONS 3-1**
> ## Assessing clients with anxiety disorders
>
> | Questions | Information gathered |
> | --- | --- |
> | *Have you noticed feelings of increased tension, worry, or unease?* | Subjective feelings of anxiety |
> | *What kind of body sensations or symptoms do you experience when you are under stress?* | Client's awareness about unique stress-related body sensations |
> | *Do you have difficulty concentrating, feel restless, or have trouble making decisions?* | Symptoms related to generalized anxiety disorder |
> | *Have you experienced severe distress in which your heart was racing, you had difficulty breathing, and you thought you may be having a heart attack?* | Symptoms related to panic disorder |
> | *Do you find yourself constantly having recurrent thoughts that are difficult to control or stop?* *Have you ever had to perform certain rituals or behaviors over and over again in order to feel calmer?* | Symptoms of obsessive thoughts or compulsive behavior, related to obsessive-compulsive disorder |
> | *Do you have severe fears of persons, places, or things that prevent you from doing what you want?* | Symptoms related to phobic disorder |
> | *Have you experienced a severe tragedy in your life that comes back to you in dreams or flashbacks?* | Symptoms related to post-traumatic stress disorder |

      6. Discuss the client's perception of current stressors or precipitating events, and determine his use of coping strategies. (See *Display 3-1, Coping strategies for stress reduction*, page 43.)

      7. Determine the impact of the client's disorder on the family, including specific role changes within the family, the degree of family involvement with the client, and the level of support provided to the client; determine whether there is a history of family abuse.

B. Nursing diagnoses

      1. Analyze the internal and external stressors affecting the client, the impact of symptoms on normal daily functioning, and the effectiveness of coping strategies and defense mechanisms. (See *Table 2-1, Common defense mechanisms*, page 26.)

      2. Establish individualized nursing diagnoses for the client (and the client's family, as needed):

        a. Disturbed personal identity

        b. Ineffective denial

       c. Ineffective role performance

       d. Posttrauma syndrome

       e. Situational low self-esteem

C. Planning and outcome identification

1. Work with the client (and his family, as needed) in setting realistic goals.
2. Establish desired outcome criteria.
   a. The client can identify specific anxiety responses.
   b. The client can identify stressors related to his current experience of anxiety-related disorder.
   c. The client decreases or controls repetitive thoughts and behaviors.
   d. The client verbalizes relief or decrease in anxiety-related symptoms.
   e. The client performs normal daily activities without an increase in anxiety or distressful symptoms.
   f. The client uses various coping strategies to reduce anxiety.
   g. The client verbalizes experiences of traumatic events.

D. Implementation

1. For clients with **generalized anxiety disorder** or **panic disorders,** see the implementation steps listed in II.D. on pages 45 and 46.
2. For clients with **obsessive-compulsive disorder,** take the following measures:
   a. Convey acceptance of the client, despite his ritualistic behaviors.
   b. Allow the client time to perform rituals; his anxiety level will increase if he cannot perform compulsive behaviors.
   c. Encourage the client to set limits on ritualistic behaviors as part of the established treatment plan.
   d. Use active listening to encourage the client to verbalize his feelings; the best time for interaction is after he completes a ritualistic behavior.
   e. Help the client to list all of the objects and places that trigger anxiety, as part of an exposure-response prevention program.
   f. Teach the client about coping measures and the medications used as part of the treatment plan.
   g. Encourage the client to use community support systems.
3. For clients with **phobic disorder,** take the following measures:
   a. Do not force the client to be in contact with a phobic object or situation.
   b. Help the client describe his feelings prior to his response to a phobic object.
   c. Help the client identify alternative coping strategies to manage his anxiety about encountering a phobic situation.
   d. Use cognitive strategies, such as reframing, to help the client put thoughts and feelings into a different perspective.
   e. Practice relaxation techniques with the client.
   f. Participate as a member of the treatment team in the established program for systematic desensitization.
   g. Teach the client about prescribed medications used in treatment.
4. For clients with **post-traumatic stress disorder,** take the following measures:
   a. Use appropriate interventions to reduce anxiety (relaxation techniques, encouraging expression of feelings, limiting caffeine and nicotine).

    b. Validate for the client that the traumatic event he experienced was highly stressful.

    c. Help the client to verbalize all aspects of the traumatic event, including his thoughts and feelings.

    d. Teach the client coping strategies to manage anxiety symptoms that accompany memories of his trauma.

    e. Encourage the client to participate in self-help or support groups.

    f. Refer the client to a specialist in chemical dependency for a formal evaluation and, if necessary, treatment for drug or alcohol abuse if this is a problem (Alcoholics Anonymous or Narcotics Anonymous is usually part of treatment).

  5. For clients with **dissociative disorder,** take the following measures:

    a. Establish a trusting relationship, and provide support during times of depersonalization, amnesia, or emergence of new personalities.

    b. Encourage the client to disclose and discuss her feelings about painful memories emerging into consciousness.

    c. Teach the client anxiety-binding techniques, which provide the client with a mechanism that can be used to reduce anxiety levels when re-experienced memories threaten to overwhelm him; one example of an anxiety-binding technique is to instruct the client to imagine that the memory is a story in a book and when anxiety gets too high, to close the book and put it on the shelf.

    d. Accurately record information about the client's various personalities as part of an interdisciplinary team approach.

    e. Encourage the client's commitment to insight-oriented therapy with an experienced therapist.

E. Outcome evaluation

  1. The client identifies his own anxiety responses.

  2. The client identifies stressors in his past or current life situation that contribute to his anxiety response.

  3. The client uses coping strategies rather than symptomatic behaviors.

  4. The client identifies and actively participates in the continued treatment plan.

Study questions

1. Selye's general adaptation theory can be used to understand the relationship between stressful events and the body's response to stress. Which of the following statements best describes this relationship?

  1. The body goes through predictable responses regardless of the type of stressor.

  2. The body's defenses become depleted from stressful events.

  3. The body reacts differently when the stress is psychological rather than physical.

  4. The body eventually adapts to any stress in a positive manner.

2. A client is pacing and complains of racing thoughts. The nurse asks the client if something upsetting happened, and the

client's response is vague and not focused on the nurse's question. The nurse assesses the client's level of anxiety as:
1. mild.
2. moderate.
3. severe.
4. panic.

3. When teaching a group of clients about antianxiety medications, the nurse explains that benzodiazapines affect which brain chemical?
1. Acetylcholine
2. Gamma-aminobutyric acid (GABA)
3. Norepinephrine
4. Serotonin

4. The nurse is assessing a client for recent stressful life events. The nurse recognizes that stressful life events are both:
1. desirable and growth-promoting.
2. positive and negative.
3. undesirable and harmful.
4. predictable and controllable.

5. When teaching stress management to clients, the nurse will most likely advocate which belief as a method of coping with stressful life events?
1. Avoidance of stress is an important goal for living.
2. Control over one's response to stress is possible.
3. Most people have no control over their level of stress.
4. Significant others are important to provide care and concern.

6. A client who only attends social events when a family member is also present exhibits behavior typical of which anxiety disorder?
1. Agoraphobia
2. Generalized anxiety disorder
3. Obsessive-compulsive disorder

4. Post-traumatic stress disorder

7. The nurse is teaching the proper insulin injection technique to a client who was recently diagnosed with diabetes. During the lesson, the client is having difficulty concentrating, her respirations are rapid, and she is fidgeting in her chair. The nurse recently performed a capillary blood glucose test, and the client's blood sugar range is normal. Which intervention is best at this time?
1. Tell the client that it is vital to pay attention because insulin injections will help provide a normal life.
2. Leave the client alone at this time, instructing her to review the literature before the next lesson.
3. Stop the insulin lesson for a while, and ask the client how things are going.
4. Tell the client to relax and that, if she does so, it will be easier to learn about injections.

8. A client is newly admitted to a psychiatric unit because of severe obsessive-compulsive behavior. Which initial response by the nurse would be most therapeutic for the client?
1. Accepting the client's ritualistic behaviors
2. Challenging the client's need for rituals
3. Expressing concern about the harmfulness of the client's rituals
4. Limiting the client's rituals that are excessive

9. The nurse is assessing a client for symptoms of post-traumatic stress disorder (PTSD). Which symptoms are typically seen with this diagnosis? Select all that apply.
1. Anger with numbing of other emotions

2. Exaggerated startle response
3. Feeling that one is having a heart attack
4. Frequent thoughts about contamination
5. Frequent nightmares
6. Survivor's guilt

10. A client with a fear of air travel is being treated in a mental health clinic for phobic disorder. The treatment method involves systematic desensitization. The nurse would consider the treatment successful if:
1. the client plans a trip requiring air travel.
2. the client takes a short trip in an airplane.
3. the client recognizes the unrealistic nature of the fear of riding on airplanes.
4. the client verbalizes a decreased fear about air travel.

11. A psychiatrist prescribes clomipramine (Anafranil) to treat a client's obsessive-compulsive behavior. The nurse understands the rational for this treatment is that the clomipramine:
1. decreases norepinephrine levels.
2. decreases GABA levels.
3. increases dopamine levels.
4. increases serotonin levels.

12. The nurse is developing a care plan for a client with post-traumatic stress disorder. Which of the following would the nurse do initially?
1. Avoid discussing the traumatic event with the client.
2. Encourage the client to verbalize thoughts and feelings about the trauma.
3. Encourage the client to put the past in proper perspective.
4. Instruct the client to use distraction

techniques to cope with flashbacks.

13. During a routine week, the community nurse sees and plans care for various clients with different types of problems. Which of the following clients would the nurse consider the most vulnerable to post-traumatic stress disorder?
1. The child with asthma who has recently failed a grade in school
2. The college student with diabetes who experienced date rape
3. The man who has recently lost his wife to cancer
4. The spouse of an individual with a severe substance abuse problem

14. Which outcome is most appropriate for a client with a dissociative disorder?
1. The client will deal with uncomfortable emotions on a conscious level.
2. The client will modify stress with the use of relaxation techniques.
3. The client will identify his anxiety responses.
4. The client will use problem-solving strategies when feeling stressed.

15. The psychiatric nurse uses cognitive-behavioral techniques when working with a client who experiences panic attacks. Which of the following techniques are common to this theoretical framework? Select all that apply.
1. Administering anti-anxiety medications as prescribed
2. Encouraging the client to restructure thoughts
3. Helping the client to use controlled relaxation breathing
4. Helping the client to examine evidence of stressors
5. Questioning the client about early childhood relationships
6. Teaching the client about anxiety and panic

Answer key

1. The answer is 1.

Selye's theory states that regardless of the stressor (whether it is chemical, physical, or psychological), the body's physiologic response is the same—an alarm reaction. If the stress continues and the body reaches the stage of exhaustion, then defenses are depleted. Adaptation may not occur if the stage of exhaustion is reached from continued stress.

2. The answer is 3.

When the client has difficulty focusing and exhibits excessive motor activity, the level of anxiety is severe. Mild anxiety is characterized by increased alertness and problem-solving ability; the client described is unable to do this. Moderate anxiety is characterized by the ability to focus on central concerns but the inability to problem-solve without assistance; the client described is unable to do this. Panic-level anxiety is characterized by complete inability to focus and reduced perceptions; the client described is not at this level.

3. The answer is 2.

Antianxiety medications stimulate the neurotransmitter GABA, which is a chemical associated with relaxation. The other neurotransmitters (acetylcholine, norepinephrine, and serotonin) are not affected by benzodiazapines.

4. The answer is 2.

The concept of stressful life events is based on the research of Holmes and Rahe, who found that both positive and negative changes result in stress. Stressful life events are not always desirable and growth promoting, nor are they always undesirable and harmful. Some stressful life events can be predictable and controllable; however, many events are entirely unpredictable.

5. The answer is 2.

When learning to manage stress, clients find it helpful to believe that they have the ability to control their response to it. It is impossible to avoid stress, which is a normal life experience. Stress can be positive and growth enhancing as well as harmful. The belief that one has some control is the significant factor in minimizing stress response. Clients who do not believe this is possible typically experience increased stress. Although significant others are important, the client's ability to help himself to cope is essential.

6. The answer is 1.

Agoraphobia is a disorder characterized by avoidance of situations in which escape may not be possible or help may be unavailable. Generalized anxiety disorder, obsessive-compulsive disorder, and post-traumatic stress disorders are anxiety disorders, but they are not typically characterized by the behavior of the client described in the question.

7. The answer is 3.

Because the client's anxiety is increased, the nurse should stop the insulin injection lesson and assess what is happening. Asking an open-ended question and conveying interest may reduce the client's anxiety and elicit information about her current concerns. Teaching is ineffective when a client is at a severe level of anxiety. Option 1 assumes the client's concerns are about having a normal life. Option 2 ignores the client's anxiety. A client experiencing severe anxiety cannot focus on relaxing; therefore, option 4 is also incorrect.

8. The answer is **1.**
It is important to accept the client's need to perform ritualistic behaviors in this situation; admission to a psychiatric unit is stressful, and this client will tend to increase rituals when anxious. Although the other responses by the nurse may be appropriate as part of an ongoing treatment plan, they are not appropriate for a newly admitted client.

9. The answer is **1, 2, 5, 6.**
These are common symptoms of PTSD. Option 3 is common in panic disorder, and option 4 is characteristic of obsessive-compulsive disorder.

10. The answer is **2.**
Systematic desensitization is a behavioral technique in which the client with a specific phobia is gradually able to work through hierarchical fears until the most fearful situation is encountered. To achieve success with this method, the client would need to do what is most fearful—riding in an airplane. The responses in options 1 and 4 may occur earlier in treatment, but they are not indicative of success. Generally, a phobic individual recognizes that his fear is disproportionate to the thing he fears.

11. The answer is **4.**
According to the psychobiologic theory, dysregulation of the neurotransmitter serotonin is thought to contribute to obsessive-compulsive behavior. Clomipramine (Anafranil) is used to increase serotonin levels, thereby decreasing the need for obsessive-compulsive behaviors.

12. The answer is **2.**
Planning care for a client with post-traumatic stress disorder would involve helping the client to verbalize thoughts and feelings about the trauma. This strategy will help the client work through the strong emotions connected with the trauma and, therefore, help foster the belief that he is able to cope. The traumatic event needs to be dealt with in a conscious way, including recognizing strong emotions; therefore, avoiding discussion and using distraction techniques would be inappropriate. Option 3 may be possible later, after the client is able to verbalize strong emotions related to trauma; however, it is inappropriate as an initial intervention.

13. The answer is **2.**
Post-traumatic stress disorder is caused by the experience of severe, specific trauma. Rape is a severely traumatic event. Although the situations in options 1, 3, and 4 are certainly stressful, they are not at the level of severe trauma.

14. The answer is **1.**
Dissociative disorders occur when traumatic events are beyond an individual's recall because these memories have been "blocked" from conscious awareness. Bringing the feelings associated with these events into conscious awareness and coping with these feelings will decrease the need for dissociation. Although the remaining options are helpful, they are not specific for a client with a dissociative disorder; they would be general outcomes for other anxiety-related disorders.

15. The answer is **2, 3, 4, 6.**
These are all appropriate techniques based on the framework of cognitive-behavioral therapy. The nurse would educate the

client, help him to use breathing techniques to interrupt anxiety, help him to examine stressors or triggers for anxiety and panic, and encourage him to change or restructure any negative or fearful thoughts. The nurse may administer antianxiety medications; however, this is not a technique of cognitive-behavioral therapy. Questioning the client about early childhood relationships may be part of a psychoanalytical approach to treatment.

4

The Mind–Body Continuum: Common Disorders

I. OVERVIEW OF MIND-BODY DISORDERS

A. Key concepts

1. Mind-body disorders are characterized by both psychological and physiologic symptoms and include somatoform disorders, sexual disorders, and eating disorders.

2. **Holistic theory** is the belief that illness and wellness are the result of complex interactions among physiologic, cognitive, emotional, and sociocultural factors.

3. **Systems theory** (the whole is greater than the sum of its parts) provides a useful perspective for conceptualizing relationships among physiologic, cognitive, emotional, and sociocultural factors in the individual, the family, and society.

   a. A **systems model** attempts to define all factors that interact to produce a particular clinical syndrome; each factor affects the others, such that behavior or activity of any one factor cannot be understood out of context from its relationship to the others.

   b. Disease develops through a disturbed balance in the relationship among all factors affecting the individual.

4. Mind-body disorders have common characteristics.

   a. Physiologic changes and symptoms may be real (as in diagnosable medical illnesses) or perceived by the individual to be actual (as in somatoform disorders).

   b. Chronic physiologic or psychological stress results from alteration of the internal physiologic environment due to the stress response and hyperfunctioning of the hypothalamic-pituitary-adrenal axis. (See pages 40 and 41.)

   c. Psychological distress either precedes, accompanies, or follows body changes and symptoms.

5. **Psychoneuroimmunology** is the study of how chronic physiologic or psychological stress alters the internal physiologic environment, including changes in hormonal levels and cellular responses.

6. **Autoimmune disorders** result from the body's inappropriate reaction to a stressor, which stimulates an immune reaction to one's own cells and organ systems. (See *Table 4-1, Medical conditions affected by stress,* page 64.)

7. Psychological, behavioral, and sociocultural factors play a potential role in the presentation or treatment of almost every general medical condition.

   a. **Psychological factors affecting general medical conditions,** which includes symptoms that do not meet the full *DSM-IV TR* criteria for an Axis I disorder, is characterized by the presence of one or more specific psychological or behavioral factors that adversely affect a general medical condition.

   b. **Psychological factors** can precipitate or exacerbate symptoms by eliciting the stress response (such as chest pain precipitated by emotional upset in a client with coronary artery disease); they can also interfere with treatment (as in a client with insulin-dependent diabetes who refuses to take insulin because of fear of injections).

   c. **Behavioral factors** can contribute additional health risks for an individual (such as failure to quit smoking despite significant hypertension).

TABLE 4-1

Medical conditions affected by stress

Immunologic Disorders
- AIDS
- Addison's disease
- Chronic hepatitis
- Graves' disease
- Type 1 (insulin-dependent) diabetes mellitus
- Multiple sclerosis
- Myasthenia gravis
- Pernicious anemia
- Rheumatoid arthritis
- Rheumatoid disorders
- Systemic lupus erythematosus

General Medical Conditions
- Cardiovascular disorders
  – Hypertension
  – Angina pectoris
- Respiratory disorders
  – Asthma
  – Chronic obstructive pulmonary disease
- Endocrine disorders
  – Thyroid disease
  – Premenstrual syndrome
- Gastrointestinal disorders
  – Peptic ulcer disease
  – Irritable bowel syndrome
- Musculoskeletal disorders
  – Acute or chronic back pain
  – Osteoporosis
- Renal disorders
  – Urinary tract infections
  – Renal calculi
- Neoplastic disorders (cancers)

---

   d. **Sociocultural factors,** such as peer pressure or media influence, can contribute to certain disorders (as in an anorexic client with a disturbed body image who idealizes thinness).

B. Causes of mind-body disorders

   1. Researchers have identified multiple physiologic, cognitive, emotional, and sociocultural factors involved in the cause of mind-body disorders.

   2. **Chronic stress,** whether from internal or external stressors, plays a major role.

      a. The central nervous system and immune system work as an integrated whole to maintain homeostasis in response to stress.

         – Communication between these systems occurs via chemical messengers, such as neurotransmitters and cytokines (cytokines, including interferons, lymphokines, and interleukins, are messengers of the immune system).

         – Release of neurotransmitters, hormones, and cytokines occurs during stress; chronic stress produces excessive stimulation of these substances, thereby upsetting homeostasis.

      b. Continued stress depletes bodily defenses, increasing the risk of physical or mental disease.

      c. Cognitive, emotional, and sociocultural stimuli are among the most potent factors activating the biologic response to stress.

   3. Increased reactivity or failure to respond to the negative feedback mechanism in the hypothalamic-pituitary-adrenal axis leads to chronic elevations of glucocorticoids; this increased reactivity can be related to several factors:

CLIENT AND FAMILY TEACHING 4-1
Guidelines for clients with mind-body disorders

Provide information about the client's specific disorder and treatment:
- The client will probably experience worsening of symptoms when under stress.

  Include information about how the family can be helpful:
- The client will be able to function despite her physical symptoms; doing things and making decisions for her will only increase dependent behavior.

- A matter-of-fact attitude is helpful to decrease emphasis on dramatic symptoms.
- Expressions of concern should be directed toward real-life problems rather than bodily symptoms.
- Encourage the client to remain with one health care provider on a long-term basis.
- Family therapy can be helpful to clarify roles, communication, and expectations within the family.

---

    a. Continuous real threat (as in chronic abuse) or continuous perceived or imagined threat (as in persistent cognitive distortions, chronic anxiety states)

    b. Genetic predisposition

    c. Learned responsiveness.

C. Treatment of mind-body disorders

1. Taking a holistic approach, treatment includes interventions directed toward both disease-specific management and stress reduction.

2. Stress-education interventions are based on the concept that the client can increase his control over symptoms by learning how to anticipate situations that are upsetting and use measures to reduce his anxiety level (such as adequate sleep, good nutrition, relaxation techniques, and planning ahead).

3. Management involves teaching an individual about his specific disorder, causative factors, reduction of risk, and medically prescribed treatments and medications. (See *Client and family teaching 4-1, Guidelines for clients with mind-body disorders.*)

4. Specific mind-body therapies include stress management training, relaxation techniques, biofeedback with relaxation training, support and self-help groups, guided imagery, art and movement therapies, meditation, and prayer.

5. **Complementary and alternative medicine (CAM)** treatments may also be used; these may rely on self-healing capabilities in which the role of the healer is more of a facilitator (See *Table 4-2, Complementary and alternative medicine treatments*, page 66.)

    a. Clients typically seek alternative therapies if traditional therapies fail to relieve their illness or symptoms or as an adjunct to traditional medicine.

    b. The National Center for Complementary and Alternative Medicine (NCCAM), a division of the National Institutes of Health, classifies CAM according to five general categories:

        – alternative medical systems

        – mind-body interventions

        – biologically based therapies

        – manipulative and body-based methods

        – energy therapies

TABLE 4-2

Complementary and alternative medicine treatments

Complementary and alternative medicine includes treatments and therapies that fall outside the mainstream of accepted medical practice. Some commonly used treatments are listed below.

Treatment	Description
Acupuncture	Identifies patterns of energy flow and energy blockage among 12 principal meridians, which roughly correspond to points along the peripheral nervous system. Ultrathin needles are inserted at points along these meridians to restore balance.
Ayurveda	Emphasizes use of body, mind, and spirit in disease prevention and treatment. Treatments include diet and herbal remedies.
Traditional Chinese medicine (TCM)	TCM is based on the concept of balanced qi (vital energy, which is believed to flow through the body). The opposing forces of yin (negative energy) and yang (positive energy) influence balanced qi. Herbal and nutritional therapy, restorative and physical exercises, meditation, acupuncture, and massage are all used in TCM.
Naturopathic medicine	Focuses on prevention of illness and use of nontoxic biologic therapies (homeopathic medicine).
Homeopathic medicine	Involves the use of small, highly diluted quantities of medicinal substances.
Chiropractic medicine	Based on the premise that the spine is the most significant factor in health. Treating misalignments of the spine by manipulation, electrical stimulation, and heat can improve health.
Herbal therapy	Involves using extracts of plant materials for various physical and mental illnesses.
Therapeutic touch	Based on the idea that illness is caused by an imbalance of the human body's energy field. Practitioners use their hands to direct energy movement.

    c. Many cultures traditionally use alternative methods based on belief systems regarding the interrelationship between mind-body-spirit; designated healers are common to many different cultures.

    d. These methods are becoming increasingly popular as consumers take a more active role in their health management.

II. SOMATOFORM DISORDERS

A. Key concepts
    1. Somatoform disorders are characterized by complaints of physical symptoms that cannot be explained by known physical mechanisms.

       a. The client typically experiences a loss or change in physical function.

       b. The symptoms are not under the client's voluntary control.

2. Somatoform disorders are also characterized by **primary gain** (anxiety relief) and **secondary gains** (special attention, relief from responsibilities); these disorders are usually **ego-syntonic** (congruent with the individual's view of self).
3. Significant impairment occurs in social or occupational functioning.
    a. The client becomes totally focused on the physical symptoms, which can severely restrict activities.
    b. Symptoms often contribute to relationship problems for the client.
4. The client generally visits multiple health care providers and may undergo exploratory and unnecessary surgical procedures.
    a. The use of multiple prescribed and over-the-counter medications is common.
    b. Dependence on pain relievers or antianxiety medications can lead to substance dependence.
    c. Denial of psychological distress and resistance to psychiatric treatment is also common.

B. Types of somatoform disorders

1. **Somatization disorder** is characterized by a history of multiple physical complaints without organic basis, occurring before age 30 and persisting for several years; it is generally associated with a combination of pseudoneurologic, gastrointestinal, genitourinary, and sexual symptoms as well as pain.
2. **Hypochondriasis** is the unrealistic fear of having a serious illness; the client's interpretation of body symptoms is without organic basis.
3. **Body dysmorphic disorder** is characterized by preoccupation with an imagined defect in a normal-appearing client; if the client actually has a defect, expressed concern is excessive.
4. **Pain disorder** is characterized by chronic pain in one or more anatomic sites; a medical condition, if present, plays a minor role in accounting for the pain.
5. **Conversion disorder** is a loss of, or change in, physical functioning that cannot be associated with any organic cause and that seems to be associated with psychosocial stressors; such a disorder is generally characterized by:
    a. **Sensory dysfunction,** such as blindness, deafness, or loss of tactile sense
    b. **Motor system dysfunction,** such as aphasia, impaired coordination, paralysis, or seizure
    c. *La belle indifference,* seeming unconcern with a fairly dramatic symptom, such as being unable to walk or move a limb

C. Causes of somatoform disorders

1. Various theories have attempted to explain the etiology of somatoform disorders.
2. According to the psychobiologic theory, the client's problem may stem from one of two causes.
    a. The client may be experiencing high levels of physiologic arousal (increased awareness of somatic sensations).
    b. The client may have **alexithymia,** which is a deficiency in the communication between brain hemispheres resulting in difficulty expressing emotions directly; consequently, distress is expressed as physical sensations.

3. Cognitive-behavioral theories focus on the way impaired thinking and learned behavior affect disease.
   a. The child learns from her parents to express anxiety through somatization; secondary gains reinforce symptoms.
   b. The individual has cognitive distortions in which benign symptoms are magnified and interpreted as serious disease.
4. Acccording to the psychoanalytic theory, the psychological source of ego conflict is denied and finds expression through displacement of anxiety onto physical symptoms.
5. Sociocultural factors may also contribute to disease.
   a. Incidence of somatoform disorders is higher among lower socioeconomic groups, rural populations, and those with limited education.
   b. Somatic symptoms are common in cultures that view direct expression of emotions as unacceptable.

D. Treatment of somatoform disorders
1. The mainstay of treatment is a long-term relationship with a specific health care provider to prevent the client from seeking multiple providers with multiple recommendations for testing, treatment, and medications.
2. Clients should avoid treatment with medications that are characterized by tolerance and dependence (antianxiety agents, analgesics).
3. Psychotherapy is generally incorporated into the treatment plan.
   a. Therapy aims to help the client express conflicts and emotions verbally.
   b. The focus should be on the client's underlying psychosocial needs.
4. Family education is also another important component of treatment; family members must be taught to avoid reinforcing secondary gains from symptoms.
5. Participation in community-based self-help group (such as Recovery, Inc.) encourages the client to learn to control distressing symptoms through specific techniques and group support.

III. SEXUAL DISORDERS

A. Key concepts
1. Human sexuality includes **gender identity** (the sense of maleness or femaleness) as well as desire for contact, warmth, tenderness, and love.
2. Sexual health involves the integration of somatic, intellectual, and social aspects of sexual being.
3. Sexual expression is influenced by a variety of factors, including:
   a. Age, health status, and physical attributes
   b. Cultural, social, and religious views
   c. Environment and personal choice of a sexual partner as a result of personality development
4. **Normal sexual behavior** is a sexual act between consenting adults that is lacking force and performed in a private setting in the absence of unwilling observers.

5. Sexual activity is **legally unacceptable** when it involves nonconsenting individuals, a child, or use of objects in such a way that bring physical or psychological harm to one of the partners.

6. The **sexual response cycle** includes phases of desire, excitement, orgasm, and resolution.

B. Types of sexual disorders

1. **Sexual dysfunctions** are characterized by a disturbance in the sexual response cycle or by pain associated with sexual intercourse; they may be classified as follows:

   a. **Sexual desire disorders:** The client has little or no sexual desire or an aversion to sexual contact.

   b. **Sexual arousal disorders:** The client cannot maintain physiologic requirements for sexual intercourse (in men, erectile dysfunction; in women, difficulty with lubrication-swelling response).

   c. **Orgasmic disorders:** The client cannot achieve orgasm.

   d. **Sexual pain disorders:** The client experiences pain before, during, or after sexual intercourse.

   e. **Sexual dysfunction due to general medical condition:** Evidence from the client's history, physical examination, or laboratory and diagnostic findings indicates that the dysfunction is due to a direct physiologic effect from a medical condition.

2. **Paraphilias** are disorders characterized by sexual fantasies, urges, or behaviors involving nonhuman objects, suffering or humiliation, children, or other nonconsenting individuals.

   a. Behaviors involving nonhuman objects include fetishism and transvestic fetishism.

   b. Behaviors involving suffering or humiliation include sexual sadism and masochism.

   c. Behaviors involving children are known as pedophilia.

   d. Behaviors involving other nonconsenting persons include voyeurism, frotteurism, and exhibitionism.

3. With **gender identity disturbance,** the client has a sense of discomfort and inappropriateness about his or her anatomic gender and wishes to be of the other sex; there is some disagreement in the medical community as to whether gender discomfort is a physical condition, a psychosocial condition, or both.

C. Causes of sexual disorders

1. **Sexual dysfunctions** may be explained by biological factors or cognitive-behavioral theory.

   a. Biological factors include altered levels of testosterone and serum prolactin; medical illness (diabetes mellitus and vascular insufficiency can cause orgasmic dysfunction); and medication (antihypertensive, antipsychotic, antidepressant, antianxiety, and anticonvulsant agents or substance abuse).

   b. The cognitive-behavioral theory suggests that strongly negative emotions become associated with sexual activity.

2. With **paraphilias,** causes may be attributed to biological factors or a host of interrelated factors (system theory).

   a. Although evidence is inconclusive at this time, researchers think that possible destruction of parts of the limbic system or disorders involving the temporal lobe may contribute to paraphilias.

   b. According to the system theory, paraphilias are the result of multiple interrelated factors, including genetics, past learning, and stress as well as physiologic, psychological, and sociocultural factors.

3. **Gender identity disorders** may result from biological or cognitive-behavioral factors.

   a. Statistics indicate that about 1 in 2,000 children are born with ambiguous-looking genitalia **(transgenderism)** each year; there is much controversy regarding how to assign sexual identity in these cases, as well as when to perform the surgical procedure to coincide with the assigned sex.

   b. According to the cognitive-behavioral theory, contributing causes include the influence of social learning on gender development in childhood and parental dynamics that encourage the child's identity with a nongender-based sex role.

D. Treatment of sexual disorders

1. Treatment of sexual disorders includes extensive evaluation of the specific problem and the client's relationship dynamics coupled with education and supportive psychotherapy.

2. Community-based treatment typically involves assessment and care of the client's physiologic and psychosocial symptoms.

3. Cognitive-behavioral therapy attempts to change the client's thinking and uses practice exercises to improve sexual activities.

4. Specialized training in **sex therapy** is advocated for professionals treating sexual disorders; the American Association of Sex Educators, Counselors, and Therapists (AASECT) provides training for certification.

IV. EATING DISORDERS

A. Key concepts

1. Eating disorders are identified as severe disturbances in eating behavior; they include anorexia nervosa and bulimia nervosa. (See *Table 4-3, Differentiating anorexia from bulimia.*)

   a. **Anorexia nervosa** is characterized by refusal to maintain minimally normal weight, intense fear of gaining weight, and significant disturbance in perception of shape or body size.

   b. **Bulimia nervosa** is characterized by repeated episodes of binge eating, followed by purging behaviors; it also includes inappropriate use of laxatives, fasting, or exercise to control weight.

2. Anorexia and bulimia are not diseases, but syndromes with multiple predisposing factors and a variety of physical and psychological characteristics. (See *Table 4-4, Comparing physical symptoms of anorexia and bulimia*, page 72.)

TABLE 4-3
Differentiating anorexia from bulimia

Anorexia nervosa
- The client's weight is less than 85% of normal for age and height.
- Although underweight, the client has an intense fear of becoming fat.
- The client has a disturbed body image (self-image related to weight).
- The client exercises strenuously and has peculiar food-handling patterns.
- The client feels a lack of control or competence in any area of life other than weight control.

Bulimia nervosa
- The client practices bingeing and purging.
   – *Binge eating* is consuming enormous quantities of food in a discrete time period; anxiety often triggers the binge.
   – *Purging* is using compensatory behaviors to rid the body of food and prevent weight gain; behaviors include self-induced vomiting or misuse of laxatives, diuretics, enemas, or other medications or substances (syrup of ipecac).
- The client fasts or exercises excessively.
- Binges commonly lead to feelings of loss of control, guilt, humiliation, and self-loathing.

    a. An individual can demonstrate symptoms of both disorders, or can revert from one to the other.

    b. Although eating disorders can exist in men, more than 90% of those with eating disorders are women.

    c. Onset generally occurs during adolescence (age 13 to 17); however, statistics indicate that children as young as 7 can have an eating disorder.

  3. **Cognitive distortions** are common among individuals with eating disorders; examples of distorted thinking include:

    a. **Selective abstraction:** "I'm still too fat...see my big hands and my big feet."

    b. **Overgeneralization:** "Only thin people get ahead in life."

    c. **Magnification:** "If I gain 2 pounds, I'll never get on the varsity team."

    d. **Superstitious thinking:** "If I gain weight, my boyfriend will leave me."

    e. **Dichotomous thinking:** "I'm not thin. I'm fat."

  4. Eating disorders are a serious health problem that can cause death; statistics indicate that eating disorders have the highest mortality rate of any mental illness—up to 20%.

  5. Eating disorders frequently coexist with other psychiatric disorders, including depression, social phobia, obsessive-compulsive disorder, panic disorder, and substance abuse.

  6. Anorexia nervosa is an **ego-syntonic** disorder (the client views her behaviors as congruent with her self-image); bulimia nervosa is an **ego-dystonic** disorder (the client views her behaviors as shameful or negative and incongruent with her self-image).

B. Causes of eating disorders

  1. Eating disorders result from a combination of factors, some of which can be traced to **biological causes** and **genetic makeup.**

    a. Changes in central nervous system pathways involving the neurotransmitters norepinephrine, dopamine, and serotonin may contribute to the development of anorexia.

TABLE 4-4

Comparing physical symptoms of anorexia and bulimia

Body changes	Anorexia nervosa	Bulimia nervosa
Weight	■ Less than 85% of normal weight for age and height	■ Normal or near-normal weight for age and height
Cardiovascular changes	■ *Bradycardia, hypotension:* related to decreased cardiac muscle mass from starvation ■ *Arrhythmias:* related to electrolyte imbalance	■ *Bradycardia, hypotension:* related to fluid deficit, possible heart muscle damage from overuse of syrup of ipecac to induce vomiting ■ *Arrhythmias:* related to electrolyte imbalance
Fluid and electrolyte imbalances	■ *Hypokalemia:* related to laxative abuse or vomiting ■ *Hypocalcemia:* related to lack of dietary intake ■ *Dehydration:* related to lack of fluid intake, vomiting, and laxative abuse	■ *Hypokalemia, hyponatremia, dehydration:* related to diuretic abuse, vomiting, and laxative abuse
Endocrine changes	■ *Amenorrhea:* starvation leads to loss of fat stores and estrogen loss, alteration in hypothalamic functioning	■ *Irregular menses, hypoglycemia:* alteration in hypothalamic functioning
Skin, hair, teeth, bone, voice changes	■ *Lanugo, dry skin, hypothermia, hair loss:* starvation and loss of subcutaneous tissue ■ *Osteoporosis:* related to loss of calcium stores	■ *Hoarseness:* irritation from vomiting ■ *Dental caries:* loss of enamel from vomiting ■ *Enlarged parotid glands:* inflammatory response from irritation related to vomiting
Gastrointestinal changes	■ *Constipation:* related to loss of bowel muscle tone and laxative abuse	■ *Constipation:* related to laxative abuse, fluid deficit, loss of bowel muscle tone ■ *Esophagitis:* irritation from vomiting

    b. Serotonin irregularities, especially in the hypothalamus where feelings of satiety are controlled, may contribute to the development of bulimia.

    c. Research about neurotransmitter irregularities is ongoing; however, it is difficult to determine whether physiochemical changes precede, accompany, or follow behavior problems.

    d. Relatives of individuals with eating disorders are 4 to 5 times more likely to have an eating disorder, suggesting a genetic predisposition to these disorders.

  2. Cognitive distortions lead to abnormal eating behaviors, which become associated with anxiety relief and are, therefore, reinforced.

  3. **Disturbed relationships** early in life can make a child vulnerable to eating disorders; these disturbances may include:

    a. **Separation-individuation conflicts:** typically occur between mother and daughter

      b. **Distorted body image:** occurs with misperception of internal needs

      c. **Anxiety control:** is dependent on control of body and biological needs

        – The client attributes or displaces anxiety to bodily function; controlling the body and its functions relieves anxiety or becomes the defense against anxiety.

        – A child or adolescent who has not successfully separated from the parent functions according to that parent's wishes or desires; the body is the only area in which the child can make decisions or exert any control.

  4. **Sociocultural influences,** such as the promotion of thinness as an ideal body image by popular culture and the media and peer pressure during adolescence (when self-perception is influenced by peer group ideals), also play a role in eating disorders.

  5. According to **family theory,** symptoms of eating disorders allow a family to avoid dealing with conflict.

      a. Family members are enmeshed, lacking clear-cut boundaries among parents and children, leading to over-involvement in the child's life.

      b. The family highly values perfection, and the child attempts to meet high standards.

      c. The eating disorder is a form of rebellion, in which the child gains a sense of control through the behavior.

C. Treatment of eating disorders

  1. A multidisciplinary approach—with collaboration among medical, psychiatric, psychological, nutritional, and nursing team members—is important.

  2. Hospitalization in an **acute-care** setting is recommended when the client has persistent symptoms despite ongoing treatment, or when severe depression with suicidal impulses is present.

      a. The priority is to maintain client safety and stabilize physiologic problems (dehydration, electrolyte imbalance, arrhythmias).

      b. A **refeeding program** is important to restore weight.

      c. **Behavioral contracting** is often used as part of treatment to reinforce appropriate eating and prevent harmful behaviors (purging).

  3. **Community-based treatment** is also important because eating disorders are often persistent and require long-term management.

      a. Collaboration and communication between providers are important to ensure continuity of care.

      b. Support groups are often helpful for the client and her family.

  4. Therapy-specific approaches may be used to treat the client.

      a. **Psychotherapy** may be used, with an individual approach focusing on issues (body image and self-esteem, self-control, and decision making) and relationships with peers and family.

      b. The **cognitive-behavioral approach** aims to reduce the client's symptoms by restructuring the faulty belief system that perpetuates the eating disorder.

      c. **Family therapy** helps family members to define appropriate boundaries, decrease controlling behaviors, and support the client in increasing self-responsibility. (See

DRUG CHART 4-1
Selected medications for treating eating disorders

Classification	Drug	Rationale for use
Tricyclic antidepressants	desipramine (Norpramin) imipramine (Tofranil)	■ Decreases frequency of binge eating and relieves anxiety and depression; affects serotonin levels ■ More effective in treating bulimia than anorexia
Selective serotonin reuptake inhibitors (SSRI)	fluoxetine (Prozac) sertraline (Zoloft)	■ Used to treat concurrent depression in eating disorders; restores serotonin levels

Client and family teaching 4-1, Guidelines for clients with mind-body disorders, page 65.)

5. Treatment may involve the use of medications (antidepressants) to reduce the frequency of binge eating; additional medications may be used to treat accompanying depression, anxiety symptoms, or obsessive/compulsive behaviors. (See *Drug chart 4-1, Selected medications for treating eating disorders*.)

NURSING PROCESS OVERVIEW

V. CARE OF THE CLIENT WITH A MIND-BODY DISORDER

A. Assessment

1. Note objective and subjective symptoms related to the client's specific diagnosis.

2. Review the client's history, and determine current internal and external stressors.

   a. Discuss the client's perception of the problem.

   b. Identify the client's self-concept and body image.

   c. Identify secondary gains from physical symptoms.

   d. Discuss significant relationship problems.

3. Ask key assessment questions to elicit information about the client's specific mind-body disorder. (See *Key questions 4-1, Assessing clients with mind-body disorders.*)

B. Nursing diagnoses

1. Determine the client's anxiety level, use of coping measures, and defense mechanisms. (See *Figure 3-2, Understanding anxiety levels and effects*, page 42, and *Display 3-1, Coping strategies for stress reduction*, page 43.)

2. Determine what the client's physical symptoms mean to her.

3. Analyze the client's insight into the relationship between physical symptoms and psychological distress.

KEY QUESTIONS 4-1
Assessing clients with mind-body disorders

Question	Information gathered
How would you rate your health: poor, fair, good, or excellent?	Self-perception; subjective data can be used in comparing to objective symptoms
Who is your primary health care provider, and how long have you been a client with this person?	Client's tendency to have multiple health care providers and to change providers frequently
What prescription and nonprescription medications are you currently taking?	Possible use of multiple prescribed and over-the-counter medications (as in somatoform disorder or in an eating disorder for weight loss) or medication-related symptoms (as in a sexual disorder)
Are you using any alternative or non-traditional treatment measures?	Use of complementary and alternative medicine treatments (as in a client with psychological factors affecting a general medical condition)
How has your illness affected your ability to function?	Possible significant impairment (usually occurs in social and occupational functioning)
Are you experiencing any problems related to sexual activity or sexual relationship?	Need for more specific questions related to sexual health
Are you satisfied with your eating patterns?	Client's perception of disturbed eating and readiness for help (direct questioning has been shown to be effective in screening for bulimia)
Are you on a strict diet?	Client's perception of disturbed eating and readiness for help (the client with anorexia may admit to dieting behavior)

4. Analyze the effect of the client's problem on her family and relationship functioning.
5. Establish individualized nursing diagnoses for the client, as needed; possible diagnoses include the following:
   a. Acute pain
   b. Anxiety
   c. Chronic low self-esteem
   d. Decisional conflict (specify)
   e. Defensive coping
   f. Disturbed body image
   g. Fatigue
   h. Health-seeking behaviors (specify)
   i. Imbalanced nutrition: Less than body requirements
   j. Ineffective coping
   k. Ineffective denial

   l. *Ineffective health maintenance*

   m. *Ineffective role performance*

   n. *Ineffective sexuality patterns*

   o. *Powerlessness*

   p. *Readiness for enhanced knowledge (specify)*

   q. *Risk for self-directed violence*

   r. *Sexual dysfunction*

   s. *Social isolation*

   t. *Spiritual distress*

   6. Establish nursing diagnoses for the client's family, as needed; possible diagnoses include the following:

   a. *Compromised family coping*

   b. *Deficient knowledge (specify)*

   c. *Ineffective family therapeutic regime management*

   d. *Interrupted family processes*

C. Planning and outcome identification

   1. Work with the client and family in setting realistic goals.

   2. For the client who has psychological factors affecting a general medical condition, establish desired outcome criteria.

   a. The client will demonstrate the ability to cope with physical illness by using stress-reduction measures.

   b. The client will use a combination of traditional and nontraditional modes of treatment.

   c. The client will identify specific stressors associated with physical illness.

   d. The client will adapt family coping to promote health.

   3. For the client or partner of a client with a **sexual disorder,** establish desired outcome criteria.

   a. The client or partner will identify the relationship between stressors and decreased sexual functioning.

   b. The client or partner will express a desire to change variant or deviant sexual behavior.

   c. The client or partner will communicate with partner about sexual issues without discomfort.

   d. The client or partner will express satisfaction with one's own sexuality pattern.

   4. For the client with a **somatoform disorder,** establish desired outcome criteria.

   a. The client will express anxiety and conflict verbally rather than with physical symptoms.

   b. The client will reduce or eliminate behavior that is demanding or manipulative in relationships with others.

   c. The client will reduce attention and other secondary gains associated with symptomatic behaviors.

   5. For a client with an **eating disorder,** establish desired outcome criteria.

   a. The client will achieve normal or near-normal weight for age and height.

   b. The client will replace maladaptive eating behaviors with stress-reduction measures.

c. The client will identify positive self-concept and realistic body image.

d. The client will state feelings of control in areas of life other than eating.

e. The client will establish open communication within the family and maintain boundaries.

D. Implementation

1. For the client with **psychological factors affecting a general medical condition,** take the following measures:

   a. Help the client to identify and use positive coping measures to handle physical illness.

   b. Encourage the client to use specific support or self-help groups.

   c. Provide the client with information related to her physical illness, the effects of stress, and the management of symptoms.

   d. Encourage client-selected alternative methods to enhance traditional treatments.

2. For the client with a **somatoform disorder,** take the following measures:

   a. Report and assess new physical complaints because organic disease is also a possibility for this client.

   b. Decrease reinforcement of secondary gains for physical symptoms. (See *Client and family teaching 4-1, Guidelines for clients with mind-body disorders*, page 65.)

   c. Avoid fostering dependency, and encourage independent behaviors.

   d. Maintain a therapeutic focus on feelings, emotional responses, and relationship problems rather than on somatic symptoms.

   e. Set limits on manipulative behaviors in a matter-of-fact manner.

   f. Help the client to identify and use positive means to meet emotional needs.

   g. Encourage the client to maintain a long-term relationship with her primary health provider.

   h. Teach and encourage the use of stress-reducing measures.

   i. Help the client to identify the relationship between stressful life events and somatic symptoms.

3. For the client with a **sexual disorder,** take the following measures:

   a. Determine self comfort level before discussing sexual issues with the client.

   b. Educate the client about normal sexual behaviors and family planning issues.

   c. Correct any misconceptions regarding sexuality and sexual functioning.

   – Explain that sexuality is a normal human response and is not synonymous with any one sexual act.

   – Also explain that complex relationships among self-concept, body image, family influence, and physical functioning all influence sexual expression.

   d. Review any prescribed medications with the client, and identify side effects associated with sexual functioning.

   e. Identify physical illness and specific effects on sexual relationships.

   f. Refer the client to a qualified counselor for sex therapy.

4. For the client with an **eating disorder,** take the following measures:

   a. Collaborate with other health team members.

    b. Reinforce the dietician's prescription for healthy eating to accomplish a realistic weight gain of 2 to 3 lb weekly, and reinforce treatment plan that establishes privileges and restrictions based on compliance.

    c. Decrease emphasis on specific "good" or "bad" foods.

    d. Weigh the client twice weekly.

    e. If the client is in an acute-care or hospital setting, remain with her during mealtimes and for 1 hour after meals.

    f. Discuss the client's fears of weight gain and loss of control, and help her identify how feelings about herself and problems are related to eating behaviors.

    g. Teach and encourage the client to use coping measures other than weight loss to maintain control and decrease anxiety.

    h. Encourage the client to verbalize her role within the family, identifying issues of dependence and independence; assist the family to redefine roles and establish open communication.

    i. Promote the client's control by having her participate in the treatment plan.

E. Outcome evaluation

1. The client identifies the relationship between specific stressors and physiologic symptoms.
2. The client verbalizes anxiety about specific problems rather than expressing anxiety with physical symptoms.
3. The client expresses satisfaction with self-concept, body image, and relationships with others.
4. The client uses stress-management techniques and follows a health-promoting lifestyle.
5. The client assumes responsibility for herself and expresses a sense of internal locus of control.
6. The client identifies and cooperates in a continued treatment plan.

Study questions

1. A client who is newly diagnosed with rheumatoid arthritis asks the community nurse how stress can affect his disease. The nurse would explain that:
   1. the psychological experience of stress will not affect symptoms of physical disease.
   2. psychological stress can cause painful emotions, which are harmful to a person with an illness.
   3. stress can overburden the body's immune system, and therefore one can experience increased disease symptoms.
   4. the body's stress response is stimulated only when there are major disruptions in one's life.

2. A client with benign essential hypertension has been referred for biofeedback training. Which of the following criteria would the nurse use to evaluate the client's success with this method?
   1. The client states that his stress level is under control.
   2. The client's blood pressure is normal while on a decreased dose of antihypertensive medication.
   3. The client uses relaxation methods on a regular basis.

4. The client follows a recommended diet and medication plan without deviation.

3. The nurse who is teaching a class on stress management is questioned about the use of alternative treatments, such as herbal therapy and therapeutic touch. She explains that the advantage of these methods would include all of the following *except:*
   1. they are congruent with many cultural belief systems.
   2. they encourage the consumer to take an active role in health management.
   3. they promote interrelationships within the mind-body-spirit.
   4. they usually work better than traditional medical practice.

4. A client is preoccupied with numerous bodily complaints even after a careful diagnostic workup reveals no physiologic problems. Which nursing intervention would be most therapeutic for this client?
   1. Acknowledge that the complaints are real to the client, and refocus the client on other concerns and problems.
   2. Challenge the physical complaints by confronting the client with the normal diagnostic findings.
   3. Ignore the client's complaints, but request that the client keep a list of all symptoms.
   4. Listen to the client's complaints carefully, and question him about specific symptoms.

5. The nurse is teaching a client about sertraline (Zoloft), which has been prescribed for depression. A significant side effect is interference with sexual arousal by inhibiting erectile function. How should the nurse approach this topic?
   1. The nurse should avoid mentioning the sexual side effects to prevent the client from having anxiety about potential erectile problems.
   2. The nurse should advise the client to report any changes in sexual functioning in case medication adjustments are needed.
   3. The nurse should explain that the client's sexual desire will probably decrease while on this medication.
   4. The nurse should tell the client that sexual side effects are expected, but that they will decrease when his depression lifts.

6. The nurse is working with a client with a gender identity disorder. The client recently started living as a member of the opposite sex. Which of the following is an *inappropriate* outcome criterion for this nurse-client relationship?
   1. The client discusses feelings about reactions expected from family and friends.
   2. The client discusses feelings and issues regarding living in another gender role.
   3. The client schedules a date for sex-change surgery as a result of the discussion.
   4. The client identifies support persons who may be helpful during the change from one gender to another.

7. The school nurse assesses for anorexia nervosa in an adolescent girl. Which of the following findings are characteristic of this disorder? Select all that apply.
   1. Bradycardia
   2. Hypotension
   3. Chronic pain in one or more sites
   4. Fear of having a serious illness
   5. Irregular or absent menses
   6. Refusal to maintain minimally normal weight

8. A nurse is planning a psychoeducational discussion for a group of adolescent clients with anorexia nervosa. Which of the following topics would the nurse select to enhance understanding about central issues in this disorder?
1. Anger management
2. Parental expectations
3. Peer pressure and substance abuse
4. Self-control and self-esteem

9. The nurse understands that a client with bulimia nervosa feels shame and guilt over binge eating and purging. This disorder is therefore considered:
1. ego-distorting.
2. ego-dystonic.
3. ego-enhancing.
4. ego-syntonic.

10. The psychoanalytic theory explains the etiology of anorexia nervosa as:
1. the achievement of secondary gain through control of eating.
2. a conflict between mother and child over separation and individualization.
3. family dynamics that lead to enmeshment of members.
4. the incorporation of thinness as an ideal body image.

11. The nurse observes a client who is hospitalized on an eating disorder unit during mealtimes and for 1 hour after eating. The rationale for this intervention is:

1. to develop a trusting relationship.
2. to maintain focus on importance of nutrition.
3. to prevent purging behaviors.
4. to reinforce the behavioral contact.

12. The initial treatment priority for a client who is hospitalized for anorexia nervosa on a special eating disorder unit is:
1. to determine the client's current body image.
2. to identify family interaction patterns.
3. to initiate a refeeding program
4. to promote the client's independence.

13. The nurse evaluates the treatment of a client with somatoform disorder as successful if:
1. the client practices self-medication rather than changing health care providers.
2. the client recognizes that physical symptoms increase anxiety level.
3. the client researches treatment protocols for various illnesses.
4. the client verbalizes anxiety directly rather than displacing it.

14. Which of the following attitudes from a nurse would hinder a discussion with an adolescent client about sexuality?
1. Accepting
2. Matter-of-fact
3. Moralistic
4. Nonjudgmental

Answer key

1. The answer is **3**.
The stress response causes stimulation of the hypothalamic-pituitary-adrenal axis, which can further compromise an immune system that has been activated by the autoimmune disorder of rheumatoid arthritis. Consequently, the client can expect disease symptoms to exacerbate when under stress. The statement that stress will not affect symptoms of physi-

cal disease is false. Experiences of emotions that are painful are not necessarily harmful to someone with an illness. In fact, learning to handle painful emotions can enhance coping. The stress response can be stimulated by major or minor disruptions in life, but the individual's perception of stress is more important than the actual problem.

2. The answer is 2.
Successful use of biofeedback enables the client to modify physiologic responses to stress, including blood pressure. A decreased need for an antihypertensive medication is an objective measurement of effectiveness. Although options 1 and 3 are outcomes of stress management, they are not specific for biofeedback. Option 4 would be a successful outcome of the client's overall medical treatment.

3. The answer is 4.
Complementary alternative medicine treatments are often used as adjuncts to traditional medical treatment. Although an individual may choose a particular alternative treatment method, there is really no current scientific proof that these methods will work better than traditional medicine. The other options are accurate regarding use of alternative treatment methods.

4. The answer is 1.
After physical factors are ruled out, somatic complaints are thought to be expressions of anxiety. The complaints are real to the client, but the nurse should not focus on them. Prompting the client to talk about other concerns will encourage expression of anxiety and dependency needs. Confronting the client as demonstrated in option 2 shows a lack of sensitivity to the unconscious nature of the problem and will increase client anxiety.

Ignoring the client's complaints merely avoids the problem. Focusing on somatic symptoms will reinforce them (increases secondary gains).

5. The answer is 2.
Clients commonly discontinue medications to avoid or correct sexual side effects, but they are less likely to do that when health professionals offer assistance with sexual issues. Generally, clients avoid discussing sexual issues unless health professionals give permission by raising the issue first. Option 1 does not promote discussion of this sensitive issue. More likely, it reflects the nurse's avoidance of uncomfortable feelings. Any impaired sexual desire would most likely be secondary to erectile dysfunction. Option 4 reflects inaccurate information; not all clients experience sexual side effects and, if experienced, they do not necessarily decrease when depression lifts.

6. The correct answer is 3.
Unless the nurse is a certified sex therapist, this would be an unexpected outcome resulting from nursing care for this client. The other options are important areas for the client to explore, and would be appropriate topics of discussion during nurse-client interactions.

7. The answer is 1, 2, 5, 6.
These are all characteristic of anorexia nervosa. Option 3 is common to someone with a somatoform pain disorder and option 4 is common in hypochondriasis.

8. The answer is 4.
Self-control and self-esteem are central issues for clients with eating disorders. Such clients typically feel a loss of control over their life and experience diminished self-esteem and severe doubts about their self-worth. They maintain their sense of

control only by controlling eating behaviors. Anger management, parental expectations, peer pressure, and substance abuse are important issues for adolescent clients, but they are not necessarily specific for clients with anorexia nervosa.

9. The answer is 2.

An ego-dystonic disorder is one in which the client views behaviors or symptoms as incongruent with self-image and therefore feels guilt, shame, and distress about the symptoms. Ego-distorting and ego-enhancing do not apply to the situation presented. An ego-syntonic disorder is one in which the client views her behaviors as congruent with her self-image (as in anorexia nervosa).

10. The answer is 2.

According to psychoanalytic theory, early mother-child dynamics lead to difficulty with a child establishing a sense of separateness from the mother. Control of eating becomes one area in which the child establishes a sense of independence. Option 1 is the behavioral view of anorexia nervosa. Option 3 reflects the family theory view of anorexia nervosa, which deals with the issue of lack of generational boundaries. Option 4 characterizes the sociocultural view of anorexia nervosa, which identifies thinness as being a culturally determined ideal.

11. The answer is 3.

The client may experience increased anxiety during treatment and, therefore, may resume behaviors designed to prevent weight gain, such as vomiting or excessive exercise. Although the other options are important areas for nursing inter-vention, they do not provide the rationale for remaining with a client for 1 hour after eating.

12. The answer is 3.

The physical need to reestablish near-normal weight takes priority because of the physiologic, life-threatening consequences of anorexia. The other options are all important aspects of treatment, but they are not the highest priority in initial treatment.

13. The answer is 4.

The client with somatoform disorder unconsciously displaces anxiety onto physical symptoms. The ability to recognize and verbalize anxious feelings directly rather than displacing them is a criterion of treatment success. The behaviors illustrated in options 1 and 3 indicate continuation of a somatoform problem. Physical symptoms generally relieve anxiety by primary gain in a client with somatoform disorder. Some clients (such as those with hypochondriasis) may have increased anxiety over a particular symptom. The statement that the client recognizes a connection between physical symptoms and anxiety would not be the best indication that treatment is successful.

14. The answer is 3.

Adolescents are not likely to feel free to ask questions and participate in a discussion if the nurse has a moralistic attitude toward sexual issues. Having an accepting, matter-of-fact, or nonjudgmental attitude will be helpful in allowing adolescents to feel comfortable discussing sexual issues.

5 *Personality Disorders*

I. OVERVIEW OF PERSONALITY DISORDERS

A. Key concepts

1. A **personality disorder** is generally defined as an inflexible, pervasive pattern of self-perception and behavior that deviates markedly from one's usual culture; it becomes established during adolescence or early adulthood and stabilizes over time, causing the individual distress or impairment.

2. Personality disorders are coded on Axis II of the multiaxial diagnostic system in *DSM-IV TR* and are clustered into three broad groups:

   a. Odd, eccentric disorders

   b. Dramatic, emotional, erratic disorders

   c. Anxious, fearful disorders

3. Personality disorders are characterized by long-standing problems in behavior, mood, perception, and relationships; behaviors typically involve self-centeredness, rigidity and inflexibility, and poor ability to self-regulate (external locus of control).

4. Individuals with personality disorders generally do not perceive a problem with their behavior; they become distressed because of other people's reactions or behavior toward them.

   a. Generally, individuals with personality disorders do not seek psychiatric treatment and usually are not hospitalized, unless they have a coexisting psychiatric disorder coded on Axis I.

   b. Although they experience problems in social and occupational functioning, individuals remain in the mainstream of society.

B. Odd, eccentric disorders

1. Individuals with odd, eccentric personality disorders generally fall into three classifications: paranoid, schizoid, or schizotypal.

2. **Paranoid personality disorder** is characterized by a pattern of distrust and suspiciousness; the individual interprets other people's motives as threatening.

3. In **schizoid personality disorder,** the individual typically lacks personal and social relationships; he is detached from others and withdraws from interactions.

4. An individual with **schizotypal personality disorder** may have behaviors similar to those of someone with schizophrenia, but psychotic episodes are infrequent; he may also be acutely uncomfortable in relationships.

C. Dramatic, emotional, erratic disorders

1. Those with dramatic, emotional, erratic personality disorders may be described as antisocial, borderline, histrionic, or narcissistic.

2. An individual with **antisocial personality disorder** has a pattern of disregard for and violation of the rights of others.

   a. The individual must be at least age 18 and must have a history of some symptoms of conduct disorder before age 15.

   b. The individual usually exhibits behavior that is hostile to the well-being of society, and therefore is frequently found in the prison system; such a person is unable to follow rules, is grossly selfish and irresponsible, and generally is manipulative in relationships with others.

3. Someone with **borderline personality disorder** is characteristically impulsive and unpredictable, having unstable moods, disturbed relationships with others, intolerance to being alone, and a chronic sense of boredom.

   a. The individual may use splitting and projecting as defense mechanisms.
   - **Splitting** is a primitive defense mechanism characterized by an "all or none" mentality (for example, in a relationship, the other person is seen as either all good or all bad; there is no recognition that a person may have both good and bad qualities).
   - **Projection** is seen when the individual is unable to recognize negative feelings or undesirable characteristics in himself and instead believes these feelings or characteristics belong to another person.

   b. Risk for self-mutilating behaviors and suicide is high with this individual.

4. **Histrionic personality disorder** is characterized by excessive emotionality and attention-seeking behaviors that are dramatic and egocentric.

5. In **narcissistic personality disorder,** the individual typically demonstrates grandiosity and the need for constant admiration by others; such a person exaggerates his importance and accomplishments.

D. Anxious, fearful disorders

1. Those with anxious, fearful disorders demonstrate avoidant, dependent, or obsessive-compulsive behavior.

2. **Avoidant personality disorder** is marked by social inhibition, feelings of inadequacy, and sensitivity to potential rejection or criticism.

3. **Dependent personality disorder** is characterized by submissive and clinging behavior associated with an excessive need to be cared for by others.

4. In **obsessive-compulsive personality disorder,** the individual has a preoccupation with orderliness, perfectionism, and the need to be in control of situations, objects, and people.

II. CAUSES OF PERSONALITY DISORDERS

A. Key concepts

1. Most theorists agree that a combination of factors, including negative childhood experiences, genetics, and environment, plays a role in the etiology of these disorders.

2. Borderline and antisocial personality disorders have been researched more than the other disorders.

B. Psychoanalytic and developmental theories

1. These theories propose that the unsuccessful mastery of tasks in early developmental stages, along with **negative early childhood experiences,** lead to the development of personality disorders (failure to establish trust in infancy as a result of inconsistent or neglectful care can be correlated with later development of paranoid personality disorder).

2. Borderline personality disorder is believed to be associated with the failure to work through the **separation-individuation** process in early toddlerhood (around age 2).

   a. The child may have been unable to separate from the mother without significant fear and anxiety (the parent rewards clinging behavior and prevents autonomy).

   b. The mother may have been perceived by the child as both strongly nurturing at times and hateful and punishing at unpredictable times.

C. Sociocultural theory

1. Research involving clients with borderline personality disorder suggests that **emotional and physical abuse** in childhood by caretakers as well as sexual abuse by noncaretakers can lead to development of a borderline personality disorder.

2. Significant predictors of developing this disorder include the following factors:

   a. Female gender

   b. Sexual abuse by a male

   c. Emotional denial by male caretakers

   d. Inconsistent treatment by female caretakers

D. Psychobiologic theory

1. There is some evidence of **genetic transmission** and presence of specific neurologic deficits in individuals with antisocial personality disorder, although no specific genes have been implicated (some clients have a history of several individuals in the same family with this disorder).

2. Some research points to **inadequate regulation of serotonin and dopamine levels** in clients with borderline personality disorder, which may be associated with the impulsive behavior and mood instability that are characteristics of this disorder.

E. Behavioral theory

1. According to theorists, the child with antisocial personality disorder **learns socially undesirable behavior from the parents,** who reward acting-out behavior by giving in rather than setting limits.

2. The child with borderline personality disorder is **rewarded for clinging, dependent behaviors.**

F. Family theory

1. According to family theorists, **significant parental deprivation** during the first 5 years of the child's life, with a chaotic home environment and inconsistent, impulsive parents can cause antisocial personality disorder.

2. An **unstable family system** leads to unstable personality development and borderline personality disorder.

   a. The **undifferentiation** of the parents is played out in the relationship to the child; for example, the conflict and instability of the parental relationship may be handled by pulling the child into the parental conflict **(triangling).**

   b. The life of the child is intensely connected and regulated by the chaotic emotional environment in the family.

III. MANAGING PERSONALITY DISORDERS

A. Acute care

1. Typically, an individual with a personality disorder is unlikely to seek help unless something has gone wrong in life (such as a failed relationship, job loss, or legal problem).
2. Hospitalization is inappropriate unless the individual has an acute coexisting psychiatric disorder coded on Axis I.
3. An individual with borderline personality disorder may exhibit suicide risk and may engage in self-mutilating behaviors; in this case, hospitalization may be recommended to reduce the risk of self-harm.

B. Community care

1. The treatment of choice for personality disorders is short-term psychotherapy focusing on solutions for specific life problems.
2. Nurses should be aware that the client with a personality disorder is not likely to be motivated for long-term treatment; his lack of motivation is related to the fact that he does not think anything is wrong with him and, therefore, he resents or resists treatment.
3. Group therapy may be appropriate if the client agrees to attend a sufficient number of sessions.

C. Medication

1. Medications are generally not recommended for personality disorders unless they are used for specific symptoms that are distressing to the client.
2. Anxiolytics and certain antidepressants (selected serotonin reuptake inhibitors) may be ordered to reduce the client's anxiety or depression.
3. Short-term, low-dose antipsychotics may be used for transient psychotic states brought on by overwhelming stress in those with personality disorders.

NURSING PROCESS OVERVIEW

 ## IV. CARE OF THE CLIENT WITH A PERSONALITY DISORDER

A. Assessment

1. Note the objective and subjective symptoms related to the client's specific diagnosis, as established and coded on Axis II.
2. Identify specific current internal and external stressors. (See *Key questions 5-1, Assessing clients with personality disorders*, page 88.)
3. Discuss the client's perception of the current or presenting problem.
   a. Identify the client's significant relationships and level of family involvement.
   b. Determine the client's willingness to accept treatment and his expectations for therapy.
4. For the client with **paranoid personality disorder,** assess for characteristics of this disorder:

> **Q KEY QUESTIONS 5-1**
> ## Assessing clients with personality disorders
>
> | Question | Information gathered |
> | --- | --- |
> | *What current problems in your life are causing you distress?* | Client's perspective of problems and degree of distress experienced |
> | *Who do you consider to be support persons in your life?* | Client's relationship system and degree of social isolation |
> | *What changes would you like to make in yourself or in your life?* | Client's perception of reality and motivation for working on self-functioning |
> | *How do you handle anxious feelings?* | Current use of defense or coping mechanisms |
> | *Have you ever done anything to hurt yourself?* | Potential risk for self-harm (self-mutilating behavior is common in clients with borderline personality disorder) |
> | *Have you ever been in trouble with the legal system?* | History of criminal behavior (clients with antisocial personality disorder often have conflicts with rules and laws in society) |

    a. Is the client suspicious and mistrustful of others?

    b. Does the client use projection as a defense mechanism?

5. For the client with **schizoid or schizotypal disorder,** assess for characteristics of this disorder:

    a. Does the client withdraw socially and act emotionally aloof?

    b. Does the client display odd mannerisms, speech, and behaviors?

    c. Does the client show little interest in having sexual experiences with another person?

    d. Does the client respond with indifference to approval from or criticism by others?

6. For the client with **borderline personality disorder,** assess for characteristics of this disorder:

    a. Does the client have unstable moods and impulsive behavior?

    b. Does the client self-mutilate?

    c. Does the client have poor self-concept and an intense fear of being alone?

    d. Does the client express contradictory ideas or feelings about others? Does the client usually view others as all good or all bad (splitting)?

    e. Does the client manipulate others in relationships?

7. For the client with **histrionic personality disorder,** assess for characteristics of this disorder:

    a. Does the client have dramatic behavior with exaggerated emotions?

    b. Does the client have frequent temper tantrums?

    c. Does the client exhibit flamboyance with sexual overtones?

    d. Does the client lack commitment in relationships?

8. For the client with **narcissistic personality disorder,** assess for characteristics of this disorder:
   a. Does the client demonstrate grandiose thinking and an exaggerated sense of self-importance?
   b. Does the client display attention-seeking behaviors?
   c. Does the client rationalize failures?
9. For the client with **antisocial personality disorder,** assess for characteristics of this disorder:
   a. Does the client behave in a manipulative and controlling manner?
   b. Does the client act extroverted and have a superficial and charming manner?
   c. Does the client lack respect for the rights of others?
   d. Does the client have an impaired conscience, with lying, cheating, and possible criminal behaviors?
   e. Does the client lack commitment to and concern for a partner in a relationship?
   f. Does the client desire immediate pleasure and gratification?
10. For the client with **avoidant personality disorder,** assess for characteristics of this disorder:
    a. Does the client respond with hypersensitivity to others' reactions and criticisms?
    b. Does the client fear rejection and failure?
    c. Does the client desire attention but withdraw socially?
    d. Does the client fear being alone?
11. For the client with **dependent personality disorder,** assess for characteristics of this disorder:
    a. Does the client lack self-confidence and have poor self-esteem?
    b. Does the client display subordination in relationships?
    c. Does the client have difficulty making decisions?
    d. Does the client devalue any personal abilities?
12. For the client with **obsessive-compulsive personality disorder,** assess for characteristics of this disorder:
    a. Does the client strive for organization, order, and perfection?
    b. Does the client behave in a controlling and demanding manner in relationships?
    c. Does the client pay great attention to detail?
    d. Does the client form rigid, moralistic, and judgmental opinions of others?
    e. Does the client convey indirect expressions of anger, such as passive-aggressive behavior (being consistently late for appointments)?

B. Nursing diagnoses

1. Nurses must analyze their own feelings and reactions to a client with a personality disorder, seeking direction from a peer or the treatment team when feelings interfere with therapeutic performance.
2. Analyze the client's predominant manner of relating to others:
   a. Withdrawn and suspicious (odd, eccentric personality disorders)
   b. Manipulative and controlling (dramatic, emotional, erratic disorders)

TABLE 5-1
Selected nursing diagnoses for personality disorders

Diagnostic category	Specific personality disorders	Nursing diagnoses
Odd, eccentric	■ Paranoid ■ Schizoid/Schizotypal	■ *Chronic low self-esteem* ■ *Disturbed thought processes* ■ *Impaired social interaction* ■ *Social isolation*
Dramatic, emotional, erratic	■ Antisocial ■ Borderline ■ Histrionic ■ Narcissistic	■ *Anxiety* ■ *Chronic low self-esteem* ■ *Ineffective coping* ■ *Risk for other-directed violence* ■ *Risk for self-directed violence*
Anxious, fearful	■ Avoidant ■ Dependent ■ Obsessive-compulsive	■ *Anxiety* ■ *Chronic low self-esteem* ■ *Decisional conflict (specify)* ■ *Impaired social interaction* ■ *Ineffective coping*

    c. Dependent (anxious, fearful disorders)

  3. Determine the client's level of self-esteem, recognizing that poor self-esteem is present despite apparent egocentricity.

  4. Establish individualized nursing diagnoses for the client and the client's family, as needed. (See *Table 5-1, Selected nursing diagnoses for personality disorders.*)

C. Planning and outcome identification

  1. Work with client and family in setting realistic goals.

  2. For the client with an **odd, eccentric personality disorder,** establish desired outcome criteria.

    a. The client will verbalize comfort in relating one-to-one with the nurse.

    b. The client will participate in group situations with support.

    c. The client will control or reduce unusual mannerisms.

    d. The client will refrain from sharing bizarre or paranoid ideas with others.

  3. For the client with a **dramatic, emotional, erratic personality disorder,** establish desired outcome criteria.

    a. The client will control impulsive behaviors, and refrain from self-destructive behaviors.

    b. The client will verbalize anxiety and angry feelings rather than act out.

    c. The client will decrease manipulative behavior and express needs in a direct manner.

    d. The client will respect the rights and needs of others, and adhere to rules and regulations in structured environments and relationships with others.

  4. For the client with an **anxious, fearful personality disorder,** establish desired outcome criteria.

       a. The client will identify positive self-statements indicating improved sense of self-esteem.

       b. The client will interact with peers in social situations.

       c. The client will manage anxiety when daily life situations are not under individual control.

       d. The client will make decisions in an independent manner.

       e. The client will tolerate lack of perfection without undue anxiety.

   5. For the **family of the client with a personality disorder,** establish desired outcome criteria .

       a. The family will maintain generational boundaries.

       b. The family will identify areas of self-functioning.

       c. The family will set consistent, appropriate limits.

       d. The family will provide positive feedback for efforts to improve functioning.

D. Implementation

   1. For the client with an **odd, eccentric personality disorder,** take the following measures:

       a. Adopt an objective, matter-of-fact manner when interacting with the client, and maintain clear, consistent verbal and nonverbal communication.

       b. Provide daily structure for activities of daily living.

       c. Maintain focus on reality and reality-based topics.

       d. Help the client to clearly identify feelings that are implied.

       e. Help the client with problem solving for life issues identified as sources of stress.

       f. Gradually involve the client in group situations, providing support when necessary, and provide positive feedback for socially appropriate behavior.

   2. For the client with a **dramatic, emotional, erratic personality disorder,** take the following measures:

       a. Prevent self-harm by observing the client frequently and developing a no-harm contract.

       b. Give immediate feedback when confronting inappropriate or manipulative behavior, and help the client to examine the consequences of appropriate and inappropriate behavior.

       c. Act as a role model for appropriate expression of feelings and negative emotions.

       d. Work with the treatment team in maintaining consistent feedback for the client, reinforcing specific treatment objectives, and avoiding manipulations of staff by the client.

       e. Avoid rescuing or rejecting the client.

       f. Set limits; reinforce consequences of manipulative behavior or disregard for rights of others.

       g. Give positive feedback for achieving goals and independent behavior.

       h. Explore the client's feelings regarding rejection, being alone, and fear of abandonment.

       i. Use a problem-solving approach to help the client explore necessary changes.

       j. Encourage the client's participation in follow-up treatment.

CLIENT AND FAMILY TEACHING 5-1
Guidelines for clients with personality disorders

Provide information about the client's specific disorder and treatment:

- Personality disorder is a problem that persists throughout life and affects important areas of the client's functioning, especially in relationships with others in social and occupational roles.
- The client with a personality disorder may be suspicious and mistrustful of others, may form dependent relationships, or may take advantage of others in relationships.
- The client with a personality disorder may lack the motivation to change aspects of self-functioning, but may respond to a problem-solving approach to specific issues.

Also provide information about ways that family functioning can improve:

- Advise the family that it may be beneficial for each family member to improve self-functioning rather than focus on changing the client.
- Stress that maintaining clear expectations of each family member's role is helpful in defining boundaries across the generations.
- Reinforce that expectations about acceptable behavior for all family members should be clearly specified and maintained.

3. For the client with an **anxious, fearful personality disorder,** take the following measures:
   a. Establish a caring, consistent therapeutic relationship and clear expectations for responsible behavior.
   b. Expect the client to make decisions, and teach him how to be assertive (or refer the client to a training program for this behavior).
   c. Encourage the client to identify positive self-attributes.
   d. Provide positive feedback when the client interacts in social situations appropriately.
   e. Teach the client to use stress-management and relaxation techniques to cope with anxiety.
4. For the **family of the client with a personality disorder,** take the following measures (see *Client and family teaching 5-1, Guidelines for clients with personality disorders*):
   a. Help family members to define and maintain generational boundaries.
   b. Provide positive feedback for efforts to define self-functioning.
   c. Encourage clear definitions of acceptable behavior for the client within the family.
   d. Encourage parents to work on areas of conflict in their own relationship.
   e. Teach family members to use stress-reduction measures to handle anxiety.

E. Outcome evaluation
1. The client maintains behavior that is appropriate in social situations.
2. The client expresses satisfaction with self-concept and relationships with others.
3. The client avoids behaviors that are manipulative or exploitative of others.

4. The client expresses angry feelings verbally rather than acting out on self or others.

5. The client respects the rights and needs of others.

6. The client tolerates areas of imperfection in life without undue anxiety.

7. The client identifies the need for follow-up treatments and agrees to cooperate with appropriate referral.

8. The family members improve self-functioning.

Study questions

1. The community nurse is following up on a client who was hospitalized with depressive disorder, not otherwise specified, following the death of her spouse. In reviewing the client's chart, the nurse notes that the client has an Axis II diagnosis of dependent personality disorder. Which behaviors would the nurse anticipate in this client?
   1. Difficulty making decisions, lack of self-confidence
   2. Grandiose thinking, attention-seeking behaviors
   3. Odd mannerisms, speech, and behaviors
   4. Unstable moods and impulsive behaviors

2. A client with an Axis II diagnosis of histrionic personality disorder behaves in a dramatic fashion and displays intense emotions when having to wait in the health clinic for an appointment. How can the nurse best respond to this situation?
   1. Call the health care provider and urge that the client be seen immediately because the behavior is disruptive to others.
   2. Directly confront the client about the unreasonable nature of the behavior and point out that other people are also waiting.
   3. Explain to the client the reason for the delay in a calm, nonthreatening manner, and offer to reschedule the appointment if the client wishes to do so.
   4. Ignore the client's behavior and avoid confrontation, which can lead to an escalation of the problem.

3. A client is hospitalized following a suicide attempt. His history reveals a previous diagnosis of schizoid personality disorder. Which of the following behaviors would be atypical of a client with this disorder?
   1. Actions designed to please the nurse
   2. Limited expressions of feelings and emotions
   3. Odd ideas and mannerisms
   4. Reluctance to join group activities

4. A client with an anxious, fearful personality has difficulty accomplishing work assignments because of her fear of failure. The client has been referred to the employee assistance program because of repeated absences from work and evidence of an alcohol problem. Which nursing diagnosis would be most appropriate?
   1. *Ineffective coping*
   2. *Decisional conflict*
   3. *Disturbed thought processes*
   4. *Risk for self-directed violence*

5. Which statement about an individual with a personality disorder is true?

1. Psychotic behavior is common during acute episodes.
2. Prognosis for recovery is good with therapeutic intervention.
3. The individual typically remains in the mainstream of society, although he has problems in social and occupational roles.
4. The individual usually seeks treatment willingly for symptoms that are personally distressful.

6. A client describes himself as "very religious, with strong opinions about what is right and what is wrong." The client is quite judgmental about beliefs and lifestyles that are "unacceptable." Which statement supports the nurse's analysis that this client's behavior is typical of someone with a personality disorder?
   1. Inflexible behaviors, along with use of rigid defense mechanisms, are characteristic.
   2. Judgmental behavior, including self-insight, is common.
   3. Religious fanatics often have personality disorders.
   4. Strong belief systems are common and can help identify evidence of instability.

7. A client has a history of conflict-filled relationships. Despite an expressed desire for friends, she acts in ways that tend to alienate people. Which nursing intervention would be important for this client?
   1. Establish a therapeutic relationship in which the nurse uses role modeling and role-playing for appropriate behaviors.
   2. Help the client to select friends who are kind and extra caring.
   3. Point out that the client acts in ways that alienate others.

4. Recognize that this client is unlikely to change and therefore intervention is inappropriate.

8. A hospitalized client with antisocial personality disorder stole money from an elderly client on the unit. Which of the following is the most appropriate for the nurse to say to this client?
   1. "Why did you take the money?"
   2. "Let's talk about how you felt when you took the money."
   3. "The consequences of stealing are loss of privileges."
   4. "This client is defenseless against you."

9. A nurse is working with clients who have personality disorders. Which of the following techniques would the nurse use to deal with her own feelings that interfere with therapeutic performance?
   1. Active listening techniques
   2. Challenging the client's assertions
   3. Forming social relations
   4. Seeking peer or supervisor direction

10. A client with borderline personality disorder is defensive and emotionally labile and often becomes suddenly and explosively angry. When interacting with this client, the nurse would:
    1. point out how angry the client is becoming, and confront the behavior.
    2. take a calm, quiet, and nonconfrontational approach, and avoid arguing with the client.
    3. tell the client to calm down and to avoid becoming explosive or restraints will be used.
    4. use gentle touch and a caring approach to calm the client.

11. A client with borderline personality disorder has a nursing diagnosis of *Risk for*

self-directed violence, which is related to the client's self-mutilation behavior (burning arms with cigarettes). Which client behavior would indicate a positive outcome of intervention?
1. The client denies feelings of wanting to harm anyone.
2. The client expresses feelings of anger toward others.
3. The client requests cigarettes at appropriate times.
4. The client tells the nurse about wanting to burn himself.

12. The nurse is working with the family of a client with a personality disorder. Which of the following should the nurse encourage the family members to work on?
1. Avoiding direct expression of problems within the family
2. Changing the client's problem behaviors
3. Improving self-functioning
4. Supporting the client's defenses

13. The nurse assesses the client with borderline personality disorder. Which of the following behaviors are common to this diagnosis? Select all that apply.

1. Intense fear of being alone
2. Evidence of self-mutilating attempts
3. Evidence of suspiciousness and mistrust of others
4. Indifferent attitude toward approval or criticism
5. Unstable moods with impulsive behaviors
6. Presence of odd mannerisms, speech, and behaviors

14. When a client with a personality disorder begins demonstrating manipulative behavior, which of the following nursing actions are most appropriate? Select all that apply.
1. Ask the client to think about the consequences of behavior.
2. Allow the client time to perform specific rituals.
3. Develop a consistent team approach to handle the client's behaviors.
4. Help the client to express anxiety verbally rather than with specific symptoms.
5. Provide immediate feedback concerning the client's specific behaviors.
6. Set limits in a clear, direct manner.

Answer key

1. The answer is 1.
The client with a dependent personality disorder typically demonstrates anxious and fearful behavior and is reluctant to make decisions. Lack of self-confidence is reflective of chronic low self-esteem. The behavior in option 2 is characteristic of someone with a dramatic, emotional, erratic personality disorder, such as narcissistic personality. The behavior in option 3 is characteristic of schizoid or schizotypal personality disorder, in which

odd, eccentric behavior is displayed. Option 4 characterizes borderline personality disorder.

2. The answer is 3.
The nurse is modeling appropriate behavior, using a calm and nonthreatening manner to avoid reinforcing the client's dramatic behavior. Offering to reschedule the client's appointment allows the client a choice, which respects the client's feelings in a nonjudgmental way. Calling the

health care provider and urging her to see the client immediately would only serve to reinforce the client's inappropriate behavior. Confronting this client would increase his anxiety and result in an escalation of dramatic behavior. The nurse should attempt to decrease, not increase, the client's anxiety. Ignoring the client's behavior would be ignoring a problem that is disruptive not only to the client, but also to other people in the clinic. The client's behavior would most likely become increasingly dramatic.

3. The answer is **1.**
A client with a schizoid personality disorder is typically detached, aloof, and socially isolated. He has no interest in seeking the approval others and would not behave in ways to please the nurse. The behaviors included in the remaining options are characteristic of someone with schizoid personality disorder.

4. The answer is **1.**
This client is experiencing difficulty in occupational functioning as well as problems with alcohol; therefore, she meets criteria for the diagnosis of *Ineffective coping*. Options 2 and 3 are incorrect because there is no evidence in this situation that the client has a conflict regarding a decision or is experiencing altered thinking. Option 4 is also incorrect because the client has not expressed thoughts of self-harm or committed any acts designed to harm herself.

5. The answer is **3.**
An individual with a personality disorder usually is not hospitalized unless a coexisting Axis I psychiatric disorder is present. Generally, these individuals make marginal adjustments and remain in society, although they typically experience relationship and occupational problems related to their inflexible behaviors. Personality disorders are chronic, lifelong patterns of behavior; acute episodes do not occur. Psychotic behavior is usually not common, although it can occur in either schizotypal personality disorder or borderline personality disorder. Because these disorders are enduring and evasive and the individual is inflexible, prognosis for recovery is unfavorable. Generally, the individual does not seek treatment because he does not perceive problems with his own behavior. Distress can occur based on other people's reaction to the individual's behavior.

6. The answer is **1.**
Individuals with personality disorder have inflexible behavior patterns and rigid defense mechanisms. They are unlikely to change over time. Such individuals generally lack self-insight and are more likely to have external locus of control thinking (blaming others for problems). Religious fanatics may be motivated by other psychodynamics (possibly psychotic states). However, strong belief systems do not necessarily mean mental instability. A mentally healthy person may have belief systems that are strong and that govern conduct.

7. The answer is **1.**
A therapeutic relationship shows acceptance, and using role modeling and role-playing can help the client to learn appropriate behaviors. Option 2 is an inappropriate and unrealistic solution to the client's problem behaviors. Option 3 is also inappropriate because the client is not likely to accept direct criticism of her behavior; such individuals do not perceive a problem with their own behavior. Option

4 ignores the client's potential for growth and improvement.

8. The answer is 3.

The most appropriate response is to reinforce the consequences of behavior that disregard the rights of others. Option 1 is incorrect because this client is likely to rationalize and excuse the behavior. Option 2 is also incorrect because the nurse should not encourage the client to provide excuses or explanations of behaviors that are clearly against the rules. A client with antisocial personality disorder is unlikely to have compassion for others and typically lacks respect for the rights of others.

9. The answer is 4.

The nurse is likely to have strong reactions to clients with personality disorders, especially those who display intense emotions and manipulative behaviors. Seeking the direction of peers and supervisors can help clarify issues and determine the best nursing responses to difficult behaviors. Active listening and challenging the client's assertions are beneficial techniques to use with clients; however, this question is asking about techniques to enhance the nurse's performance. Forming social relationships would not help in dealing with feelings that interfere with therapeutic performance.

10. The answer is 2.

The best way to respond to the client with angry behavior is a calm, nonconfrontational, nonargumentative approach. This will avoid further escalating the client's behavior. Confronting the client's behavior could exacerbate anger and trigger explosive behavior. Telling the client to calm down minimizes the client's problems, and the mention of restraints may be perceived as threatening to the client. Touch may also be perceived as threatening; it is not recommended for a client who may become explosive.

11. The answer is 4.

The fact that the client directly tells the nurse about wanting to self-mutilate, rather than acting on these feelings, is evidence of his responding to nursing intervention. Option 1 does not indicate that self-mutilating behavior is decreasing, and options 2 and 3 do not address the established nursing diagnosis.

12. The answer is 3.

Family members typically benefit from working on ways to improve self-functioning. This facilitates ownership of problems among individuals involved in ongoing relationship difficulties. The direct expression of problems is helpful and therefore should not be avoided. It would be impossible to change the client's behavior; encouraging family members to do so would frustrate them. The client's defenses are likely to be quite strong, and this client is likely to blame others for problems; consequently, supporting his blaming others is not helpful.

13. The answer is 1, 2, 5.

These are all common characteristics of an individual with borderline personality disorder. Suspiciousness and mistrust of others (option 3) is characteristic of paranoid personality disorder. Options 4 and 6 are characteristic of someone with schizoid personality disorder, who is generally aloof in relationships and has unusual speech and mannerisms.

14. The answer is 1, 3, 5, 6.

These interventions allow the nurse to immediately confront the client's manipulative behavior and provide consistent structure (through limit-setting and a team approach). Option 2 is appropriate for the client with obsessive-compulsive behavior; option 4, for someone with a somatatization problem.

6 Mood Disorders and Suicidal Behavior

I. OVERVIEW OF MOOD DISORDERS AND SUICIDAL BEHAVIOR

A. Key concepts

1. **Mood disorders** are characterized by disturbances in feelings, thinking, and behavior that tend to occur on a continuum, ranging from severe depression to severe mania (hyperactivity). (See *Figure 6-1, Understanding the mood swing continuum.*)

2. **Depression** is an emotional state characterized by sadness, discouragement, guilt, decreased self-esteem, and feelings of helplessness or hopelessness.

3. **Mania** is an emotional state characterized by elation, high optimism, increased energy, and an exaggerated sense of importance and invincibility.

4. **Unipolar depression** is a mood disturbance with only depression, but no occurrence of mania.

5. **Bipolar disorder** is a mood disturbance in which the symptoms of mania have occurred at least one time; an episode of depression may or may not have occurred.

6. **Grief** is a normal response to a loss (death of a significant other, divorce, illness or hospitalization, job loss, or loss of personal possessions); grief is differentiated from depression by the following factors:

   a. **Acute grieving** may occur up to 3 months after a significant loss.

   b. **Grief resolution** is characterized by the grieving person's ability to remember, comfortably and realistically, both the pleasures and disappointments associated with the loss. Grief resolution may take up to 3 years.

FIGURE 6-1
Understanding the mood swing continuum

Mood disorders are characterized by mood swings—episodic changes in an individual's feeling, thinking, and behavior—that range from elation to despair. Bipolar disorders consist of one or more manic episodes or one or more depressive episodes. Cyclothymia consists of both hypomanic (elevated or irritable) and dysthymic (chronically sad or depressed) mood swings. Situated between the extreme moods is a normal mood.

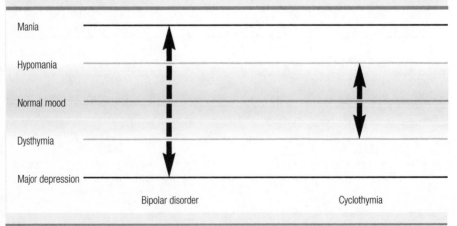

      c. **Maladaptive grief response** can lead to a mood disorder; the response may be delayed, inhibited, prolonged, or exaggerated.

      d. Loss of self-esteem in the grieving person is not characteristic of normal grieving, and may indicate a mood disorder.

    7. **Suicidal behavior** involves thoughts of taking one's own life.

      a. A **suicidal threat** is defined as a suicidal intent that is usually accompanied by behavior changes; the threat includes a plan and the means to execute the plan.

      b. A **suicidal gesture** refers to a self-destructive act that does not involve serious injury; however, it may be followed by a more serious attempt.

      c. A **suicidal attempt** is a self-destructive act that has a potential outcome of death.

B. Impact of mood disorders

    1. Mood disorders, especially depression, may become chronic and incapacitating without appropriate intervention.

    2. Many individuals with a mood disorder are not diagnosed or are misdiagnosed. (See *Table 6-1, Common risk factors associated with mood disorders and suicidal behaviors.*)

TABLE 6-1

Common risk factors associated with mood disorders and suicidal behaviors

Risk factor	Mood disorders	Suicidal behaviors
Sex	▪ Depression twice as likely in women as men (2:1)	▪ Increased risk in men
Age	▪ Higher in young women and older men	▪ Risk increases with age (but adolescents make more attempts)
Marital status	▪ Higher in married women and single men ▪ Lower in married men	▪ Risk lower among married men and women
Family history	▪ Higher risk among first-degree relatives	▪ Higher risk among family members of suicide victims

Precipitators (recent life events)	▪ Birth in family within 6 months
	▪ Loss of significant other
	▪ Job problems
	▪ Separation or divorce
	▪ Physical illness
		▪ Increases with:
		  – solitariness (living alone)
		  – unemployment
		  – recent loss
		  – recent surgery or childbirth
		  – social disgrace

Other factors	▪ Seasonal pattern: depression higher in fall and winter	▪ High risk with alcohol and drug abuse ▪ Increased risk in those with mood or thought disorders

      a. Estimates suggest that 10 to 14 million Americans are afflicted with some form of mood disorder.

      b. Only 16% to 23% of persons who meet *DSM-IV TR* criteria for mood disorders actually seek mental health care.

  3. About 18.8 million American adults (about 9.5% of the U.S. population) have a **depressive disorder**; it is estimated that about 1 in 6 people will experience a depressive disorder in their lifetime.

      a. Nearly twice as many women as men (12% vs. 6.6%) are affected each year; some research indicates that social and cultural factors may account for the increased rate in women.

      b. Adolescents (between ages 9 and 17) have a 4.9% incidence of major depression.

      c. An estimated 2 million Americans over age 65 have a depressive disorder, indicating that depression is a significant problem for elderly individuals.

      d. Between 50% and 85% of those with a major depressive disorder will experience more than one episode of depression; the average is four episodes within a lifetime.

      e. A depressive episode is typically first experienced between ages 25 and 44; however, individuals born after World War II typically have an earlier age of onset.

  4. Bipolar disorder affects about 1% of the U.S. population.

      a. Persons with this disorder will typically experience 10 episodes across a lifetime; about 30% begin having symptoms before age 25.

      b. Bipolar disorder affects men and women equally, although women may have depression as their first experience of this disorder.

C. Family and cultural considerations

  1. Family members of individuals with a mood disorder are severely affected.

      a. Changes in energy levels, role functioning, and socialization that occur in an individual with a mood disorder affect every aspect of family life.

      b. Children of depressed mothers have increased vulnerability for emotional problems.

  2. African Americans have a lower rate of mood disorders than Whites and Hispanic Americans.

  3. People of Asian descent manifest more somatic symptoms (general fatigue and unexplained body aches), while people from Western cultures typically have mood and cognitive symptoms (depressed mood and decreased ability to concentrate).

II. TYPES OF MOOD DISORDERS

A. Major depressive disorder

  1. Characterized by at least 2 weeks of a depressed mood or loss of interest in pleasure and activities, major depressive disorder also includes at least four of the following symptoms of depression:

      a. Increase or decrease in appetite

           b. Increase or decrease in sleep

           c. Psychomotor agitation or retardation

           d. Fatigue and loss of energy

           e. Decreased ability to think and concentrate

           f. Recurrent thoughts of suicide

    2. *DSM-IV TR* **specifiers**, or subtypes, of major depressive disorder include the following:

        a. **Melancholic features:** the client experiences either anhedonia in relation to all activities or lack of mood reactivity to usually pleasurable activities; this specifier is also characterized by waking early in the morning, feeling worse in the morning, and excessive guilt.

        b. **Atypical features:** the client exhibits mood reactivity (ability to respond to positive environmental stimuli), increased levels of anxiety, changes in appetite and sleep, and increased sensitivity to interpersonal rejection.

        c. **Psychotic features:** the client's depression is accompanied by delusions and hallucinations; the theme of the psychotic symptoms is usually mood congruent with depression.

        d. **Postpartum onset:** onset of symptoms occurs within 4 weeks of delivery (affects 1 in 10 new mothers), and symptoms are similar to that of a typical major depressive disorder; however, psychotic features may also be present.

        e. **Seasonal pattern specifier:** although **seasonal affective disorder (SAD)** is currently not classified as a diagnostic category in *DSM-IV TR,* it is included as a specifier.

           – SAD commonly occurs in the fall and winter and is associated with the decrease in sunlight.

           – Common symptoms include hypersomnia, overeating and carbohydrate craving, and weight gain.

B. Dysthymia

    1. Dysthymia is characterized by a chronically depressed mood occurring most of the day, more days than not, for at least a 2-year period; during periods of depressed mood, at least two or more of the other symptoms of depression (see II. A.) must be present.

    2. This disorder usually does not affect social or occupational functioning.

C. Bipolar disorder

    1. **Bipolar I disorder** is characterized by one or more manic or mixed episodes, usually accompanied by a major depressive episode; symptoms of a **manic episode** include the following:

        a. Inflated self-esteem or grandiosity

        b. Decreased need for sleep

        c. Increased or pressured speech

        d. Flight of ideas

        e. Distractibility

        f. Increased involvement in goal-directed activities

        g. Excessive involvement in pleasurable activities that have a high potential for painful consequences (charging expensive items on a credit card that is already at maximum limit; sleeping with multiple partners without regard to safe sex practices).

2. **Bipolar II disorder** is characterized by one or more major depressive episodes accompanied by at least one hypomanic episode. A **hypomanic episode** is one in which at least three or more of the symptoms of mania are present.

D. Cyclothymia is characterized by at least 2 years of several periods of hypomanic symptoms not as severe as those in a manic episode.

E. Pseudodementia is a disorder associated with depression in elderly clients.

1. The clinical presentation of depression is similar to symptoms associated with a cognitive impairment disorder.

2. Treatment of depression that is successful in eliminating the symptoms of dementia will establish this diagnosis.

III. CAUSES OF MOOD DISORDERS

A. Key concepts

1. Although the exact cause of mood disorders has not been established, the current consensus is that these disorders result from complex interactions among a variety of factors.

2. Implicating factors include genetic predisposition, neurochemical imbalances (affecting neurotransmission and neuroendocrine regulation), certain medications, medical conditions, and psychosocial and environmental processes.

B. Genetic predisposition

1. **Major depressive disorder** is up to 3 times more common among first-degree biological relatives.

   a. Twin studies reveal a higher rate of concordance in monozygotic twins than dizygotic twins, indicating a genetic component.

   b. Researchers are currently investigating a defective gene on chromosome 4; those with this defective gene are 26 times more likely to be hospitalized for severe depression and suicide attempt; research is also focused on genes on chromosomes 11, 18, and 21.

2. The risk of developing **bipolar disorder** increases 4% to 24% in first-degree relatives of people with bipolar disorder.

   a. Twin studies of monozygotic twins indicate a 65% concordance rate.

   b. Early research describing the location of genetic markers on specific genes has not been replicated, although research is ongoing.

C. Neurotransmission dysregulation

1. According to the **biogenic amine theory**, norepinephrine and serotonin are deficient in individuals with a depressive disorder, whereas these neurotransmitters are increased in those with a bipolar disorder; changes in quantity and sensitivity of receptor sites are also important.

2. According to the **Kindling theory**, external environmental stressors activate internal physiologic stress responses, which trigger the first episode of a mood dis-

order; the first episode then creates electrophysiologic sensitivity to future episodes so that less stress is required to evoke another episode.

D. Neuroendocrine dysregulation

1. Laboratory findings involving the **hypothalamic-pituitary-adrenal (HPA) axis** indicate that some individuals with depressive disorders exhibit increased cortisol levels, resistance of cortisol to suppression by dexamethasone (dexamethasone suppression test), and blunted adrenocorticotropin hormone response to corticotropin-releasing factor challenge as compared to normal controls; elevated corticotropin-releasing factor has also been found in cerebrospinal fluid.
2. **Subclinical hypothyroidism** has been found in some individuals with depressive disorders, especially women. Blunting of response of thyroid-stimulating hormone to thyrotropic-releasing factor has been found in about 25% of euthyroid individuals with depressive disorders.
3. **Circadian rhythm changes** have also been studied, indicating abnormal sleep EEG activity in many individuals with mood disorders.

E. Medication use and medical conditions

1. The following medications are known to produce depression as a side effect:
    a. Hormones (oral contraceptives, glucocorticoids)
    b. Cardiovascular drugs (beta-blockers, calcium channel blockers, thiazide diuretics, and digitalis preparations)
    c. Psychotropics (benzodiazepines, neuroleptics)
    d. Anti-inflammatory and anti-infective drugs (nonsteroidal anti-inflammatory drugs, antituberculosis drugs, and sulfonamides)
    e. Antiulcer medications (cimetidine, ranitidine).
2. Clinically significant depressive symptoms occur in up to 36% of individuals with a nonpsychiatric general medical condition, including:
    a. Cerebrovascular accident
    b. Cognitive impairment disorders (dementia)
    c. Diabetes
    d. Coronary artery disease
    e. Cancer
    f. Chronic fatigue syndrome
    g. Acquired immune deficiency syndrome (AIDS).

F. Psychosocial and environmental factors

1. According to psychoanalytic theory, depression results from inward-directed anger and aggression over a significant loss **(object loss)**.
2. Beck's theory proposes that depression is a problem of cognitive patterns that have developed in an individual over time.
    a. The individual holds negative views of self, the world, and the future.
    b. He views himself as unattractive and incompetent, the outward environment as demanding and unyielding, and the future as hopeless. (See *Table 6-2, Common negative cognitions*, page 106.)
3. Environmental factors (recent loss of family member through death, divorce, or separation; lack of social support system; or significant health problem) are as-

TABLE 6-2

Common negative cognitions

Negative cognition	Description	Example
Overgeneralization	Believing that everything will go wrong because of a single negative occurrence (blowing things out of proportion); key words include "never" and "always"	After scoring a low grade in algebra, a student says, "I will never learn this stuff."
All-or-nothing thinking	Viewing everything in extremes—either "black or white," with no middle ground	John takes pictures of his friend's wedding. All but three of the pictures are perfect. John is dissatisfied because all the pictures are not perfect and considers himself a failure at photography.
"Should" statements	Using "should," "shouldn't," "must," and "ought to" statements to establish standards for self and others; "should" statements generally lead to frustration; those directed toward oneself lead to guilt; those directed at others lead to anger and resentment	John (from previous example) says to himself, "I should have taken all of the pictures right."
Labeling	Applying negatively loaded labels to oneself or others	Unable to comprehend a 300-page section of her nursing text, a student says, "I'm an idiot."
Mind reading	Jumping to conclusions regarding another person's reactions without checking those reactions with the other person	Pat is having an enjoyable lunch with a friend, but the friend looks dejected. Pat asks what the problem is. After coaxing, the friend says, "I know you think that I'm a bad person."
Fortune telling	Being absolutely convinced that things will not turn out right, regardless of evidence to the contrary	Ellen has received several letters of commendation from her boss, but when it's time to apply for a promotion, she states, "I'd better not apply; my boss will never give me a promotion. I only perform mediocre work."

sociated with the onset of mood disorder; sleep deprivation has been associated with the occurrence of another manic episode in individuals with a history of bipolar disorder.

IV. MANAGING MOOD DISORDERS

A. Key concepts

1. Clients may receive treatment in various settings, including acute psychiatric hospitals, community-based treatment in outpatient programs, or private psychotherapy with a primary practitioner.
2. Resources for clients and families include:
   a. Community support groups, such as Depressives Anonymous and Recovery, Inc.
   b. National Depressive and Manic Depressive Association, which provides information and assistance
   c. National Alliance for the Mentally Ill, which provides information, support groups, and political action for legislative efforts on behalf of the mentally ill and their families

B. Acute, psychiatric, hospital-based care

1. This setting may be recommended when a client's mood disorder is severe or danger for self-harm exists.
2. Clients with suicidal behavior require hospitalization for protection, so they can receive:
   a. Supportive psychotherapy and milieu management
   b. Cognitive-behavioral therapy
   c. Medication with antidepressants, neuroleptics (if psychotic-level symptoms occur), or mood-stabilizing agents. (See *Drug chart 6-1, Selected medications for treating mood disorders*, page 108.)
3. Electroconvulsive therapy may be recommended for severe depression that is unresponsive to antidepressant therapy. (See page 259.)

C. Community-based treatment

1. **Primary prevention** may be accomplished through identification of at-risk populations and teaching self-care measures to decrease occurrence of mood disorders; self-care measures may include:
   a. Adequate exercise and rest
   b. Good nutrition
   c. Stress management
   d. Use of support systems
   e. Verbalizing rather than internalizing feelings
   f. Assertiveness training programs.
2. **Case finding** occurs when health care practitioners identify individuals in the community who have symptoms of a mood disorder but are not in treatment.
   a. Case finding can promote early intervention and decrease chronicity.
   b. Nurses can educate clients and families about:
      - The nature and course of the disorder
      - Recognizing individual symptom patterns
      - Self-monitoring for symptom return and seeking prompt treatment
      - Self-care measures.

DRUG CHART 6-1
Selected medications for treating mood disorders

Classification	Drug	Rationale for use
Antidepressants		
Tricyclic antidepressants (TCAs)	amitriptyline (Elavil) clomipramine (Anafranil) desipramine (Norpramin) nortriptyline (Pamelor)	Act by blocking reuptake of neurotransmitters at presynaptic neuron; provide elevation of mood, increased activity level, and appetite stimulation.
Monoamine oxidase inhibitors (MAOIs)	isocarboxazid (Marplan) phenelzine (Nardil) tranylcypromine (Parnate)	Act by inhibiting the enzyme monoamine oxidase. When enzyme is inhibited, increased amounts of neurotransmitters remain at the synapse and act to elevate mood and increase activity level.
Selective serotonin reuptake inhibitors (SSRIs)	fluoxetine (Prozac) fluvoxamine (Luvox) paroxetine (Paxil) sertraline (Zoloft)	Act specifically on serotonin, preventing its reuptake; because they are selective, SSRIs do not have the side effects of TCAs and MAOIs (related to increasing norepinephrine levels at synapses).
Atypical antidepressants	bupropion (Wellbutrin) mirtazapine (Remeron) nefazodone (Serzone) trazodone (Desyrel) venlafaxine (Effexor)	Act similar to TCAs. Antidepressant effects are not yet well understood; however, these drugs produce fewer side effects than TCAs.
Herbal remedies	*Hypericum perforatum* (St. John's wort)	May relieve mild-to-moderate depression; however, research has not consistently supported this result.
Mood stabilizers		
Antimanic	lithium carbonate (Eskalith, Lithobid, Lithonate)	Acts by interfering with a neuropathway (phosphoinositide second messenger system) in the limbic system, which helps to stabilize neurochemical regulation in the brain, thereby stabilizing mood.
Anticonvulsants	carbamazepine (Tegretol) gabapentin (Neurontin) lamotrigine (Lamictal) topiramate (Topamax) valproic acid (Depakote)	Act by affecting sodium and calcium channels, thereby decreasing release of neurotransmitters; thought to inhibit the process of kindling.
Atypical antipsychotic		
	olanzapine (Zyprexa)	Acts as a mood stabilizer; the FDA recently approved this drug for use in bipolar disorder.

3. **Crisis intervention services** should be used for those individuals with suicidal behavior.

4. **Medication management** may include the use of antidepressants, mood stabilizers, or antipsychotics (see *Drug chart 6-1, Selected medications for treating mood disorders*); ultraviolet light therapy may also be used for those with seasonal affective disorder. (See page 259.)

5. **Cognitive-behavior therapy** is the recommended type of psychotherapeutic approach for a client with a mood disorder.

   a. In some studies, it has been found to be as effective as antidepressant therapy.

   b. This approach includes identifying and challenging the accuracy of the client's negative cognitions, reinforcing more accurate perceptions, and encouraging behaviors that are designed to counteract the depressive symptoms.

NURSING PROCESS OVERVIEW

V. CARE OF THE CLIENT WITH A MOOD DISORDER

A. Assessment

1. Review the client's history for precipitating stressors and significant data; include the following information:

   a. Genetic-biologic vulnerability (family history)

   b. Stressful life events and recent losses

   c. Results of standardized assessment tools for depression (Beck Depression Inventory, Hamilton Rating Scale of Depression, Geriatric Depression Scale, Self-Rating Depression Scale)

   d. Past episodes of mood disorder or suicidal behaviors

   e. Medication history

   f. Drug and alcohol use

   g. Education and employment history.

2. Note the client's characteristic physiologic, cognitive, emotional, and behavioral responses. (See *Table 6-3, Comparing assessment data in mood disorders*, page 110.)

3. Assess the client's awareness of the disorder, and determine current stressors and coping behaviors. (See *Key questions 6-1, Assessing clients with mood disorders*, page 111.)

4. Assess for the following suicidal risk factors and the lethality of the client's suicidal behavior. (See *Display 6-1, Quick assessment of suicide risk factors*, page 112, and *Table 6-1, Common risk factors associated with mood disorders and suicidal behaviors*, page 101.)

   a. The **client's intent** (to relieve stress, as a solution to difficult problems)

   b. The **suicidal plan**, including whether the client has an organized plan and the means to carry out the plan

   c. The client's **mental state** (presence of thought disorder, level of anxiety, severity of mood disorder)

   d. **Support systems** available

TABLE 6-3

Comparing assessment data in mood disorders

Characteristics	Depressive disorders	Bipolar (manic) disorders
Physiologic responses	■ Altered appetite (increased or decreased) ■ Altered sleep patterns (hypersomnia or insomnia) ■ Constipation (due to dietary factors)	■ Reduced appetite (due to hyperactivity) ■ Little sleep (due to excess energy) ■ Constipation (possible) ■ Boundless energy leading to physical exhaustion ■ Ignored physiologic responses
Cognitive responses	■ Indecisiveness ■ Reduced concentration and attention span ■ Rumination (constant preoccupation with same thoughts), somatic delusions, poverty of thought	■ Impaired judgment ■ Reduced concentration and attention span, distractibility, flight of ideas ■ Grandiose beliefs and delusions, tangential thinking
Emotional responses	■ Sadness, despondency ■ Anger, agitation, resentfulness ■ Guilt, feelings of worthlessness ■ Hopelessness, helplessness ■ Apathy	■ Euphoria, elation ■ Anger, irritability, rage ■ Lack of guilt, narcissism ■ Exaggerated sense of ability ■ Emotional lability
Behavioral responses	■ Poor personal hygiene ■ Psychomotor retardation ■ Decreased motivation ■ Anhedonia ■ Frequent complaints and demands ■ Lack of spontaneity ■ Lack of exercise ■ Fatigue ■ Somatic complaints ■ Restless and undirected activity	■ Poor personal hygiene ■ Psychomotor agitation ■ Impulsiveness, lack of inhibition ■ Hypersexuality, increase in high-risk sexual behavior ■ Manipulativeness, domineering personality ■ Inappropriate singing, dancing, and joking ■ Undirected hyperactivity

     e. **Current stressors** affecting the client, including other illnesses (both psychiatric and medical), recent losses, and history of substance abuse.

    5. Assess the family support system and the client or family's knowledge of specific mood disorder symptoms, medications and treatment recommendations, signs of relapse, and self-care measures.

B. Analysis and nursing diagnosis

    1. Analyze the client's predominant mood, anxiety level, degree of self-esteem, and severity of symptoms.

       a. Determine the client's risk for suicide, understanding that an individual with a mood disorder is at increased risk (suicide is most likely when going into or coming out of a depression).

       b. Determine the level of family support available.

KEY QUESTIONS 6-1
Assessing clients with mood disorders

Questions	Information gathered
Client with depression	
Can you describe what your depression feels like to you? How long have you felt this way?	Client's experience of depression
How would you rate your feeling of depression on a scale of 1 to 10, with 10 being the worst depression?	Severity of depressive symptoms
What activities or things in your life give you pleasure?	Presence of anhedonia
Do you sleep excessively or have difficulty sleeping?	Disturbed sleep patterns
Have you lost weight recently or have a poor appetite?	Altered appetite and need for dietary follow-up
Have you experienced any losses or changes in your life?	Maladaption to changes in the client's life
Are you experiencing thoughts of suicide? Do you have a specific suicide plan?	Suicide intent and need for intervention
Client with mania	
Have you experienced racing thoughts or find that you can't speak your thoughts quickly enough?	Presence of flight of ideas or pressured speech
What projects or activities have you recently been doing?	Hyperactivity
Have you completed the things you have started?	Inability to complete tasks
Have you become impatient or easily angered with others?	Irritability, impulsiveness
How many hours a night do you sleep?	Altered sleep patterns
How would you describe your mood?	Presence of elation, euphoria

2. Establish individualized nursing diagnoses for the client or family with a depressive disorder, bipolar disorder, or suicidal behaviors; prioritize the following diagnoses as needed:
   a. *Anxiety*
   b. *Chronic low self-esteem*
   c. *Compromised family coping*
   d. *Deficient knowledge (specify)*

DISPLAY 6-1

Quick assessment of suicide risk factors

- Sex (men more than women)
- Age (adolescent or older than age 50)
- Previous attempt (increases risk)
- Alcohol or substance abuse
- Presence of thought disorder

- Lack of support system
- Unmarried, divorced, or widowed
- Presence of physical illness (especially chronic)
- Organized plan

---

    e. Disturbed sleep pattern

    f. Disturbed thought process

    g. Dysfunctional grieving

    h. Hopelessness

    i. Imbalanced nutrition: Less than body requirements

    j. Ineffective coping

    k. Ineffective sexuality patterns

    l. Interrupted family processes

    m. Powerlessness

    n. Risk for self-directed or other-directed violence

    o. Social isolation

    p. Spiritual distress.

C. Planning and outcome identification

  1. Work with the client in setting realistic goals.

  2. Establish desired outcome criteria for a client with a mood disorder.

    a. The client will demonstrate decreased anxiety.

    b. The client will identify aspects of self-control over his current life situation.

    c. The client will proceed through the grieving process, verbalizing feelings to supportive persons.

    d. The client will reestablish sleep patterns, including at least 6 to 7 hours of uninterrupted sleep nightly.

    e. The client will eat nutritious meals, either three meals or six smaller meals a day.

    f. The client will verbalize positive, realistic self-statements.

    g. The client will report increased hope for the future.

    h. The client will identify thoughts that are not reality-based.

    i. The client will interact in social situations, reporting satisfaction and feelings of belonging.

    j. The client will agree to report feelings of wanting to harm himself to treatment staff in a timely manner.

    k. The client will refrain from any acts of harm to himself or others.

    l. The client will reestablish normal sexual patterns.

  3. Establish desired outcome criteria for the client's family.

    a. The family will express feelings about individual concerns.

Guidelines for clients with mood disorders

Provide information about the client's specific disorder:

- Depression is characterized by sadness, feelings of hopelessness, and decreased self-esteem. No single cause has been established, but research indicates genetics, chemical imbalance in the brain, and life changes (losses) are involved.
- Mania is characterized by elation, feelings of boundless energy, and a belief that one is superior and gifted. An individual with mania may be too busy to sleep or eat and may spend money wildly or engage in risk-taking behaviors. No single cause has been established, but research indicates genetics, chemical imbalance in the brain, and life changes are involved.
- An individual with a mood disorder generally experiences thoughts of suicide. Times of increased risk include going into or coming out of a depression.

Provide information about treatment measures:

- Medications (antidepressants for depression, mood-stabilizing agents for mania) are commonly used.
- Taking medication as prescribed is very important.

- Antidepressants may not have an immediate effect; the client may not see any noticeable mood improvement for 2 to 4 weeks.
- Checking blood levels regularly is important for clients taking mood-stabilizing agents.
- Talk therapy can also be an effective treatment, along with medication.

Include information about how the family can be helpful:

- Attempts to cheer up a depressed client or to bring down a manic client are not helpful.
- Matter-of-fact acceptance of the client's current mood is helpful.
- Reassurance that the mood will improve with treatment is supportive.
- Encourage the client to maintain regular activity and rest patterns (balance of both).
- Talk about suicide should be taken seriously; contact the client's health care provider when this occurs.

---

b. The family will verbalize knowledge about mood disorders, the client's treatment plan, signs of relapse, and symptom management. (See *Client and family teaching 6-1, Guidelines for clients with mood disorders*.)

D. Implementation

1. For the client with a **depressive disorder**, take the following measures:
   a. Accept the client, avoiding any action that could be interpreted as criticism.
   b. Facilitate adequate nutrition, considering the client's food preferences.
   c. Implement suicide precautions according to assessments about the client's intent.
   d. Avoid excessive cheerfulness, sympathy, or superficiality.
   e. Help the client to develop a daily schedule that includes activities and rest.
   f. Promote sleep with bedtime relaxation interventions (quiet time, back rubs, music or relaxation tapes, or guided imagery).
   g. Encourage participation and social interaction, offering support as needed.
   h. Help the client to identify feelings and reduce negative cognitions. (See *Table 6-2, Common negative cognitions*, page 106.)
   i. Encourage success in achieving goals by helping the client structure simple, manageable tasks.
   j. Question or express doubt about the client's negative self-statements.
   k. Facilitate movement through the grieving process by accepting the client's expressed feelings.

    l. When a client expresses delusional beliefs, use reality reinforcement techniques. (See page 132.)

✋ *m.* Administer medications as prescribed, monitoring laboratory study findings and blood levels (for mood-stabilizing medications).

    n. Monitor the client for therapeutic effects and side effects of medications.

    o. Teach the client about the disorder, including the etiology, symptom identification and management, treatment recommendations, medications, and long-term self-management.

    p. Provide the client with activities (art, music, dance therapy) that allow him to express his feelings; collaborate with other health team members, especially activity therapists.

    q. Encourage the client to participate in self-help or other support groups in the community.

2. For the client with a **bipolar disorder** (manic behaviors), use the interventions listed above for depressive disorder in addition to the following:

    a. Promote adequate nutrition by providing high-calorie foods that can be eaten on the run.

    b. Remove the client from excessively stimulating environments when hyperactivity escalates.

    c. Promote rest periods, and encourage use of quiet activities if the client is unable to rest.

    d. Take a matter-of-fact, consistent approach in describing acceptable behaviors and realistic limits.

    e. Help the client to think through the consequences of impulsive behaviors.

    f. Refrain from laughing or otherwise encouraging inappropriate behaviors.

✋ *g.* Provide a safe environment, and monitor the client to prevent accidents and injury.

    h. Provide the client with simple tasks that focus attention and yield successful completion.

    i. Help the client to identify realistic goals and future plans.

3. For the client with **suicidal behavior**, take the following measures:

    a. Establish a supportive relationship aligned with the part of the client that wishes to live.

    b. Monitor the client closely, following suicide precautions established by agency protocol.

    c. Question the client directly about suicide, asking about a specific plan and a means to accomplish the plan. (*Note:* Asking the client does not increase the risk.)

    d. Remove dangerous and potentially lethal materials or objects, according to agency protocol.

    e. Encourage the client to discuss stressors and feelings of pain, anger, and anguish.

    f. Encourage the client to agree to a no-suicide contract as part of his behavioral agreement.

    g. Assist the client with the problem-solving process when specific problems are identified.

E. Outcome evaluation

1. The client verbalizes decreased anxiety and normal mood.
2. The client does not harm himself, and reports wanting to live.
3. The client eats nutritious meals each day, maintaining a normal weight.
4. The client exhibits normal sleep patterns, allowing for adequate energy during the day.
5. The client verbalizes feeling able to cope with current life changes and is able to identify specific ways for coping.
6. The client voices positive self-statements.
7. The client expresses hope for the future.
8. The client expresses satisfaction with improved social interaction and identifies available support systems.
9. The client demonstrates clear thinking patterns, with no evidence of delusions, excessive guilt, or flight of ideas.
10. The client and family use knowledge about the disorder, treatment program, medications, and symptoms to manage the disorder on an ongoing basis.

Study questions

1. Using cognitive-behavioral therapy, which treatment would be appropriate for a client with depression?
   1. Challenging negative thinking
   2. Encouraging analysis of dreams
   3. Prescribing antidepressant medications
   4. Using ultraviolet light therapy

2. While assessing a client diagnosed with bipolar disorder, the nurse would expect to find a history of:
   1. a depressive episode followed by prolonged sadness.
   2. a series of depressive episodes that reoccur periodically.
   3. symptoms of mania that may or may not be followed by depression.
   4. symptoms of mania that include delusional thoughts.

3. A client completing requirements for student teaching reports to the nurse an incident in which a student was rude and disrespectful. The client states, "None of the students respects my teaching ability." The nurse identifies this as an example of which common negative cognition?
   1. Labeling
   2. Fortune telling
   3. Overgeneralization
   4. "Should" statement

4. Which of the following behaviors in a client with a diagnosis of bipolar disorder, single manic episode, would the nurse expect to assess?
   1. Apathy, poor insight, and poverty of ideas
   2. Anxiety, somatic complaints, and insomnia
   3. Elation, hyperactivity, and impaired judgment
   4. Social isolation, delusional thinking, and clang associations

5. A manic client is creating considerable chaos in a day-treatment program, behaving in a dominating and manipulative way. Which nursing intervention is most appropriate?
   1. Allow the peer group to intervene.
   2. Describe acceptable behavior and set realistic limits with the client.
   3. Recommend that the client be hospitalized for treatment.
   4. Tell the client that his behavior is inappropriate.

6. According to the biogenic amine theory, an individual with depression has a deficiency in which neurotransmitters?
   1. Dopamine and thyroxin
   2. GABA and acetylcholine
   3. Cortisone and epinephrine
   4. Serotonin and norepinephrine

7. The nurse is teaching a client and her family about the causes of depression. Which of the following causative factors should the nurse emphasize as the most significant?
   1. Brain structure abnormalities
   2. Chemical imbalance in the brain
   3. Social environment
   4. Recessive gene transmission

8. When evaluating for imminent suicide risk, which information given by the client would be most significant?
   1. At least a 2-year history of feeling depressed more days than not
   2. Divorced from spouse 6 months ago
   3. Feeling loss of energy and appetite
   4. Reference to suicide as best solution to identified problems

9. A client in an acute psychiatric hospital unit tells a nurse about his plans for suicide. The nurse's priority is to:
   1. allow the client time alone for reflection.
   2. encourage the client to use problem solving.
   3. follow agency protocol for suicide precautions.
   4. stimulate the client's interest in activities.

10. Which mood disorder is characterized by the client feeling depressed most of the day for a 2-year period?
    1. Cyclothymia
    2. Dysthymia
    3. Melancholic depressive disorder
    4. Seasonal affective disorder

11. The community nurse is speaking to a group of new mothers as part of a primary prevention program. Which self-care measures would be most helpful as a strategy to decrease the occurrence of mood disorders?
    1. Keeping busy, so as not to confront problem areas
    2. Medication with antidepressants
    3. Use of crisis intervention services
    4. Verbalizing rather than internalizing feelings

12. The husband of a client who has recently lost her job tells the clinic nurse that the client's moods are constantly changing from extremely happy and elated to sadness and crying. As part of an immediate assessment of the family situation, the nurse should question the husband and wife about which of the following?
    1. The client's academic and work history
    2. The specific history of psychopathology in the client's family
    3. The client's specific symptoms, duration of the symptoms, and the impact of the symptoms on the family
    4. The quality of the couple's marital relationship

13. During a daily community meeting, a client with bipolar disorder, manic type, begins pacing around the room and speaking rapidly in a loud voice. Which nursing intervention is most appropriate?
1. Ask the client to accompany the nurse and move to a quieter room.
2. Allow the community group to handle the client's behavior.
3. End the community meeting at this time.
4. Offer the client an antianxiety medication.

14. The nurse teaches the family of a client with major depression disorder. Which of the following information should be included in the teaching? Select all that apply.
1. Depression is characterized by sadness, feelings of hopelessness, and decreased self-worth.
2. It is common for a pressed individual to have thoughts of suicide.
3. Attempts to cheer up a person with depression are often helpful.
4. Talk therapy, along with antidepressant medications, is usually the treatment.
5. Someone with depression may be preoccupied with spending money and too busy to sleep.
6. Encourage a person with depression to keep a regular routine of activity and rest.

Answer key

1. The answer is 1.
Cognitive-behavioral therapy includes identifying and challenging a client's negative cognitions. The belief is that these negative thoughts influence the feelings and behaviors in depression. Dream analysis would be used in psychoanalytic psychotherapy. Antidepressant medication could be part of a treatment program for an individual with depression; however, this would not be considered cognitive-behavioral therapy. Ultraviolet light therapy would be a somatic approach to treatment for seasonal affective disorder.

2. The answer is 3.
The definition of bipolar disorder is a mood disturbance in which the symptoms of mania have occurred at least one time. Depression may or may not occur as a separate episode in bipolar disorder. None of the other options indicate a correct understanding of bipolar disorder.

3. The answer is 3.
The client in this situation is overgeneralizing the response of one particular student, inferring that the entire class has this attitude and blowing the incident out of proportion. Labeling is the application of negative labels to oneself or others. Fortune telling is the conviction that things will not turn out right, despite evidence to the contrary. "Should" statements refer to statements establishing standards for self and others.

4. The answer is 3.
A client with bipolar disorder, manic episode, would demonstrate flight of ideas and hyperactivity as part of the increased psychomotor activity. The mood is one of elation and the feeling is that one is invincible; therefore, judgment may be quite impaired. The symptoms in option 1 would be more characteristic of an individual with long-term schizophrenia. The symptoms in option 2 would be more

characteristic of someone with an anxiety disorder, although a manic individual may also not sleep because of excessive energy. The symptoms in option 4 are more characteristic of schizophrenia.

5. The answer is 2.

In this situation, it would be appropriate for the nurse to suggest alternative behaviors in place of unacceptable ones to help the client gain self-control. The peer group is not responsible for monitoring the client's behavior. The client's behavior does not warrant hospitalization. Option 4 is inappropriate because the client is told only what is unacceptable and is not given any alternatives.

6. The answer is 4.

The biogenic amine theory of depression describes deficiencies in the neurotransmitters serotonin and norepinephrine. Antidepressant medications increase the levels of these neurotransmitters and therefore help to relieve depressive symptoms. According to current research, dopamine, thyroxin, GABA, acetylcholine, cortisone, and epinephrine are not directly related to depression.

7. The answer is 2.

Chemical imbalance of neurotransmitters in the brain is the most significant factor in depression. However, the exact cause has not been established, so other factors may also be involved. Although genetic transmission certainly may be a factor, no definite pattern of transmission has been identified. A person's social environment, including lack of support systems, may also increase the risk of depression.

8. The answer is 4.

An individual who talks about suicide as a solution to problems is at high risk. This client's suicidal threats need to be taken seriously because he does not see any other viable solutions to problems in living. All of the factors included in the other options would increase the client's risk for depression; however, actual statements about suicidal intent are red flags indicating imminent danger.

9. The answer is 3.

The nurse must act to safeguard the client from danger, including self-harm. Implementing the specific agency protocol for suicidal precautions would best protect the client. A client with suicidal intent should not be left alone. One-to-one observations are generally part of suicide precautions. Encouraging the client to use problem solving and stimulating his interest in activities would be helpful for someone with depression; however, the nurse's priority is to protect the client by initiating suicide precautions.

10. The answer is 2.

Dysthymia is characterized by at least a 2-year history of depression, occurring most of the day for more days than not. Cyclothymia is characterized by at least 2 years of several periods of hypomanic symptoms. Melancholic depressive disorder is characterized by either anhedonia in relation to all activities or lack of mood reactivity to usually pleasurable stimuli. Seasonal affective disorder is characterized by depressed feelings in fall and winter, associated with loss of sunlight.

11. The answer is 4.

Individuals who develop mood disorders often have difficulty expressing feelings, especially feelings of anger toward significant others. Internalizing those feelings can contribute to loss of self-esteem and guilt, and therefore negative cognitions and depression. Ignoring problems is not a helpful strategy. Recognizing problems and using problem-solving methods will contribute to mental health. Antidepressants are certainly necessary in the treatment of the mood disorder of depression; however, they are not used in primary prevention. Crisis intervention would be a useful strategy in handling the immediate needs of someone experiencing a crisis; it is not a tool of primary prevention.

12. The answer is 3.

Assessment of the current family situation would include identifying the client's symptoms, duration of symptoms, and the unique impact on this particular family. The assessment data related to options 1 and 2 would be important, but the immediate assessment would be more specific to the current family crisis. The quality of the marital relationship would be one aspect of the entire family situation.

13. The answer is 1.

The most appropriate intervention when a client's mania begins to escalate is to remove him from an overstimulating environment (the community meeting) and lead him to a quieter setting, thereby help-ing him regain self-control. This is the least restrictive intervention and should be offered prior to the use of antianxiety medication (a form of chemical restraint). In this situation, the community group may be intimidated by the client's behavior and reluctant to intervene; also the nurse is responsible for limit setting and intervention when client behavior is inappropriate. The community meeting is an important forum for client participation and should not be terminated because one client is upset.

14. The answer is 1, 2, 4, 6.

These statements about major depressive disorders provide correct information and will be helpful to the client's family. Option 3 is incorrect; it is better to acknowledge the client's sad mood and offer reassurance that his mood will improve. Option 5 is more characteristic of someone in a manic phase of bipolar disorder.

7 Schizophrenic Disorders

I. OVERVIEW OF SCHIZOPHRENIC DISORDERS

A. Key concepts

1. **Schizophrenic disorders** encompass a group of psychotic reactions that affect multiple areas of an individual's functioning, including thinking and communicating, perceiving and interpreting reality, feeling and demonstrating emotion, and behaving in a socially acceptable manner.

2. According to the criteria identified in *DSM-IV TR*, the disturbance lasts for at least 6 months and includes at least 1 month of active-phase symptoms involving two or more of the following:

   a. Delusions

   b. Hallucinations

   c. Disorganized speech

   d. Grossly disorganized or catatonic behavior

   e. Negative symptoms (affective flattening, alogia, or avolition).

3. Other definitive criteria must also be met.

   a. Social and occupational dysfunction are present.

   b. Schizoaffective disorders and mood disorder with psychotic features have been ruled out.

   c. The disturbance is not caused by the physiologic effect of a substance or a general medical condition.

4. The nodal age at onset for men is between 18 and 25; for women, between 25 and mid-30s.

5. The course of schizophrenia is variable and remissions may occur; some clients recover completely, whereas others have a chronic, unremitting disorder.

B. Common symptoms of schizophrenia

1. Symptoms of schizophrenia can be classified as positive or negative; most clients with this disorder have a mixture of both types of symptoms. (See *Table 7-1, Common symptoms of schizophrenia*.)

TABLE 7-1
Common symptoms of schizophrenia

Thinking and communicating	Perceiving and interpreting	Behaving and interacting
■ Loose associations	■ Delusions	■ Relationship withdrawal*
■ Alogia*	■ Hallucinations	■ Motor hyperactivity or hypoactivity
■ Concrete thinking	■ Illusions	
■ Lack of insight	■ Depersonalization	■ Ambivalence
	■ Attending to irrelevant stimuli	■ Anhedonia*
Feeling and affect	■ Poor reality testing	■ Avolition*
■ Flat*		■ Poor personal hygiene
■ Blunted		
■ Inappropriate		

*Indicates negative symptoms.

[handwritten annotations:]

alogia: lack of pleasure or The capacity to experience it. not simple disinterest

avolition: lack of desire, drive or motivation to pursue meaningful goals.

flat affect: lack of emotional reactivity

anhedonia: lack of pleasure

alogia: The inability to speak because of mental deficiency, mental confusion or aphasia.

DISPLAY 7-1
Common delusions in schizophrenia

- **Delusions of reference:** Everything occurring in environment has direct significance to oneself
- **Delusions of persecution:** People or institutions are plotting against or attacking oneself
- **Delusions of external influences:** One is controlled by others or outside forces

- **Somatic delusions:** Appearance or functioning of one's body is altered
- **Grandiose delusions:** Inflated self-worth, power, knowledge, or identity

   a. **Positive symptoms** include hallucinations, delusions, loose associations, and bizarre or disorganized behavior.
   b. **Negative symptoms** include restricted emotion (flat affect), anhedonia, avolition, alogia, and social withdrawal.
  2. Common symptoms include the following:
   a. **Delusions** are fixed false beliefs that cannot be discounted by use of logic. (See *Display 7-1, Common delusions in schizophrenia*.)
   b. **Loose associations** refer to the lack of logical relationships between thoughts and ideas, which may be reflected in a variety of symptoms. (See *Table 7-2, Symptoms of loose associations*.)
   c. **Hallucinations** are false sensory perceptions involving any of the five senses; in schizophrenia, auditory hallucinations are most common.
   d. **Illusions** are misinterpretations of environmental stimuli.
   e. **Depersonalization-derealization** is a feeling that the "self" has been fundamentally changed or altered.
   f. **Affective flattening** refers to the absence of emotional response; affect can also be described as *blunted* (dulled response) or *inappropriate* (opposite of what is expected in a situation).
   g. **Ambivalence** is the presence of conflicting or opposite emotions leading to difficulty making a choice or a decision.
   h. **Avolition** is the lack of motivation to persist in goal-directed activity.
   i. **Alogia** refers to a decreased speech pattern or poverty of speech.
   j. **Echopraxia** is the senseless copying of another's actions.
   k. **Anhedonia** is the lack of pleasure in activities and things that the individual would normally perceive as pleasurable or enjoyable.
   l. **Concrete thinking** is the literal interpretation of another's communication, reflecting a problem with abstract thought; it may be tested by asking the client to interpret a common proverb.

C. Types of schizophrenia
  1. **Paranoid schizophrenia** is characterized by systematized delusions or auditory hallucinations; the individual may be suspicious, argumentative, hostile, and aggressive.
   a. The individual's behavior is less regressive with this type, and he is not as socially impaired.
   b. Prognosis is better than that of other types.

TABLE 7-2
Symptoms of loose associations

Symptom	Description
Neologism	Making up new words (such as *"potlomp"* or *"lemopty"*)
Word salad	Words in a sentence that may seem connected but do not compose coherent thought (such as *"The blue isn't silly eating upwards time."*)
Illogical or paralogical thinking	Syllogistic thinking that defies logic (such as *"Blessed Mary is a virgin. I am a virgin. Therefore, I am Blessed Mary."*)
Echolalia	Senseless repetition of the words of another person
Echopraxia	Senseless copying of another person's behavior or actions
Clang association	Words that rhyme are put together for their sound association, without coherent thought (such as *"sky and pie"* or *"my and dye"*)

   2. **Disorganized schizophrenia** involves disorganized speech and behaviors as well as flat or inappropriate affect; associative disturbances are common.
       a. The individual may have odd mannerisms, exhibit extreme social withdrawal, or neglect hygiene and appearance.
       b. Onset usually occurs before age 25, and the course may be chronic.
       c. The individual demonstrates regressive behavior, with poor social interaction and poor reality contact.
   3. **Catatonic schizophrenia** is characterized by marked psychomotor disturbances, which may involve immobility or excessive activity.
       a. An individual with **catatonic stupor** may exhibit inactivity, negativism, and waxy flexibility (abnormal posturing).
       b. **Catatonic excitement** involves extreme agitation and may be accompanied by echolalia and echopraxia.
   4. In **undifferentiated schizophrenia,** the essential features are delusions, hallucinations, incoherent speech, and disorganized behaviors; this classification is used when criteria for other types are not met.
   5. **Residual schizophrenia** is identified by the current absence of acute symptoms, but a history of past episodes; negative symptoms (marked social isolation, withdrawal, and impaired role functioning) may be present.

II. IMPACT OF DISEASE

A. Key concepts
   1. Although a small percentage of the population has schizophrenia, the disease has enormous implications for the individual, family, and society.

      a. About 1% of the population will experience schizophrenia in their lifetime; for many schizophrenics, the disease is lifelong.

      b. More than 50% of people with schizophrenia have substance problems, which may represent an attempt to self-medicate the distressing symptoms.

      c. An estimated 33% to 50% of homeless people in the United States suffer from schizophrenia.

      d. Schizophrenic clients occupy 25% of inpatient hospital beds.

  2. Individuals with schizophrenia have a shorter life expectancy than the general population; unhealthy behaviors and lifestyles, including obesity, smoking, and substance abuse, may contribute to this.

B. Perception of reality and communicative patterns

  1. The psychotic thinking and communicative patterns in clients with a schizophrenic disorder indicate severe impairment in perception of reality or a disturbance in ego function.

  2. Individuals affected may not perceive any abnormality and may have difficulty developing any insight into problems; an individual who has insight would question his perceptions of reality, acknowledge the illness, and understand the necessity for medications and the periodic assistance of others.

  3. Affected individuals have a poor sense of identity and lowered self-esteem.

  4. Affected individuals may also have difficulty filtering out extraneous environmental stimuli, resulting in an inability to focus on tasks and conversations.

C. Interpersonal and family relationships

  1. Schizophrenics generally withdraw from interactions **(ego protection)**.

  2. They have a fear of interactions (reflects a poor sense of identity).

  3. They suffer from a basic feeling of rejection and lack of trust.

  4. Family members of individuals with schizophrenia are also severely affected by this disorder, and living with a person who suffers from schizophrenia can be very difficult; these families experience stress and are required to cope with a variety of problems.

  5. The National Alliance for the Mentally Ill (NAMI) provides support for the family and advocacy for the severely mentally ill.

III. CAUSES OF SCHIZOPHRENIA

A. Key concepts

  1. Although the exact cause of schizophrenia remains unclear, the current consensus is that these disorders result from complex interactions among a variety of factors.

  2. Factors that have been studied and implicated include genetic predisposition, neurodevelopmental abnormalities, brain structural abnormalities, neurochemical imbalances, and psychosocial and environmental processes.

B. Genetic predisposition

  1. Although genetics provide a significant risk factor, a single genetic marker has not been identified; it is likely that multiple genes may be involved.

2. Research shows that combinations of genes can result in an individual inheriting schizophrenia even if there is no direct family history.
3. Risk of developing schizophrenia with a family history is as follows:
    a. One affected parent: 12% to 15% risk
    b. Both parents affected: 35% to 39% risk
    c. Sibling affected: 8% to 10% risk
    d. Dizygotic twin affected: 15% risk
    e. Monozygotic twin affected: 50% risk.

C. Neurodevelopmental abnormalities

1. Research indicates that the development of minor fetal malformations during early gestation may play a role in later manifestation of schizophrenia.
2. Factors that can affect neurodevelopment and that may increase the risk of disease include:
    a. Influenza infection (maternal) during the second trimester
    b. Trauma or injury at birth
    c. Abuse or trauma during infancy or early childhood.

D. Brain structural abnormalities and chemical imbalances

1. In some subgroups of schizophrenic clients, brain imaging techniques (computed tomography, magnetic resonance imaging, positron emission tomography) have shown abnormalities in the structure of the brain, including:
    a. Enlarged ventricles
    b. Decreased cortical blood flow, especially in prefrontal cortex
    c. Decreased metabolic activity in certain brain areas
    d. Cerebral atrophy.
2. Early research focused on the **dopamine hypothesis,** which stated that excessive dopamine activity in cortical areas of the brain was related to the positive symptoms of schizophrenia.
3. Current research indicates the importance of other neurotransmitters, including serotonin, norepinephrine, glutamate, and GABA.
4. Homeostasis, or the relationship between neurotransmitters, may be more important than relative amounts of specific neurotransmitters.
5. Receptor sites for specific neurotransmitters are also important.
    a. Changes in the numbers and types of receptors can affect the level of neurotransmitters.
    b. Psychotropic medications can affect neurotransmitter receptor sites as well as the neurotransmitters.

E. Psychosocial and environmental factors

1. Developmental theorists, such as Freud, Sullivan, and Erikson, proposed that the lack of warm, nurturing attention in the earliest years of life contributes to the lack of self-identity, reality misinterpretation, and relationship withdrawal in the individual with schizophrenia.
2. The role of the family in the development of schizophrenia has not been validated by research; however, one area of family functioning that has been implicated in increased relapse rates of individuals with schizophrenia is **high expressed emo-**

tion (HEE); families with this characteristic are described as emotionally over-involved, hostile, and critical.

3. Consistently, research indicates a strong association between schizophrenia and low socioeconomic status.

4. An interactive **stress-vulnerability model** suggests that those with schizophrenia have a genetic, biologically based vulnerability for schizophrenia; this vulnerability, when accompanied by exposure to life stressors, can produce symptoms in the individual.

IV. MANAGING SCHIZOPHRENIA

A. Key concepts

1. Continuity of care is important; clients may receive treatment in various settings, including acute psychiatric hospitals, long-term psychiatric hospitals, and community-based programs.

2. Level of care depends on the severity of symptoms as well as availability of family and social supports; treatment is generally provided in the least restrictive setting possible.

3. A **case management** approach is important because client care is generally long-term, requiring collaboration with multiple care providers to ensure services are provided in a coordinated manner.

4. **Assertive Community Treatment (ACT),** a model of a team treatment approach that is particularly effective for persons with serious mental illness, focuses on comprehensive rehabilitation and social support.

B. Short-term psychiatric hospitalization

1. Brief hospitalization on a psychiatric unit is used to manage acute symptoms and to provide a safe, structured environment.

2. Various treatments include:
   a. Administration of antipsychotic medications (See *Drug chart 7-1, Selected antipsychotic medications for treating schizophrenia.*)
   b. Milieu management
   c. Supportive therapy, which is generally reality-oriented, with use of a cognitive-behavioral approach
   d. Psychoeducation for the client and family
   e. Discharge planning to ensure continuity of care.

C. Long-term psychiatric hospitalization

1. Long-term hospitalization is used for clients with persistent symptoms who may pose a danger to themselves or others.

2. The goal is to stabilize and transfer the client as soon as possible to a less restrictive setting.

D. Community-based treatment

1. The goal of community-based treatment is to provide comprehensive client and family services.

⊘ DRUG CHART 7-1
Selected antipsychotic medications for treating schizophrenia

Classification	Drug	Rationale for use
Typical antipsychotics	chlorpromazine (Thorazine) fluphenazine (Prolixin) haloperidol (Haldol) molindone (Moban) thioridazine (Mellaril) thiothixene (Navane) trifluoperazine (Stelazine)	Act by blocking selected dopamine receptors in both striatal and limbic areas of brain. Also affect other receptors, including those for histamine, acetylcholine, and serotonin. Provide antipsychotic effect, decreasing positive symptoms of schizophrenia.
Atypical antipsychotics	clozapine (Clozaril) olanzapine (Zyprexa) quetiapine (Seroquel) risperidone (Risperdal) sertindole (Serlect) ziprasidone (Geodon)	Produce selective dopamine and serotonin receptor blocking in limbic system. Provide antipsychotic effect (positive symptoms) and decrease negative symptoms. Produce fewer side effects than typical antipsychotics.
Dopamine-system stabilizers	aripiprazole (Abilify)	Thought to balance dopamine systems. Acts as either dopamine agonist or antagonist in different areas of the brain. Good side effect profile.

2. **Supportive housing** includes transitional-living halfway houses, cooperative living arrangements, crisis community residences, foster care, and board-and-care homes.
3. **Day-treatment programs** offer group therapy, social skills training, medication management, and socialization and recreation.
4. **Supportive therapy** involves the services of a case manager and therapists for the client and family.
5. **Psychoeducational programs** exist for the client, family, and community groups.
6. **Outreach services** provide case-finding and preventive treatment programs for individuals and families at increased risk.

E. Psychosocial rehabilitation
1. Psychosocial rehabilitation emphasizes development of skills and supports necessary for successful living, learning, and working in the community.
2. Clubhouse programs, modeled after the Fountain House Clubhouse in New York City, can be part of a comprehensive treatment program.
   a. Clubhouses operate on a partnership model, empowering members with day-to-day operation and decision-making.
   b. Clients gather to work together, socialize, and learn job skills.

V. CARE OF THE CLIENT WITH A SCHIZOPHRENIC DISORDER

A. Assessment

1. Review the client's history for precipitating stressors and significant data, including the following information:
   a. Genetic-biologic vulnerability (family history)
   b. Stressful life events
   c. Results of mental status examination
   d. Past psychiatric history and treatment compliance
   e. Medication history
   f. Drug and alcohol use
   g. Education and employment history.

2. Assess the client for characteristic symptoms of schizophrenia. (See *Table 7-1, Common symptoms of schizophrenia*, page 121, and *Key questions 7-1, Assessing clients with schizophrenia.*)

3. Assess family and community support systems, including:
   a. Current living arrangements and degree of supervision
   b. Family involvement and support
   c. Case management or therapy
   d. Participation in community treatment programs.

4. Assess the client's and family's understanding of the client's specific schizophrenic disorder, medications and treatment recommendations, relapse signs, and stress-reducing measures. (See *Client and family teaching 7-1, Guidelines for clients with schizophrenia*, page 130.)

5. Assess the client for side effects of antipsychotic medications, including:
   a. Extrapyramidal effects (use specific tools, such as the AIMS scale or Simpson neurologic scale, to make assessment)
   b. Anticholinergic effects
   c. Cardiovascular and other effects (See *Table 15-1, Managing common side effects of psychotropic drugs*, page 262.)

B. Nursing diagnoses

1. Determine the client's positive and negative symptoms.
2. Analyze the client's strengths and weaknesses, including:
   a. Self-care ability
   b. Socialization
   c. Communication
   d. Reality testing
   e. Job skills
   f. Support systems.
3. Analyze the client's risk factors for acting-out behavior, including:
   a. Agitation
   b. Anger

Q KEY QUESTIONS 7-1
Assessing clients with schizophrenia

Questions	Information gathered
Do you believe you have an illness? What is your explanation of your illness?	Reality perception and level of insight
Have you been in treatment before? What was helpful for you at that time?	Past history
What do you think are your strengths? What do you think are your problem areas?	Level of self-esteem; identification of stressful life events; knowledge base regarding illness
Do you hear voices that others do not hear or see things that others do not see? Do you believe that someone or some group is plotting against you or trying to harm you?	Presence of hallucinations or delusions
What medications do you take? Do you have any problems with your medications?	Compliance with medication regimen; knowledge of, and problems with, medications
Who do you consider a support person in your life?	Level of supportive relationships
What are your activities during a typical day? What activities and events do you enjoy?	Cognitive and communicative ability; presence of anhedonia; self-care ability

      c. Suspiciousness

      d. Presence of threatening hallucinations.

    4. Establish and prioritize individualized nursing diagnoses for the client and his family; appropriate diagnoses may include:

      a. Altered role performance

      b. Chronic low self-esteem

      c. Deficient knowledge (specify)

      d. Disturbed sensory perception (Specify: visual, auditory, kinesthetic, gustatory, tactile, olfactory)

      e. Disturbed thought processes

      f. Impaired home maintenance

      g. Ineffective coping

      h. Ineffective family therapeutic regimen management

      i. Ineffective therapeutic regimen management

      j. Interrupted family processes

CLIENT AND FAMILY TEACHING 7-1
Guidelines for clients with schizophrenia

Provide information about the client's specific schizophrenic disorder:
- Schizophrenia is a brain disorder that affects all aspects of functioning.
- No single cause has been found, but research indicates genetics, changes in brain structure and chemicals, and stress-related factors are involved.
- Symptoms can include hearing voices (hallucinations), beliefs that are false (delusions), communicating in ways that are difficult to understand, and poor occupational and social functioning.
- Symptoms may improve and can also recur throughout life.
- The client will need to take antipsychotic medication as prescribed. Many medications have side effects that can be managed if reported promptly to the health care provider.
- Follow-up treatment with a case manager or therapist is vital.

Provide information about how the family can be helpful:
- Identify events that are typically upsetting to the client, and provide extra support as needed.

- Note when the client is becoming upset, and encourage measures to reduce anxiety (time outs, relaxation techniques, balanced rest and activity, and proper diet).
- Note which symptoms the client exhibits when ill. When these recur, encourage the client to contact his health provider (if he becomes resistant, contact the health provider on your own).
- Do not support (agree with) hallucinations or delusions. Point out reality, but do not argue with the client.
- Encourage the client to take medications, as prescribed.
- Be aware that side effects are common, but are manageable. Side effects should be reported promptly to the health care provider.
- Encourage the client to follow up with all treatments and appointments.
- Dealing with a schizophrenic individual can be very difficult. Remember to look after your own needs and to share your feelings and concerns with the health care provider.
- Consider joining a community support group, such as the National Alliance for the Mentally Ill.

---

  k. Noncompliance

  l. Risk for directed or other-directed violence

  m. Self-care deficit (specify).

C. Planning and outcome identification

  1. Work with the client in setting realistic goals; initially, goals may be limited, depending on the client's degree of impairment.

  2. Establish desired outcome criteria for a client with schizophrenia.

   a. The client will demonstrate decreased anxiety level.

   b. The client will interact on one-to-one basis with the nurse or treatment team member.

   c. The client will maintain personal hygiene and activities of daily living.

   d. The client will decrease or refrain from behaviors that are considered bizarre or inappropriate.

   e. The client will differentiate between thoughts and feelings that are self-generated and those that are from the external environment.

   f. The client will increase appropriate social interaction.

   g. The client will identify positive "self" statements.

   h. The client will cooperate with the established treatment plan and agree to follow up with community care recommendations.

      i. The client will verbalize knowledge about the disorder, treatment plans, medications, relapse signs, and stress management techniques.

      j. The client will perform role functions in an appropriate manner.

  3. Establish desired outcome criteria for the client's family as well.

      a. The family will express feelings about individual concerns.

      b. The family will verbalize knowledge about the client's disorder, treatment plans, medications, relapse signs, handling crises, and symptom management.

D. Implementation

  1. For a **withdrawn and isolated client,** take the following measures:

      a. Establish a therapeutic relationship with the client.

      b. Initiate planned, short, frequent, and undemanding interactions.

      c. Plan simple one-on-one activities.

      d. Maintain consistency and honesty in interactions.

      e. Gradually encourage the client to interact with peers in nonthreatening situations.

      f. Provide social skills training.

      g. Use measures to enhance self-esteem.

  2. For **the client exhibiting regressive or unusual behaviors,** take the following measures:

      a. Assume a matter-of-fact approach to bizarre behaviors (do not reinforce these behaviors).

      b. Treat the client as an adult, despite regression.

      c. Monitor the client's eating patterns; encourage and assist when necessary.

      d. Assist with hygiene and grooming, performing these tasks only when the client is unable to.

      e. Be cautious with touch because it may be perceived as threatening.

      f. Establish a routine schedule of activities of daily living.

      g. Give simple choices of two items for the ambivalent client.

  3. For **the client with unclear communication patterns,** take the following measures:

      a. Communicate in a clear, unambiguous manner.

      b. Ensure that communication is verbally and nonverbally congruent.

      c. Clarify any ambiguous or unclear meanings related to the client's communication. (See *Display 7-2, Clarifying communication,* page 132.)

      d. Use appropriate therapeutic communication techniques. (See pages 8 and 9.)

  4. For a **highly suspicious and hostile client,** take the following measures:

      a. Establish a professional relationship; overfriendliness may be perceived as threatening to the client.

      b. Be cautious with touch because it may be perceived as threatening.

      c. Allow the client as much control and autonomy as possible within the limits of the therapeutic setting.

      d. Work on establishing trust through short interactions that communicate interest and respect.

      e. Explain any treatments, medications, and laboratory tests before initiating them.

DISPLAY 7-2
Clarifying communication

Schizophrenic clients often have difficulty communicating because of disorganized speech and cognitive problems, as illustrated below:

Client: "The skirts in the sky are flying high and I'm not going with them."
Nurse: "You are trying to tell me something, but I don't understand what it is. Can you tell me in a different way?"
Client (pointing to a nurse walking briskly down the hall): "They are all in a hurry..."

Nurse: "You're telling me that the nurses are very busy and that you feel left out?"
Client: "Yes, I need help with my bath."

Interpretation
In this example, the client is using highly symbolic language to try to communicate. The nurse indicates that she does not understand what is being said. When the client tries again, the nurse thinks she understands and repeats, directly to the client, the message she thinks the client is trying to communicate. The client then confirms the message.

    f. Avoid focusing on or reinforcing suspicious thoughts or delusions.

    g. Identify and respond to emotional needs underlying suspicious thoughts or delusions. (See *Display 7-3, Responding to suspicious thoughts or delusions.*)

    h. Intervene when the client shows signs of increased anxiety and of potential acting-out behavior.

    i. Be careful not to behave in a manner that can be misinterpreted by the client.

5. For the **client with hallucinations or delusions,** take the following measures:

    a. Do not focus attention on the client's hallucinations or delusions; interrupt the hallucinatory experience by initiating one-to-one interaction that is reality-based.

    b. Point out that you do not share the client's perception ("I do not hear the voices you say you hear."), but validate that you believe the hallucination is real to the client.

    c. Avoid arguing with the client about hallucinations or delusions.

    d. Respond to the client's feelings communicated during hallucinatory or delusional experiences ("You seem frightened.").

    e. Redirect and focus the client on a structured activity or reality-based task.

    f. Move the client to a more quiet, less stimulating environment.

    g. Wait until the client's hallucinations or delusions stop before initiating a teaching session about them.
   - Explain that hallucinations or delusions are symptoms of psychiatric disorders.
   - Point out that anxiety or increased stimuli from the environment may stimulate hallucinations.

    h. Help the client control hallucinations by focusing on reality and by taking prescribed medications.

    i. If hallucinations persist, help the client learn to ignore them and to act in an appropriate manner despite the hallucinations.

    j. Teach cognitive strategies and tell the client to use **self-talk** ("The voices are not reasonable") and **thought stopping** ("I won't think about this").

DISPLAY 7-3
Responding to suspicious thoughts or delusions

When responding to a schizophrenic client who is suspicious or expresses a delusion, present reality in a nonconfrontational manner and listen closely for clues to his underlying needs.

Client (furtively standing by the nurse's station, looking at the tape recorder on the desk): "That tape recorder is used to record my thoughts. People here are against me."
Nurse: "It doesn't seem to me that this is so. The night nurse uses this tape recorder to make the evening report. I believe that you are safe here."
Client: "I don't feel safe here. Can I stay by the desk while you are here?"

Nurse: "Yes. I'll be here for 5 more minutes, until the lunch trays come. Here's a newspaper for you to read."
Client: "I'll stay here and read the paper."

Interpretation
In this example, the client misinterprets the environment by drawing an unwarranted conclusion about the tape recorder kept at the nurses' station. The nurse responds by presenting reality to the patient in a matter-of-fact manner. Similarly, the nurse responds to the underlying meaning of the client's communication by saying that the client is safe and can remain close by. Then, the nurse refocuses the client on another environmental object, the newspaper.

6. For **the client with agitated behavior and potential for violence,** take the following measures:
   a. Observe behavior for early cues of agitation; intervene before the client begins acting out.
   b. Provide a safe, quiet environment; decrease stimuli when the client becomes agitated.
   c. Avoid retaliating when the client is verbally hostile; use a quiet, calm tone of voice, provide personal space, and avoid physical contact.
   d. Encourage the client to talk about, rather than act out, feelings.
   e. Offer medications, as needed (p.r.n.), to the agitated client.
   f. Isolate the client from general milieu if agitation increases.
   g. Set limits on unacceptable behavior, and consistently follow institutional protocol for intervention.
   h. Follow institutional protocol for responding to the client exhibiting acting-out behavior.
   i. Ensure that an adequate number of experienced staff members is available when attempting to subdue a violent client; follow institutional (and legal/ethical) guidelines if seclusion and restraint become necessary (these measures are used only as a last resort when least restrictive measures are ineffective).
7. For the **family of the client with a schizophrenic disorder,** take the following measures:
   a. Encourage family members to discuss their feelings and needs.
   b. Help the family to define basic rules about respecting each other's privacy and living together.
   c. Encourage interaction for each family member with a wider social environment.
   d. Encourage family members to become involved in support groups.

    e. Assist members to identify anxiety-producing situations and to plan specific coping strategies.

    f. Teach the family about schizophrenia and its management. (See *Client and family teaching 7-1, Guidelines for clients with schizophrenia,* page 130.)

E. Outcome evaluation

1. The client identifies internal feelings of anxiety and uses learned coping measures to decrease anxiety.
2. The client independently maintains personal hygiene.
3. The client follows a routine schedule for activities of daily living.
4. The client demonstrates appropriate behavior in social situations.
5. The client communicates without evidence of loose, dissociated thinking.
6. The client differentiates between thoughts and feelings that are stimulated from within himself and those that are stimulated from the external environment.
7. The client exhibits decreased or controlled magical thinking, delusions, hallucinations, and illusions.
8. The client demonstrates improved social interaction with others.
9. The client displays affect that is appropriate to a given feeling, thought, or situation.
10. The client exhibits decreased suspiciousness, negativity, and anger.
11. The client identifies positive aspects of self.
12. The client participates in the treatment plan and agrees to follow up in community treatment.
13. The client and family demonstrate their understanding of the client's disorder, treatment program, medications, symptoms, and crisis management on an ongoing basis.
14. Family members use effective coping strategies to handle anxiety-producing situations.

Study questions

1. Which behaviors would the nurse most likely assess in a client with a diagnosis of disorganized schizophrenia?
   1. Absence of acute symptoms, impaired role function
   2. Extreme social withdrawal, odd mannerisms and behaviors
   3. Psychomotor immobility, presence of waxy flexibility
   4. Suspiciousness toward others, increased hostility

2. In planning care for a client with schizophrenia who has negative symptoms, the nurse would anticipate a problem with:
   1. auditory hallucinations.
   2. bizarre behaviors.
   3. ideas of reference.
   4. motivation for activities.

3. The family of a schizophrenic client asks the nurse if there is a genetic cause of

this disorder. To answer the family, which fact would the nurse cite?

1. Conclusive evidence indicates a specific gene transmits the disorder.
2. Incidence of this disorder is variable in all families.
3. There is little evidence that genes play a role in transmission.
4. Genetic factors can increase the vulnerability for this disorder.

4. Which of the following nursing interventions would be most appropriate for a client with schizophrenia, paranoid type?

1. Establishing a nondemanding relationship
2. Encouraging involvement in group activities
3. Spending more time with the client
4. Waiting until the client initiates interaction

5. A client tells the nurse that psychotropic medicines are dangerous and refuses to take them. Which intervention should the nurse use first?

1. Ask the client about any previous problems with psychotropic medications.
2. Ask the client if an injection is preferable.
3. Insist that the client take medication as prescribed.
4. Withhold the medication until the client is less suspicious.

6. Upon a client's admission for acute psychiatric hospitalization, the nurse documents the following: *Client refuses to bathe or dress, remains in room most of the day, speaks infrequently to peers or staff.* Which nursing diagnosis would be the priority at this time?

1. *Anxiety*
2. *Decisional conflict*
3. *Self-care deficit*
4. *Social isolation*

7. Which statement is correct about a 25-year-old client with newly diagnosed schizophrenia?

1. Age of onset is typical for schizophrenia.
2. Age of onset is later than usual for schizophrenia.
3. Age of onset is earlier than usual for schizophrenia.
4. Age of onset follows no predictable pattern in schizophrenia.

8. Which factor is associated with increased risk for schizophrenia?

1. Alcoholism
2. Adolescent pregnancy
3. Overcrowded schools
4. Poverty

9. An appropriate nursing strategy for dealing with a schizophrenic client's withdrawal would be:

1. To avoid establishing a relationship with the client.
2. To make group interactions the main focus of therapy.
3. To hold in-depth, one-on-one counseling sessions.
4. To keep interactions short, frequent, and nondemanding.

10. When evaluating care of a client with schizophrenia, the nurse should keep which point in mind?

1. Frequent reassessment is needed and is based on the client's response to treatment.
2. The family does not need to be included in the care because the client is an adult.

3. The client is too ill to learn about his illness.
4. Relapse is not an issue for a client with schizophrenia.

11. A male client tells the nurse that the FBI is monitoring and recording his every movement and that microphones have been planted in the unit walls. Which action would be the most therapeutic response?
   1. Confront the delusional material directly by telling the client that this simply is not so.
   2. Tell the client that this must seem frightening to him but that you believe he is safe here.
   3. Tell the client to wait and talk about these beliefs in his one-on-one counseling sessions.
   4. Isolate the client when he begins to talk about these beliefs.

12. Which of the following client behaviors documented in a client's chart would validate the nursing diagnosis of *Risk for other-directed violence*?
   1. The client's description of being endowed with super powers
   2. Frequent angry outbursts noted toward peers and staff
   3. Refusal to eat cafeteria food
   4. Refusal to join in group activities

13. The nurse educates the family about symptom management for when the schizophrenic client becomes upset or anxious. Which of the following would the nurse state is helpful?
   1. Call the therapist to request a medication change.
   2. Encourage the use of learned relaxation measures.
   3. Request that the client be hospitalized until the crisis is over.

4. Wait until the anxiety worsens before intervening.

14. A client who has had auditory hallucinations for many years tells the nurse that the voices prevent his participation in a social skills training program at the community mental health center. Which intervention is most appropriate?
   1. Have the client analyze the content of the voices.
   2. Advise the client to participate in the program when the voices cease.
   3. Advise the client to take his medication as prescribed.
   4. Teach the client to use thought-stopping techniques.

15. The nurse assesses for evidence of positive symptoms of schizophrenia in a newly admitted client. Which of the following symptoms are considered positive evidence? Select all that apply.
   1. Anhedonia
   2. Delusions
   3. Flat affect
   4. Hallucinations
   5. Loose associations
   6. Social withdrawal

16. A client with schizophrenia is referred for psychosocial rehabilitation. Which of the following are typical of this type of program? Select all that apply.
   1. Analyzing family issues and past problems
   2. Developing social skills and supports
   3. Learning how to live independently in a community
   4. Learning job skills for employment
   5. Treating family members affected by the illness
   6. Participating in in-depth psychoanalytical counseling

Answer key

1. The answer is 2.

Disorganized schizophrenia is characterized by regressive behavior with extreme social withdrawal and frequently odd mannerisms. The absence of acute symptoms and impaired role function are more characteristic of residual-type schizophrenia. Psychomotor immobility and presence of waxy flexibility are more indicative of catatonic schizophrenia. Suspiciousness toward others and increased hostility is more characteristic of paranoid schizophrenia.

2. The answer is 4.

In a client demonstrating negative symptoms of schizophrenia, avolition, or the lack of motivation for activities, is a common problem. All of the other symptoms listed are the positive symptoms of schizophrenia.

3. The answer is 4.

Research shows that family history statistically increases the risk for development of schizophrenia. However, no single gene has yet been identified. Options 2 and 3 are both incorrect because genetics plays a role in the etiology of schizophrenia.

4. The answer is 1.

A nonthreatening, nondemanding relationship helps decrease the mistrust that is common in a client with paranoid schizophrenia. Encouraging involvement in group activities and spending more time with the client would be threatening for a client who is suspicious of other people's motives. This client is unlikely to initiate interaction; the nurse is responsible for initiating a relationship with the client.

5. The answer is 1.

The nurse needs to clarify the client's previous experience with psychotropic medication in order to understand the meaning of the client's statement. Asking the client if an injection is preferable may add to the client's suspicion and feeling threatened. Withholding medication prescribed to relieve delusional beliefs will likely intensify paranoid thinking. Insisting that the client take medication can be a violation of his right to refuse treatment.

6. The answer is 4.

These behaviors indicate the client's withdrawal from others and possible fear or mistrust of relationships. There is no indication of *Anxiety* or *Decisional conflict* in the information provided. Although the client refuses to bathe or dress, *Self-care deficit* would not be the priority nursing diagnosis in this situation.

7. The answer is 1.

The primary age of onset for schizophrenia is late adolescence through young adulthood (ages 17 to 27). Paranoid schizophrenia may sometimes have a later onset. All of the other options are incorrect.

8. The answer is 4.

Low socioeconomic status or poverty is an identified environmental factor associated with increased incidence of schizophrenia. Although alcoholism, adolescent pregnancy, and overcrowded schools may be stressful, research does not show they increase the risk for schizophrenia.

9. The answer is 4.

The nurse must proceed slowly, building trust gradually with a client who is withdrawn and initiating brief, undemanding contact (such as by showing interest in the client's daily activities and hygiene). Not attempting to establish a relationship suggests ignoring the client, which is inappropriate. Making group interactions the main focus of therapy or having in-depth, one-on-one counseling sessions may be potentially overwhelming to a withdrawn client.

10. The answer is 1.

Because clients respond to treatment in different ways, the nurse must constantly evaluate the client and his potential. Premorbid adjustment must also be considered. Most clients with schizophrenia go home, and the family should be involved and supported. The client can learn about the illness if information is provided gradually and in easy-to-understand terms. Relapse is common in schizophrenia.

11. The answer is 2.

The nurse must realize that these perceptions are very real to the client. Acknowledging the client's feelings provides support; explaining how the nurse sees the situation in a different way provides reality orientation. Confronting the delusional material directly will not work with this client and may diminish trust. Telling the client to wait and talk about these beliefs in his one-on-one counseling session will reinforce the delusion. Isolation will increase anxiety. Distraction with a radio or activities would be a better approach.

12. The answer is 2.

Anger is an important factor that indicates the potential for acting out. Because the client is angry with both peers and staff, any acting out would probably be directed toward others. The client's description of being endowed with super powers and his refusal to eat cafeteria food indicate that he may have delusional beliefs, but not necessarily a risk for violence. Refusal to join in group activities indicates discomfort with a group; however, no threat of violence is apparent.

13. The answer is 2.

The client with schizophrenia can learn relaxation techniques, which help reduce anxiety. The family can be supportive and helpful by encouraging the client to use these techniques. Anxiety is a common experience for everyone, and is no reason to change medication. Handling anxiety is a learned skill that is important to reinforce. There is no indication that the client is in crisis. It is much easier to intervene early in anxiety rather than waiting until escalation occurs.

14. The answer is 4.

Clients with long-lasting auditory hallucinations can learn to use thought-stopping measures to accomplish tasks. Analyzing the content of the voices may be indicated when hallucinations first occur to establish whether the voices are threatening to the client or instructing him to harm others. However, focusing on their content at this point would reinforce this symptom. The voices have lasted many years; the client should participate despite the voices. There is no indication that the client is not taking medication as prescribed.

15. The answer is 2, 4, 5.

These are considered positive symptoms of schizophrenia. Options 1, 3, and 6 are considered negative symptoms.

16. The answer is 2, 3, 4.

The goal of psychosocial rehabilitation as a treatment method is to help the client develop the skills and supports necessary for successful living, learning, and working in the community. Analysis of family issues and past problems and treatment of family members are not commonly part of this type of program. The emphasis of psychosocial rehabilitation is on the client's development of skills in the here and now; consequently, psychoanalytic counseling is not part of the approach.

8 *Substance-Related Disorders*

I. OVERVIEW OF SUBSTANCE-RELATED DISORDERS

A. Key concepts

1. **Psychoactive substances** are drugs or chemicals that alter one or several of the following: perception, awareness, consciousness, thinking, judgment, decision-making, insight, mood, or behavior.

2. **Substance abuse** is the misuse of a substance with significant and recurrent adverse consequences related to repeated use.

3. Commonly abused substances include alcohol, amphetamines, caffeine, cannabis, cocaine, hallucinogens, inhalants, nicotine, opioids, phencyclidine, barbiturates, nonbarbiturate sedative-hypnotics, and anxiolytics.

   a. Alcohol is the most commonly abused substance in the United States, with 13.4 million persons classified with alcohol abuse or dependence.

   b. Cocaine and heroin use continue to be a major problem as well.

   c. Marijuana (most widely used illicit drug), MDMA (ecstasy), and oxycontin also continue to be used by significant numbers.

4. **Substance dependence** is a cluster of cognitive, behavioral, and physiologic symptoms indicating continued use of a substance despite significant life problems related to its use; diagnosis of substance dependence requires at least three of the following symptoms occurring over 12 months:

   a. **Tolerance:** the need for greatly increased amounts of a substance to obtain the desired effect; or a diminished effect with continued use of the same amount of the substance

   b. **Withdrawal:** the behavioral, physiologic, and cognitive symptoms that occur when blood or tissue concentrations of a substance abruptly decline

   c. Compulsive drug-taking behavior

   d. Inability to reduce substance use

   e. Excess time spent obtaining drugs

   f. Impairment in social or occupational functioning or recreational activities

   g. Continued substance use despite negative consequences.

5. **Polysubstance abuse** is the use of more than one abusive substance; of the 16.6 million persons with substance dependence or abuse in the United States, about a half million were classified as dependent on both alcohol and illicit drugs.

6. **Substance intoxication** is the development of a reversible substance-specific syndrome induced by ingestion or exposure to a substance that produces physiologic effects on the central nervous system (CNS).

7. **Dual diagnosis** refers to the assignment of another psychiatric diagnosis for an individual with a substance-specific disorder; studies have identified associations between alcohol use and anxiety disorder, depression, schizophrenia, eating disorder, and antisocial personality disorder.

8. **Cross-tolerance** (addiction) is demonstrated when a person dependent on one substance requires higher doses of another substance in the same general category; for example, an individual who develops tolerance to alcohol—a CNS depressant—will require higher-than-normal doses of another CNS depressant (such as benzodiazepine) to achieve the desired effect.

9. **Codependence** is the enabling behaviors of individuals in the family or social system of a person who is substance-dependent; these behaviors inadvertently promote continued use by protecting the individual from the consequences of his actions.

10. **Substance withdrawal** is the development of a substance-specific syndrome due to stopping or decreasing the substance use.

11. **Detoxification** is controlled withdrawal from an abusive substance in a medically prescribed program using gradually tapered sedation, a controlled environment, and nutritional supplements.

B. Classification of commonly abused drugs

1. Commonly abused substances are classified according to several major categories, largely based on their effects. (See *Table 8-1, Classification of common abusive substances.*)

TABLE 8-1
Classification of common abusive substances

CNS depressants
Alcohol
- beer
- wine
- liquor

Barbiturates
- pentobarbital (Nembutal)
- secobarbital (Seconal)
- amobarbital (Amytal)

Nonbarbiturate sedative/hypnotics
- methaqualone (Quaalude)
- ethchlorvynol (Placidyl)
- glutethimide (Doriden)
- chloral hydrate (Noctec)

Anxiolytics (benzodiazepines)
- diazepam (Valium)
- chlordiazepoxide (Librium)
- oxazepam (Serax)
- aprazolam (Xanax)
- lorazepam (Ativan)

Inhalants
- hydrocarbon solvents (found in gasoline, glue, paint thinners, cleaning fluids)
- aerosol propellants (found in spray cans)
- anesthetic gases (chloroform, nitrous oxide)

CNS depressants *(continued)*
Opioids (narcotic analgesics)
- heroin, opium
- morphine and derivatives (MS Contin, Roxanol)
- codeine
- oxycodone (in Percodan)

Synthetics
- meperidine (Demerol)
- methadone (Dolophine)
- propoxyphene (Darvon)
- pentazocine (Talwin)

CNS stimulants
Amphetamines
- dextroamphetamine (Dexedrine)
- methamphetamine (Desoxyn)
- amphetamine sulfate (Benzedrine)

Nonamphetamine stimulants
- methylphenidate (Ritalin)
- pemoline (Cylert)
- phenmetrazine (Preludin)
- cocaine (crack, coke)

Nicotine
- cigarettes
- chewing and pipe tobacco
- snuff

CNS stimulants *(continued)*
Caffeine
- coffee
- cola
- tea

Hallucinogens
- mescaline (in peyote cactus)
- psilocybin (in *Psilocybe* mushrooms)
- lysergic acid (LSD)
- phencyclidine (PCP)

Cannabinoids
- cannabis (marijuana)
- hashish (hash)
- tetrahydrocannabinol (Marinol)

Club drugs
Stimulants and hallucinogens
- MDMA (ecstasy)

CNS depressants
- gamma hydroxybutyrate (GHB)

Benzodiazepine-like substances
- flunitrazepam (Rohypnol) ("date rape" drug)

Anesthetic and CNS depressant
- ketamine

2. **CNS depressants** produce their effects by stimulating inhibitory neurotransmitters (gamma-aminobutyric acid; GABA) or altering excitatory neurotransmitters (dopamine and norepinephrine).
   a. Chronic use of CNS depressants may reduce the production and supply of inhibitory neurotransmitters.
   b. Neuroexcitation occurs when CNS depressants are abruptly withdrawn; rebound norepinephrine and dopamine stimulation accounts for the withdrawal symptoms.
3. **CNS stimulants** produce their effects by increasing the release of dopamine and norepinephrine from presynaptic neurons and preventing their reuptake.
   a. This presynaptic blockade eventually causes catecholamine depletion and, therefore, increases the need for the stimulating substance.
   b. When CNS stimulants are abruptly withdrawn, excitatory neurotransmitters are profoundly depleted and severe dysphoria and depression occur.
4. **Opioids** are both CNS depressants and powerful analgesics.
   a. Opioids are thought to block release of substance P and attach to endorphin receptors to relieve pain; they stimulate the opioid receptors in the nucleus ceruleus and suppress noradrenergic neurotransmitters.
   b. When opioids are abruptly withdrawn, rebound release of large amounts of norepinephrine occurs.
5. **Hallucinogens** excite presynaptic receptors in the pontine nuclei and produce visual, proprioceptive, and perceptual disturbances.
   a. The hallucinogen phencyclidine (PCP) acts at several neurotransmitter sites, thereby releasing dopamine, norepinephrine, and serotonin as well as inhibiting GABA.
   b. Withdrawal of hallucinogens produces unpleasant effects (anxiety, insomnia, panic) related to neurotransmitter imbalances.
6. **Cannabinoids** are difficult to categorize; they are related to hallucinogens (effects include alteration in perceptions) and to CNS depressants (depression of higher brain centers).
   a. Other effects include euphoria, short-term memory loss, and decreased concentration.
   b. Withdrawal of cannabinoids can produce effects of excess stimulation because the depressant action of the substance is stopped.
7. **Inhalants** act as CNS depressants and rapidly cross the blood-brain barrier.
   a. They are particularly dangerous because the dosage of an inhalant cannot be controlled.
   b. Inhalants do not produce withdrawal symptoms when abruptly stopped.
8. **Club drugs** is a collective term used for drugs that are associated with "raves" and all-night dance parties.
   a. These drugs can act as CNS depressants, CNS stimulants, or hallucinogens or can mimic the properties of benzodiazepines, depending on the specific drug.
   b. Commonly used club drugs include MDMA (ecstasy), GHB (gamma hydroxybutyrate), RoHypnol ("date rape" drug), LSD, methamphetamine, and ketamine.

C. Factors affecting substance abuse

1. **Gender** is an important factor in substance abuse.
   a. Men are more than twice as likely to abuse drugs as women.
   b. Certain factors place women at high risk for drug abuse, including:
      - Chaotic family life in childhood
      - Victimization (abuse) in childhood
      - Decreased level of self-esteem.
2. Because alcohol has religious, social, and cultural significance, different **cultural groups** use alcohol in markedly different ways, thus affecting the abuse rate in various groups.
   a. Asian cultures have an overall low prevalence of alcohol-related disorders; this may be related to genetic inheritance factors that regulate alcohol metabolism in this cultural group.
   b. Black and white Americans have nearly identical rates of alcohol abuse and dependence.
   c. Hispanics have a somewhat higher rate of alcohol-related disorders.
   d. Native Americans have a high incidence of alcohol-related disorders.
3. Certain common **personality traits** have been identified among substance abusers, although there is some controversy over whether the traits or the abuse occurs first; these traits include:
   a. Dominant and critical behavior toward others (which masks self-doubt and passivity)
   b. Personal insecurity and diminished self-esteem
   c. Rebellious attitude toward authority
   d. Difficulty with intimate relationships and tendency toward narcissism.
4. **Defense mechanisms** are common in those who abuse substances.
   a. Denial is manifested when an individual fails to acknowledge how destructive the substance use has become and the effect of use on the individual's problems.
   b. Other common defense mechanisms used by substance abusers include rationalization and projection. (See *Table 2-1, Common defense mechanisms*, page 26.)

D. Family influences

1. About half of all families in the United States have problems related to the abuse of substances.
2. The family system can become chaotic and disorganized, especially when a parent is a substance abuser.
3. Children of a substance abuser exhibit stress, guilt, and difficulties in relationships with others; they may attempt to compensate for the parent by adopting various roles (caretaker, scapegoat).
4. Adolescents in families with a substance-abusing parent have been found to have low levels of warmth, increased anger and rebelliousness, and difficulty with trust and intimacy.
5. **Codependent or enabling behavior** is common among family members of the substance abuser

    a. Family members characteristically alternate blaming and rescuing the abuser; rescuing the abuser may permit the abuser to avoid the consequences of addiction.

    b. Codependent family members develop behavioral patterns that present problems in many areas of life; for example, codependent family members tend to become caretakers in friend or work relationships, ignoring their own needs to fulfill the needs of others, which can result in bitterness, anger, resentment, and depletion of emotional and physical energy.

    c. Incidence of depression is high among these family members.

E. Nursing profession and substance abuse

  1. Nurses and other health professionals have the same risk factors as others for addiction; however, workplace stress, work-related injuries, and easy access to prescription drugs place nurses at great risk for substance abuse.

  2. Practicing nurses must identify and report nurses who may be suffering from chemical dependency; most state nurse practice acts include provisions for mandatory reporting of impaired nurses.

  3. Many state nursing associations, supported by national nursing organizations, have established peer support systems to help nurses who abuse substances.

  4. A typical recovery program for nurses requires the nurse with substance abuse to stop practicing and enter a 12-step program (Alcoholics Anonymous or Narcotics Anonymous); following initial treatment, a monitoring program (including total abstinence from addictive chemicals, continued treatment, random drug testing, worksite professional monitoring, and 12-step meeting attendance) may be implemented.

F. Laboratory testing for abusive substances

  1. Blood and urine levels are used to detect recent use of substances.

  2. For most psychoactive drugs (opioids, CNS depressants and stimulants) urinalysis can detect evidence 2 to 4 days after use; it can detect hallucinogens up to 1 month after use.

II. TYPES OF ABUSED SUBSTANCES

A. Alcohol

  1. Acute alcohol intoxication causes slurred speech, lack of coordination, unsteady gait, and impaired attention and memory; high doses can cause stupor and coma.

  2. Chronic use causes multisystem dysfunction.

    a. Gastrointestinal effects include gastritis, pancreatitis, and cirrhosis of the liver.

    b. CNS effects are related to the effect of thiamin (vitamin B_1) deficiency.

      – **Wernicke's syndrome** is an acute confusional state characterized by ataxia, delirium, and peripheral neuropathy; treatment with thiamin can reverse this disorder.

      – **Korsakoff's syndrome** is a chronic cognitive impairment (dementia) characterized by cerebral atrophy and memory loss; this disorder is treated in a supportive manner as with other disorders of dementia. (See pages 208 and 209.)

c. Cardiovascular problems include anemia, cardiomyopathy, and clotting disorders.

d. **Blackouts** (antegrade amnesia) occur with chronic alcohol use and are characterized by loss of short-term memory; the individual functions during a blackout in social situations but later has no memory of what occurred during this time.

e. Reproductive problems include fetal alcohol syndrome (FAS) in infants of impaired mothers; low birth weight, abnormal facial features, microcephaly, mental retardation, cardiac and genital abnormalities, and vision and hearing problem are characteristic of FAS.

3. **Blood alcohol level (BAL)** is important in the legal definition of intoxication and the determining criteria for driving under the influence (DUI); in 2004, a BAL of 0.08 became the nationwide standard for determining the legal limit for DUI.

a. BAL peaks within 50 minutes to 3 hours after heavy drinking ends.

b. Coma generally occurs with a BAL of 0.4 g/dl and severe respiratory depression with a BAL of 0.5 g/dl.

c. An individual who has developed tolerance can have an increased BAL with minimal behavioral changes and can, therefore, be at risk for severe withdrawal.

4. Withdrawal symptoms can occur within hours to days after a person's last drink.

a. **Alcohol withdrawal syndrome (AWS)** can occur 6 to 8 hours after the last drink and is characterized by anxiety, agitation, tremors, anorexia, nausea, sweating, and increased pulse and blood pressure.

b. **Alcohol withdrawal delirium** (formerly called **delirium tremens**) usually occurs 2 to 3 days after the last drink, but may appear as many as 14 days after the last drink; it is characterized by increased temperature, pulse, and blood pressure; severe diaphoresis; auditory, visual, and tactile hallucinations; agitation; confusion; and seizures.

B. **Barbiturates, nonbarbiturates, sedative-hypnotics, and benzodiazepines (anxiolytics)**

1. These drugs are usually consumed orally.

2. Acute effects include euphoria, impaired attention and memory, sedation, psychomotor retardation, facial flushing, bradycardia, and hypotension; high doses can cause respiratory depression, coma, and death.

3. Chronic use can cause psychological effects (depression, paranoia), depending on the specific substance and its effects on body systems.

4. The effects of CNS depressants are additive (synergistic) with one another and also with alcohol; therefore, the depressant effects are compounded when more than one substance in this group is taken; results are unpredictable and may often be fatal.

5. Most **overdoses** of CNS depressants are mixtures of drugs, commonly alcohol and barbiturates, or possibly benzodiazepines or barbiturates and opiates (such as heroin or oxycontin).

    a. An opiate-blocking drug, naloxone (Narcan), is often used as an **antidote** in case an opiate was part of the mix.

    b. There is no direct antidote to barbiturates or alcohol, so respiratory support is provided until the drugs are removed from the system; drugs to alkalinize the urine help speed the excretion of barbiturates.

    c. Flumazenil (Mazicon) is used for treatment of benzodiazepine overdose; this drug acts as an antagonist of GABA receptors.

    d. Activated charcoal (Liqui-Char) may be used to minimize systemic absorption of drugs (useful if given within 4 hours of ingestion).

6. Withdrawal symptoms are similar to those of alcohol withdrawal.

    a. Withdrawal occurs 24 to 72 hours after the last dose. In substances with long half-life (such as diazepam), withdrawal symptoms may not occur for up to 1 week.

    b. Withdrawal is characterized by anxiety, tremors, insomnia, anorexia, nausea, and vomiting; more severe symptoms, such as hypertension, tachycardia, delirium, and hallucinations, can also occur.

    c. Treatment of withdrawal may include one or more medications, depending on the substance and symptoms. (See *Table 8-2, Treatment of withdrawal from abusive substances*, page 148.)

C. Opioids (CNS depressants and analgesics)

1. The most common methods of use include oral ingestion, smoking, snuffing, and injection.

2. Acute effects include euphoria, agitation, apathy, decreased sensation of pain, impaired attention and memory, sedation ("nodding out"), psychomotor retardation, pinpoint pupils, nausea, and vomiting; more severe effects include decreased blood pressure, hypothermia, respiratory depression, and death.

3. Chronic use can cause physical problems and greatly impair social and occupational functioning.

    a. Gastrointestinal effects include a slowing of peristalsis and chronic constipation.

    b. Individuals who abuse heroin intravenously may develop multiple skin abscesses on their extremities as well as darkened, hardened, and scarred veins ("tracks").

    c. Use of contaminated needles may lead to multiple infectious diseases, including hepatitis B, C, and D and acquired immunodeficiency syndrome (AIDS).

    d. A heroin abuser's lifestyle is characterized by **drug-seeking behaviors** to the exclusion of other activities of living; such individuals seldom maintain a steady job that will support their habit and commonly obtain funds illegally (stealing, prostitution).

4. Opioid overdose is a medical emergency that places an individual in danger of respiratory arrest.

    a. Naloxone (Narcan), an opioid antagonist, is given I.V. to reverse the overdose; it is short acting and must be given in repeat doses, and the client must be closely observed for hypotension.

    b. Volume replacement is used to treat hypotension.

TABLE 8-2
Treatment of withdrawal from abusive substances

Substance	Treatment	Rationale
CNS depressants		
Alcohol Barbiturates Nonbarbiturate sedative/hypnotic Benzodiazepines	Benzodiazepines (diazepam, chlordiazepoxide, lorazepam, oxazepam) administered in scheduled doses with gradual tapering of frequency and amount over a 5- to 10-day period.	Restore depleted gamma-aminobutyric levels and prevents neuroexcitation response to withdrawal of CNS depressants.
	Anticonvulsants (phenytoin, carbamazepine)	Prevent seizures that can occur with excessive neuroexcitation during severe withdrawal.
	Nutritional supplements (multivitamins, folic acid, and thiamine)	Restore depleted nutrients (thiamine is important for alcohol abusers, who generally develop thiamine deficiency).
	Nonsteroidal anti-inflammatory drug (Ascriptin)	Provides analgesia for common complaints of headache, muscle soreness.
Opioids	Central-acting anti-adrenergic agent (clonidine)	Stimulates alpha-adrenergic receptors in CNS, which reduces norepinephrine rebound when opioid is stopped.
	Synthetic opioid (methadone)	Decreases opiate dependence when administered in scheduled doses with gradual tapering over 14- to 28-day period; can also be administered as long-term maintenance therapy to replace dependence on illegal opioids.
	Narcotic antagonist (buprenorphine)	Suppresses acute opioid withdrawal symptoms.
CNS stimulants		
Amphetamines Cocaine	Dopamine agonists (bromocriptine, amantadine)	Restore dopamine, which is depleted by chronic use of CNS stimulant.
	Antidepressant (desipramine)	Restores serotonin, which is depleted by chronic use of CNS stimulant, and counteracts severe depression occurring from withdrawal.
	Antipsychotic (haloperidol)	Treats psychotic symptoms, which may occur.
Hallucinogens		
LSD PCP	Benzodiazepines (diazepam, lorazepam)	Treat panic response, which can occur during withdrawal.
	Antipsychotic (haloperidol)	Treats psychotic symptoms by counteracting excessive dopamine release caused by hallucinogenic substance.
Cannabis	Calm environment, supportive care	Physiologic withdrawal symptoms do not occur.

5. Fetal exposure to opioids has been associated with an increased rate of prematurity and a 5- to 10-times higher risk of sudden infant death syndrome (SIDS); newborns of addicted mothers suffer withdrawal symptoms (noise sensitivity, sweating, irritability, tremors, nasal congestion, and feeding difficulties).
6. Withdrawal symptoms may occur 6 to 24 hours after last dose.
    a. Symptoms are distressing, but medically benign, and include nausea, vomiting, muscle aches, cramping, lacrimation, rhinorrhea, piloerection, sweating, fever, and insomnia.
    b. Tachycardia and hypertension can also occur from norepinephrine rebound.
    c. Treatment of withdrawal may include a narcotic antagonist or other medication. (See *Table 8-2, Treatment of withdrawal from abusive substances.*)

D. Inhalants
1. The usual method of use involves inhalation of the substance's fumes through the nose and mouth.
2. Acute effects include euphoria, dizziness, ataxia, uninhibited behavior, the sensation of floating, and perceptual changes (including hallucinations); inhalants can cause respiratory and cardiac depression, leading to sudden death.
3. Chronic use may lead to kidney, liver, and brain damage.
4. Although inhalant use is widespread and dangerous, only a small percentage of users become dependent; adolescents are the most common users, often engaging in inhalant use as a part of peer group activity and pressure.
5. Although a withdrawal syndrome has not been well established, symptoms (including sleep disturbances, tremor, irritability, diaphoresis, nausea, and fleeting illusions) have been documented 24 to 48 hours after last dose.

E. Amphetamines and related drugs (CNS stimulants)
1. The most common methods of use include oral ingestion, smoking, and injection.
2. Acute effects include increased energy, euphoria, extreme vigilance, hostility, impaired judgment, increased blood pressure, tachycardia, dilated pupils, insomnia, decreased appetite, nausea, and vomiting.
3. Amphetamine intoxication is characterized by euphoria, hyperactivity, anxiety, impaired judgment, tachycardia, arrhythmias, myocardial infarction, hypertension, and seizures.
    a. Treatment is supportive and based on specific physiologic symptoms.
    b. A protective environment may be necessary to prevent injury or suicide.
4. Chronic use of amphetamines may cause paranoia and malnutrition.
    a. I.V. use can lead to infectious diseases, such as hepatitis B, C, and D and AIDS.
    b. Individuals who are chronic users are at increased risk for cerebrovascular and cardiovascular accidents.
    c. Individuals who are amphetamine abusers may have binges followed by a period of exhaustion, depression, and withdrawal ("crash").
5. MDMA (ecstasy) can cause death when combined with high levels of physical activity (such as at a rave dance); death results from hyperthermia, hypertension, muscle breakdown, and kidney failure.

6. **Caffeine** and **nicotine** are currently the most widely used stimulants in the United States.

   a. An intake of 500 to 600 mg/day of caffeine (equivalent to 4 cups of coffee) can cause anxiety, insomnia, and depression; tachycardia and arrhythmias may also occur.

   b. Nicotine continues to affect roughly 30% of the U.S. population; besides the well documented overall health risks (lung cancer, emphysema), nicotine causes tachycardia and increased blood pressure.

7. **Withdrawal symptoms** for amphetamines and related substances occur within a few hours to several days after cessation of the drug.

   a. Withdrawal is characterized by depression, fatigue, vivid and unpleasant dreams, insomnia or hypersomnia, paranoia, and psychomotor retardation or agitation.

   b. Withdrawal from caffeine has not been included in the *DSM-IV TR;* however, symptoms documented include headache, fatigue, anxiety or depression, nausea, and vomiting.

   c. Nicotine withdrawal causes depression, insomnia, irritability, anxiety, bradycardia, and increased appetite; treatment of withdrawal includes use of nicotine gum (Nicorette) or nicotine patch (Nicotrol) in gradually decreasing doses over a period lasting from 3 weeks to 3 months.

F. Cocaine

1. The usual methods of use include sniffing, smoking, or injecting the drug.

2. Acute effects following use of cocaine (a CNS stimulant) include euphoria, anxiety, anger, impaired thinking and judgment, and hypervigilance.

   a. More severe physical effects include tachycardia, cardiac arrhythmias, pupil dilation, elevated blood pressure, confusion, and seizures.

   b. Death can occur as a result of cardiac arrhythmias or intracranial hemorrhage caused by severe hypertension.

3. Chronic effects include perforated nasal septum (from snorting the drug), lung damage, and chronic infectious diseases (hepatitis B, C, D, and AIDS) caused by I.V. transmission; cocaine produces extreme euphoria and can, therefore, cause psychological dependence after initial use.

4. Overdose is characterized by euphoria, grandiosity, anger, combativeness, and impaired judgment; in addition, tachycardia, hypertension, nausea and vomiting, seizures, arrhythmias, hyperthermia, and death may occur.

   a. Treatment is supportive and based on specific symptoms.

   b. Ventilatory support may be needed.

5. Fetal exposure to cocaine during the first trimester is associated with neurologic damage, leading to learning and behavior problems; after birth, these infants experience abnormal sleep patterns, tremors, seizures (occasionally), irritability, and feeding difficulties.

6. Withdrawal symptoms are similar to withdrawal from other stimulants. (See II.E.7 for a discussion of withdrawal symptoms; also see *Table 8-2, Treatment of withdrawal from abusive substances*, page 148.)

G. Hallucinogens

1. The most common methods of use include oral ingestion, injection, smoking, and sniffing.
2. Acute effects include intensified perceptions, including heightened response to color, textures, and sounds.
   a. Illusions and hallucinations, anxiety, and depression may also occur; some drugs in this group (LSD, PCP) can cause dilated pupils and tachycardia.
   b. Effects produced by these drugs are unpredictable and may be related to the specific drug and dosage as well as the individual's mental state.
   c. A **panic reaction** ("bad trip") is characterized by an intense level of anxiety, fear, and paranoia.
3. Chronic use may result in **flashbacks** (transient spontaneous repetition of a previous hallucinogenic experience occurring in the absence of substance use), psychotic disorders with delusions, and mood and anxiety disorders.
4. PCP use and dependence can lead to such symptoms as belligerence, assaultiveness, impulsive behaviors, psychomotor agitation, and impaired judgment; physical responses include hypertension, tachycardia, and decreased pain responsiveness.
5. Withdrawal symptoms include lethargy, depression, and possible panic attacks. (See *Table 8-2, Treatment of withdrawal from abusive substances*, page 148.)

H. Cannabis (CNS depressant and hallucinogen)

1. The most common methods of use are oral ingestion and smoking.
2. Acute effects include altered sensory perceptions, euphoria, impaired coordination, social withdrawal, conjunctival irritation, increased appetite, dry mouth, and tachycardia.
3. Chronic use may lead to lethargy and mild depression; paranoid reactions are possible.
   a. Chronic use may cause chronic cough and an increased risk for chronic lung diseases, such as emphysema and cancer.
   b. Decreased testosterone levels also occur.
   c. Cannabis crosses the placenta and is associated with low birth weight and small head circumference.
4. The major psychoactive ingredient in cannabinoids is tetrahydrocannabinol (THC).
   a. The drug is used medicinally to counter chemotherapy-induced nausea and vomiting; it is also used in treating multiple sclerosis, glaucoma, epilepsy, and chronic pain.
   b. Debate regarding legislation of the drug's medicinal use is ongoing at both the state and federal levels.
5. Withdrawal symptoms include restlessness, irritability, insomnia, tremors, and nausea; treatment of withdrawal is usually supportive. (See *Table 8-2, Treatment of withdrawal from abusive substances*, page 148.)

III. CAUSES OF SUBSTANCE ABUSE

A. Key concepts
1. The exact cause of substance abuse remains unclear.
2. Research points to a variety of possible factors, including:
   - a. Genetic factors
   - b. Biochemical mechanisms
   - c. Environmental factors
   - d. Interpersonal factors
   - e. Cultural attitudes about substances and their use.

B. Genetic theory
1. Evidence indicates a genetic component involved in substance abuse; however, most of this research has been done on alcohol abuse.
2. Alcohol metabolism has a genetic component, which helps to explain differing rates of alcoholism among various cultural groups.
3. The risk of becoming an alcoholic for first-degree relatives of alcoholics can be as high as 40% to 60%.
4. Identical twins of alcoholic parents have a more than 50% chance of becoming alcoholics; fraternal twins, less than a 30% chance.

C. Psychobiologic theory
1. According to researchers, addictive substances activate neurotransmitters in the mesolimbic dopaminergic reward pathways in the brain.
   - a. Stimulation of these pathways leads to the reinforcing properties of "highs."
   - b. An imbalance in neurotransmitters promotes the continued need for the addictive substance.
2. Research has also demonstrated a strong correlation between stress and drug use, especially in relation to relapse.

D. Psychosocial and environmental theories
1. According to psychodynamic theory, the individual has an ego impairment and a disturbance in sense of self.
   - a. Reliance on a substance enhances self-esteem and improves the person's ability to interact with others.
   - b. Feelings of guilt and shame are allayed by continued use of the substance.
2. Family theory implicates a dysfunctional family system, particularly characterized by enmeshed families in which children feel increased dependency and turn to substances for **pseudoseparation** (rebellion).
3. According to sociocultural theorists, substances are used to relieve the feeling of hopelessness experienced with poverty and chronic unemployment; the need for drugs is promoted and reinforced by society.
   - a. Societal ambivalence about substance use is seen when the predominant message from advertising is that taking medicine (drugs) solves problems.
   - b. For example, popular magazines and newspapers carry advertising for anti-anxiety agents and antidepressants; the advertisements indicate that people

who experience anxiety in daily life and social situations should take medicine.

4. Cognitive-behavioral theorists believe that substance abuse is a learned response
to stressful stimuli; the response is reinforced because substance use temporar-
ily decreases anxiety and increases a feeling of well-being.

IV. MANAGING SUBSTANCE ABUSE

A. Key concepts

1. Treatment decisions, including the client's recommended care, depend on several overriding factors, including:
   a. Type of substance abused and the severity of dependence
   b. Risk for withdrawal symptoms
   c. Current social and occupational functioning
   d. Number of previous relapses
   e. Willingness of the client to accept help.
2. Treatment may include admission to a hospital or residential program, various
community-based programs, preventive measures, pharmacological management, and family support.

B. Hospital-based or residential programs

1. These programs are usually recommended for clients with severe substance dependence or failure to achieve success in community-based programs; follow-up
care is recommended after treatment in an inpatient setting.
2. **Medical detoxification units** located in community hospitals provide detoxification for several days to 1 week; a referral is then made for another residential
program or a community-based follow-up program.
3. **Chemical dependency units** located in psychiatric hospitals or special residential treatment centers provide short-term (3 to 6 weeks) programs; treatment
is usually based on a 12-step program, as recommended by Alcoholics Anonymous (AA) and Narcotics Anonymous (NA) models.
4. **Long-term residential programs** (3 to 6 months) may be recommended for individuals with a long history of substance abuse and multiple problems resulting from that abuse; such programs provide a therapeutic community setting for
treatment of abuse as well as training in life skills.

C. Community-based programs

1. These kinds of programs are more common in today's managed care environment, which emphasizes cost containment and treatment in the least restrictive
setting.
2. **Partial-hospitalization programs** may provide treatment for up to 20 hours
weekly, with therapeutic group support and education regarding substance abuse,
coping skills, and building self-esteem.
3. **Outpatient counseling** may be provided by an individual therapist, a group therapy program, or a specific drug and alcohol counselor employed by local drug
and alcohol clinics or mental health centers.

TABLE 8-3
Self-help treatment programs

Self-help programs are typically based on the original 12-step model developed by Alcoholics Anonymous (AA), which reinforces the disease concept of substance abuse and emphasizes recovery occurring one day at a time. AA and Narcotics Anonymous (NA) groups rely on help from members who are also substance abusers but who have been successful in the recovery process. A special one-to-one relationship with a sponsor who has been successful in recovery is recommended.

12-step model groups
- AA
- NA
- Alanon (for spouse or significant others of alcoholics and substance users)
- Alateen (for adolescent children of alcoholics)
- Adult Children of Alcoholics

---

4. **Self-help groups,** such as AA and NA, provide support and a specific program designed to establish and maintain sobriety and drug-free lifestyles. (See *Table 8-3, Self-help treatment programs.*)

D. Prevention
1. Community educational programs target vulnerable groups as well as the general population.
2. Members of the health care team, including community nurses, serve as speakers and use written materials for education.
3. Elements of prevention programs include:
   a. Teaching the concept of substance abuse and dependence, including symptoms and warning signs
   b. Teaching about the consequences of substance abuse and the effect of substances on the body and general life functioning
   c. Teaching about the options available for assistance and treatment
   d. Teaching alternative coping mechanisms to avoid substance abuse.

E. Pharmacological management
1. Methadone maintenance programs attempt to replace a client's reliance on heroin with the use of a medically controlled dose of methadone (or other synthetic opioid).
   a. Methadone provides a noneuphoric state that frees the addicted person from the physiologic craving for heroin. (See *Drug chart 8-1, Medications for treating alcohol and heroin dependence.*)
   b. Methadone programs have been controversial because of their failure to bring about drug-free states in heroin-dependent clients.
2. Several pharmacological alternatives are currently available for alcoholics. (See *Drug chart 8-1, Medications for treating alcohol and heroin dependence.*)

F. Family support
1. Family members of a substance abuser are encouraged to define and maintain responsible self-functioning, thus decreasing codependent behaviors.
2. Support groups, such as Alanon, Alateen, and Adult Children of Alcoholics (ACOA), provide support to families using the 12-step program; these programs focus on

DRUG CHART 8-1
Medications for treating alcohol and heroin dependence

Drug	Rationale for use
For alcohol dependence	
disulfiram (Antabuse)	▪ Inhibits complete alcohol breakdown in the body; when alcohol is taken with disulfiram, acute hypersensitivity occurs. ▪ Symptoms include flushing, severe nausea and vomiting, dizziness, and hypotension. Acts as a psychological deterrent to prevent client from using alcohol. (*Note:* Client must refrain from taking alcohol in any form, including nonbeverage alcohol (cough syrups or extracts).
naltrexone (ReVia)	▪ Opioid receptor antagonist; blocks brain reward pathway activated by alcohol; reduces pleasurable response to drinking and therefore limits urge to drink.
acamprosate (Campral)	▪ Opioid receptor antagonist; acts similarly to naltrexone.
For heroin dependence	
methadone (Dolophine)	▪ Synthetic opioid; provides noneuphoric state, freedom from physiologic craving for heroin.
buprenorphine (Buprenex)	▪ Synthetic opioid; acts similarly to methadone.
levomethadyl acetate (LAAM)	▪ Synthetic opioid with longer half-life than methadone; administered 3 times per week rather than daily.

family members changing their own behavior rather than trying to change the behavior of the substance abuser.

NURSING PROCESS OVERVIEW

V. CARE OF THE CLIENT WITH A SUBSTANCE-RELATED DISORDER

A. Assessment

1. Assess the client for any known substance abuse problem. (See *Key questions 8-1, Assessing clients with substance-related disorders*, page 156.)

   a. Identify symptoms of acute intoxication.

   b. Identify withdrawal symptoms.

   c. Question the client regarding patterns of use, including types of substances used, frequency of use, amount used, and route of administration. *(Note:* Clients with a history of substance abuse tend to underestimate use.)

   d. Perform a general physical assessment to determine the client's health status and to check for signs of physical problems related to abuse.

Q KEY QUESTIONS 8-1
Assessing clients with substance-related disorders

Questions	Information gathered
What substances do you use? How much and how often do you use? What is the method of use (oral ingestion, smoking, inhaling, injecting)?	Specific substances used and an estimate of how severe use has become *(Note:* Underestimation of use is common.)
Have you ever experienced withdrawal symptoms? Have you been treated for this in the past?	Presence of physiologic dependence; history of previous treatment
Do you believe you have a problem with substance use?	Client's ability or willingness to acknowledge problem or use
Have you had any periods in your life when you did not use substances? How long did this last?	History of drug-free periods; ability to maintain abstinence
Have you experienced any legal problems, job losses, or relationship problems associated with substance use?	Losses incurred; extent of effect on social and occupational functioning
Have you ever attempted to harm yourself or another when using substance?	Potential for suicide or acting-out

    e. Review the client's past history for presence of previously diagnosed mental illness.

2. When screening the client with undetected alcohol problems, use an established screening questionnaire, such as CAGE:

    a. Have you ever felt you ought to cut down on your drinking?

    b. Have people annoyed you by criticizing your drinking?

    c. Have you ever felt bad or guilty about your drinking?

    d. Have you ever had a drink in the morning ("eye opener") to steady your nerves or get rid of a hangover?

3. Assess the effect of substance abuse on the client's functioning, including losses incurred (relationships, jobs, finances, self-respect) and legal problems (DUI, disorderly conduct, selling or using illegal substances).

4. Assess the client's treatment history, including previous hospitalizations, counseling, and attendance of self-help groups.

5. Assess the client for typical emotional responses associated with substance abuse, including:

    a. Feelings of anxiety, anger, guilt, shame, despair, and depression.

    b. Use of common defense mechanisms, including denial (of substance abuse problem), rationalization about use, and projection of blame.

CLIENT AND FAMILY TEACHING 8-1

Guidelines for clients with substance-related disorders

Provide information about substance abuse and the client's specific substance-related disorder:
- Substance abuse is a disease, not a moral weakness.
- Substance abuse, when present, affects all family members, not just the person with the disorder.
- Symptoms commonly include a compulsive need for the substance, increasing the amount of a substance over time with an inability to reduce use, and using a substance despite multiple problems associated with use.
- Withdrawal symptoms can occur when the client's substance intake is reduced or stopped.

Include information about how the family can be helpful:
- The client can be helped prior to reaching "rock bottom."
- Options for treatment range from hospital-based programs (to handle withdrawal and teach skills necessary for living without substances) to community-based therapy (with a special drug and alcohol counselor or self-help groups, such as AA and NA).
- Although you can encourage the client to seek treatment, you cannot make this happen—only the client can.
- Reality-based statements, such as "You were unable to work 3 days last week because of your drinking," will help confront the client's denial.
- Protecting the substance abuser from consequences of his behavior (calling him out sick for work, making excuses to friends) is not helpful and is evidence of codependency.
- Report any signs of increasing depression or suicidal thoughts by the client or any other family members to the mental health provider.
- Maintain responsibility for keeping yourself healthy and functioning in your usual roles.
- Seek help from support groups (Alanon, Alateen) or individual counseling.
- Learn and use appropriate ways to manage stress.

---

6. Assess the effect of the client's substance use on family members, including the extent of family involvement with the client, the willingness of the family to participate in the client's treatment, and the family's knowledge of problems with substance abuse. (See *Client and family teaching 8-1, Guidelines for clients with substance-related disorders.*)

B. Nursing diagnoses

1. Analyze the client's response to screening questionnaires; when substance abuse is suspected, use follow-up assessments.
   a. Analyze the extent to which substances have affected the client's social and occupational functioning and general health status.
   b. Analyze the potential for adverse consequences related to withdrawal symptoms.
   c. Analyze the level of depression and potential for suicidal behaviors.
2. Establish individualized nursing diagnoses for the client, including the following, as needed:
   a. *Chronic low self-esteem*
   b. *Defensive coping*
   c. *Deficient knowledge (specify)*
   d. *Hopelessness*
   e. *Imbalanced nutrition: Less than body requirements*
   f. *Impaired adjustment*
   g. *Impaired social interaction*
   h. *Ineffective coping*
   i. *Ineffective denial*

    j. Ineffective role performance

    k. Powerlessness

    l. Spiritual distress.

  3. Establish nursing diagnoses for the family, as needed; diagnoses may include the following:

    a. Dysfunctional family processes: alcoholism

    b. Interrupted family processes.

C. Planning and outcome identification

  1. Work with the client and his family in setting realistic goals.

  2. Establish desired outcome criteria for the client with a substance-related disorder.

    a. The client will acknowledge dependence on abusive substance(s).

    b. The client will safely detoxify from substance(s).

    c. The client will participate in the treatment program as recommended (in either the hospital or the community).

    d. The client will verbalize increased knowledge regarding the effect of substances on health and functioning in family and societal roles.

    e. The client will maintain sobriety or a drug-free state.

    f. The client will use adaptive coping measures for handling life stress rather than turning to substances(s).

    g. The client will maintain participation in a self-help group (AA, NA), accepting feedback and input from the sponsor.

    h. The client will establish a lifestyle that is healthy and free from abusive substances.

    i. The client will seek assistance at the first signs of relapse.

  3. Establish desired outcome criteria for the family.

    a. Family members will verbalize increased knowledge regarding substances and specific effects on individual and family functioning.

    b. Family members will seek help from support groups (Alanon, Alateen) or a counselor (family therapy).

    c. Family members will avoid codependent behaviors.

    d. Family members will maintain individual functioning in social and occupational roles despite the client's success or lack of success with treatment.

D. Implementation

  1. During detoxification and withdrawal (see *Table 8-2, Treatment of withdrawal from abusive substances*, page 148), take the following measures:

    a. Monitor the client's vital signs; increased pulse and blood pressure indicate undermedication with benzodiazepine, and decreased blood pressure indicates overmedication with benzodiazepine.

    b. Administer scheduled and as-needed (p.r.n.) medications for detoxification.

    c. Monitor the client's intake and output for possible I.V. fluid replacement.

    d. Encourage adequate fluids and nutritious foods.

    e. Maintain standard seizure precautions as indicated by the severity of the client's problem.

2. Maintain an accepting attitude and a nonjudgmental approach when interacting with the client; be aware of personal biases that will affect nursing care.
3. Teach the client and his family about substance abuse. (See *Client and family teaching 8-1, Guidelines for clients with substance-related disorders*, page 157.)
   a. Inform them about the symptoms of abuse and its consequences on functioning and general health.
   b. Provide information about the progressive course of dependence.
   c. Educate them about relapse, including warning signs (increased anger and frustration, excuses for poor behavior, increased relationship problems, denial of substance problem, and return to associations with other substance users).
   d. Inform them about the dangers of I.V. drug use, including contracting hepatitis B, C, and D and AIDS.
   e. Emphasize personal responsibility for effecting behavioral change.
   f. Provide information about possible treatment options.
4. Encourage the client and family to use self-help groups for support and ongoing assistance. (See *Table 8-3, Self-help treatment programs*, page 154.)
5. Help the client to verbalize and express feelings covered up by the use of substances.
6. Review lifestyle changes necessary to maintain abstinence or sobriety.
7. Teach and encourage the use of stress management and coping measures.
8. Use appropriate measures to enhance the client's self-esteem.
   a. Give appropriate praise and encouragement.
   b. Show respect, and maintain the client's dignity.
   c. Help the client to identify and use personal strengths.
   d. Project optimism to counteract feelings of helplessness and powerlessness.

E. Outcome evaluation
1. The client admits to having a substance abuse problem and safely detoxifies from the abusive substance.
2. The client participates in a recommended initial treatment program and subsequent follow-up measures.
3. The client maintains a substance-free lifestyle.
4. The client uses adaptive coping measures rather than substance abuse in handling life stress.
5. The client attends an appropriate self-help group and follows the 12-step program.
6. The family uses appropriate support programs and reports increased coping of individual members.

Study questions

1. The nurse understands that the essential difference between substance abuse and substance dependence is that substance *dependence:*
   1. includes characteristics of tolerance and withdrawal.
   2. includes characteristics of adverse consequences and repeated use.
   3. produces less severe symptoms than that of abuse.
   4. requires long-term treatment in a hospital-based program.

2. The sister of a client with a substance-related disorder tells the nurse that she calls out sick for the client occasionally when he has too much to drink and cannot work. This behavior can be described as:
   1. caretaking.
   2. codependent.
   3. helpful.
   4. supportive.

3. When a client abuses a CNS depressant, withdrawal symptoms will be caused by which of the following?
   1. Acetylcholine excess
   2. Dopamine depletion
   3. Serotonin inhibition
   4. Norepinephrine rebound

4. The general classification of drugs belonging to the opioid category is analgesic and:
   1. depressant.
   2. hallucinogenic.
   3. stimulant.
   4. tranquilizing.

5. The community nurse practicing primary prevention of alcohol abuse would target which groups for educational efforts?
   1. Adolescents in their late teens and young adults in their early twenties
   2. Elderly men who live in retirement communities
   3. Women working in careers outside the home
   4. Women working in the home

6. A staff nurse has observed a coworker arriving to work drunk at least three times in the past month. Which action by the nurse would best ensure client safety and obtain necessary assistance for the coworker?
   1. Ignore the coworker's behavior, and frequently assess the clients assigned to the coworker.
   2. Make general statements about safety issues at the next staff meeting.
   3. Report the coworker's behavior to the appropriate supervisor.
   4. Warn the coworker that this practice is unsafe.

7. A client being treated in a chemical dependency unit tells the nurse that he only uses drugs when under stress and therefore does not have a substance problem. Which defense mechanism is the client using?
   1. Compensation
   2. Denial
   3. Suppression
   4. Undoing

8. The nurse is teaching a community group about substance abuse. She explains that a genetic component has been implicated with which of the following commonly abused substances?

1. Alcohol
2. Barbiturates
3. Heroin
4. Marijuana

9. The nurse recommends that the family of a client with a substance-related disorder attend a support group, such as Alanon or Alateen. The purpose of these groups is to help family members understand the problem and to:
 1. change the problem behaviors of the abuser.
 2. learn how to assist the abuser in getting help.
 3. maintain focus on changing their own behaviors.
 4. prevent substance problems in vulnerable family members.

10. The nurse is assessing a client who is a chronic alcohol abuser. Which problems are related to thiamin deficiency?
 1. Cardiovascular symptoms, such as decreased hemoglobin and hematocrit levels
 2. CNS symptoms, such as ataxia and peripheral neuropathy
 3. Gastrointestinal symptoms, such as nausea and vomiting
 4. Respiratory symptoms, such as cough and sore throat

11. When assessing a client who abuses barbiturates and benzodiazepine, the nurse would observe for evidence of which withdrawal symptoms?
 1. Anxiety, tremors, and tachycardia
 2. Respiratory depression, stupor, and bradycardia
 3. Muscle aches, cramps, and lacrimation
 4. Paranoia, depression, and agitation

12. When teaching an adolescent health class about the dangers of inhalant abuse, the nurse warns about the possibility of:
 1. contracting an infectious disease, such as hepatitis or AIDS
 2. recurrent flashback events
 3. psychological dependence after initial use
 4. sudden death from cardiac or respiratory depression

13. Which medication is commonly used in treatment programs for heroin abusers to produce a noneuphoric state and to replace heroin use?
 1. diazepam
 2. carbamazepine
 3. clonidine
 4. methadone

14. The nurse administers bromocriptine (Parlodel) to a client undergoing detoxification for amphetamine abuse. The rationale for this medication is to:
 1. aid in GABA inhibition.
 2. prevent norepinephrine excess.
 3. restore depleted dopamine levels.
 4. treat psychotic symptoms.

15. The nurse is teaching a client about disulfiram (Antabuse), which the client is taking to deter his use of alcohol. She explains that using alcohol when taking this medication can result in:
 1. abdominal cramps and diarrhea.
 2. drowsiness and decreased respiration.
 3. flushing, vomiting, and dizziness.
 4. increased pulse and blood pressure.

16. During an initial assessment of a client admitted to a substance abuse unit for detoxification and treatment, the nurse asks questions to determine patterns of use of substances. Which of the following questions are most appropriate at this time? Select all that apply.

1. How long have you used substances?
2. How often do you use substances?
3. How do you get substances into your body?
4. Do you feel bad or guilty about your use of substances?
5. How much of each substance do you use?
6. Have you ever felt you should cut down substance use?
7. What substances do you use?

Answer key

1. The answer is 1.
Tolerance (the need to increase the amount of a substance to obtain desired effect) and withdrawal (symptoms occurring when a substance is decreased or stopped) are the essential criteria in establishing substance dependence. Both abuse and dependence produce adverse consequences and are characterized by repeated use. Dependence would cause symptoms that are more severe. Option 4 is not necessarily true; after the initial detoxification period, community-based treatment may be appropriate.

2. The answer is 2.
Enabling behaviors that inadvertently promote continued use of a substance by the person abusing substances is known as codependency. The sister's behavior is not an example of caretaking or support. She is taking responsibility for the client's behavior and allowing him to avoid the consequences of his abuse problem. The behavior is unhelpful and unsupportive.

3. The answer is 4.
CNS depressants, when abused, cause depletion of stimulating neurotransmitters. When the CNS depressant is stopped, the result is a rebound of excitatory or stimulating neurotransmitters, such as norepinephrine. Acetylcholine, dopamine, and serotonin are not significant factors in the symptoms of withdrawal from a CNS depressant.

4. The answer is 1.
Opiates are both analgesics and CNS depressants because they decrease the effect of neurotransmitters that are excitatory or stimulating. Hallucinogenic and stimulant are categories that do not apply to opiates. Although an opiate can provide a tranquilizing effect, the general category would be that of a depressant.

5. The answer is 1.
High-risk groups for alcohol abuse include individuals between ages 18 and 25 and the unemployed. There is no evidence that elderly men in retirement communities have increased rates of alcohol abuse. Men have a 2 to 3 times increased risk than women of abusing alcohol.

6. The answer is 3.
The nurse is obligated by ethical considerations of client safety, as well as by nurse practice acts in many states, to report substance abuse in health care workers. Most health care facilities have an employee assistance program to help workers with substance abuse problems. Ignoring the coworker's behavior would be a form of enabling behavior (codependency) on the staff nurse's part. Making general statements about safety in a staff meeting

avoids dealing with the problem. Warning the coworker is inadequate; it does not ensure client safety or help him receive necessary help.

7. The answer is **2.**
Individuals who have substance problems often use denial. Compensation, suppression, and undoing are incorrect and do not fit the situation described.

8. The answer is **1.**
Several chromosomes (1, 3, and 7) have been implicated in increased vulnerability to alcohol abuse. Statistics have shown that risk for alcohol abuse in first-degree relatives of alcohol abusers is as high as 40% to 60%. Most of the genetic research has been done related to alcohol. Definitive data regarding genetic transmission is not available at this time for barbiturates, heroin, and marijuana.

9. The answer is **3.**
Family support groups, such as Alanon and Alateen, emphasize the importance of changing one's own behavior rather than trying to change the behavior of the individual with a substance abuse problem. Trying to change the abuser's behavior or learning ways to find help for the abuser would be viewed as codependent behaviors, and thus would not be advocated by family support groups. Learning about substance abuse may help a vulnerable family member to avoid this problem; however, that is not the purpose of these groups.

10. The answer is **2.**
Wernicke's encephalopathy is a CNS disorder caused by acute thiamin deficiency in people who abuse alcohol. Other symptoms, besides ataxia and peripheral neuropathy, are acute confusion or delir-

ium. Cardiovascular and gastrointestinal symptoms are associated with alcohol abuse; they are not caused by thiamin deficiency. Respiratory problems are not usually directly related to alcohol.

11. The answer is **1.**
Barbiturates and benzodiazepine are CNS depressants; therefore, withdrawal symptoms are related to CNS stimulation caused by the rebounding of neurotransmitters (norepinephrine). Symptoms include increased anxiety, tremors, and vital sign changes (such as tachycardia and hypertension). Respiratory depression, stupor, and bradycardia are typically associated with an overdose—not withdrawal—of barbiturates or benzodiazepine. Muscle aches, cramps, and lacrimation are most commonly associated with withdrawal from opiates. Paranoia, depression, and agitation are usually associated with withdrawal from CNS stimulants, such as amphetamines or cocaine.

12. The answer is **4.**
Inhalants are CNS depressants; if taken in an excess amount, they can cause cardiac and respiratory depression. It is impossible to control the inhalant dosage; therefore, death can occur. Contracting an infectious disease, recurrent flashback events, and psychological dependence after initial use are not associated with inhalant abuse.

13. The answer is **4.**
Methadone maintenance programs are used to provide a heroin-dependent individual with a medically controlled dose of methadone to produce a noneuphoric state that will prevent withdrawal symptoms. This method of treatment is advocated to help heroin abusers avoid crim-

inal activities associated with obtaining heroin; it also prevents diseases associated with I.V. use of heroin. Diazepam and carbamazepine may be used for withdrawal from alcohol, barbiturates, and benzodiazepines. Clonidine can be used in acute withdrawal from heroin to avoid norepinephrine rebound when opiates are stopped.

14. The answer is 3.
Amphetamine abuse depletes the neurotransmitter dopamine. When withdrawing from amphetamines, dopamine depletion causes depression, insomnia, and intense craving for the drug. Bromocriptine (Parlodel) is a dopamine agonist that will help restore this neurotransmitter. GABA inhibition, prevention of norepinephrine excess, and treatment of psychotic symptoms are incorrect rationales for the use of this medication.

15. The answer is 3.
Disulfiram (Antabuse) prevents complete alcohol metabolism in the body. Therefore, when alcohol is consumed, the client has a hypersensitivity reaction. Flushing, vomiting, and dizziness are associated with the incomplete breakdown of alcohol metabolites. Abdominal cramps, diarrhea, drowsiness, decreased respiration, and increased pulse and blood pressure are not associated with the use of disulfiram along with alcohol.

16. The answer is 1, 2, 3, 5, 7.
These questions will elicit information about the client's pattern of use of substances. Options 4 and 6 are questions related to CAGE, a tool for screening suspected substance abusers.

9 Physical Abuse, Sexual Abuse, and Family Violence

165

I. OVERVIEW OF ABUSE AND VIOLENT BEHAVIOR

A. Key concepts

1. **Violence** is the physical force exerted for the purpose of violating or damaging another person; it is an unjust exercise of power, often resulting in physical injury.

2. **Abuse** is the willful infliction of physical injury, mental anguish, or both.

3. An **abuser,** or **perpetrator,** is the person who inflicts violence or abuse on another; the **victim** is the person who is the scapegoat, target, or recipient of the abuse or violence.

4. **Family violence** is a pattern of coercive behavior of one family member (or significant other) by another; it includes physical abuse, neglect, psychological abuse, economic abuse, and sexual abuse.

   a. Family violence is a primary public health issue in the United States; it is estimated that 50% of all Americans have experienced violence in their families.

   b. Family violence occurs across many boundaries, affecting all socioeconomic levels, genders, geographic areas, races, religions, and occupations.

   c. It also occurs across the lifespan; the victim may be a fetus, an infant, a child, an adolescent, an adult, or an elderly person.

5. Child abuse and abuse of women are serious problems in the United States.

   a. Recent statistics indicate that about 12 out of every 1,000 children are abused each year, and the rate of abuse has increased in each year surveyed since 2000; about 1,400 children died from abuse in 2002.

   b. According to recent surveys, about 1.3 million women are physically assaulted annually, about 20% resulting from abuse by an intimate partner.

   c. Up to 54% of women who visit emergency departments have been assaulted by partners; during their prenatal visit, about 23% of pregnant women report an abusive situation.

   d. It is estimated that 1 out of every 3 women will be raped or sexually assaulted in her lifetime.

6. Child sexual abuse profoundly affects development, causing low self-esteem, self-hatred, difficulty trusting, and poor control of aggressive impulses.

   a. There is a high correlation between childhood sexual abuse and adult psychiatric disorders (dissociative disorders, substance abuse disorders).

   b. Victims of child sexual abuse often experience symptoms of post-traumatic stress disorder (PTSD).

   c. The World Health Organization (WHO) indicates that rates of child sexual abuse range from 7% to 36% in girls and 3% to 29% in boys (ages neonate to 15 years).

B. Types of abuse

1. **Physical abuse** may be characterized by beating, hitting, cutting, shooting, burning, or raping.

2. **Neglect** is characterized by withholding or failing to provide personal care, personal needs (food, water, shelter), cleanliness, health care, social contact, or the education and supervision of children.

3. **Psychological abuse** includes:

   a. Verbal assaults and threats of physical harm, usually to intimidate or manipulate

   b. Sarcasm, humiliation, devaluing, and criticism

   c. Inconsistent communication patterns, including withdrawal and silence

   d. Isolation of the victim (such as preventing the victim from interaction and communication with family and friends)

   e. Violation of personal rights (such as refusing to allow the victim contact with family, friends, and others).

4. **Sexual abuse** is pressured or forced sexual activity, including sexually stimulated talk or actions, inappropriate touching or intercourse, rape, and incest (sexual behavior between blood relatives).

   a. A sexual perpetrator is typically male, between the ages of 25 and 44, and married or cohabiting at the time of the offense.

   – If the sexual perpetrator has a history of criminal behavior, it generally involves crimes against property rather than people.

   – Most perpetrators do not have a history of mental illness but may demonstrate common maladaptive behaviors. (See *Display 9-1, Characteristics of an abuser or violent perpetrator*.)

   b. A victim of a sexual assault typically experiences an overwhelming sense of violation and helplessness following the crime.

   – The immediate effect may be either an **expressed response pattern,** in which the victim expresses feelings of fear, anger, and anxiety, or a **controlled response pattern,** in which the defense mechanism of denial allows the victim to be calm, composed, or subdued.

   – Long-term effects can include symptoms of PTSD, difficulties with intimate relationships, depressive disorders, and even suicide.

5. **Elder abuse** involves the abuse, neglect, or victimization of an older person who is under the care of another person.

   a. Since the late 1980s, there has been a 150% increase in the number of reported cases of elder abuse; however, some experts believe that only 1 in 14 cases is reported, and therefore the full scope of this problem is unknown.

DISPLAY 9-1

Characteristics of an abuser or violent perpetrator

The following characteristics are typical of abusers and violent perpetrators:
- Abused as a child (in many cases)
- Low self-esteem
- Extreme jealousy and possessiveness
- Social isolation

- Poor impulse control
- Poor coping skills
- Drug or alcohol abuse
- Rigid, obsessive views about control issues
- Narcissistic personality

      b. Elder abuse victims generally depend on their abusers and have little possibility of leaving the situation.

      c. Elder abuse victims suffer severe emotional distress and an increased mortality rate as well as increased rates of depression.

  6. Economic abuse (financial exploitation) includes:

      a. Stealing of the victim's money or assets

      b. Denying the victim access to personal finances

      c. Inappropriate use of the victim's money or property.

C. Legal issues affecting family violence

  1. Nurses, like other professional health care workers, are required by law to report suspected incidents of child abuse; failure to report is accompanied by civil or criminal penalties (or both).

  2. All states have laws that allow courts to issue **protection from abuse orders;** however, the definition of domestic violence and how the laws help protect victims varies greatly from one jurisdiction to another.

      a. A growing trend within the scope of **family violence protection acts** allows police to charge a perpetrator without the victim's consent.

      b. When an abuser uses a weapon (such as a gun or knife) to injure a woman, the health care provider must report the act of abuse to the police, regardless of the woman's intent to seek legal remedies for the abuse.

TABLE 9-1
Physical signs of abuse

Nurses may use the information below as a guide to physical signs of abuse in children, women, and elderly clients.

Child victim

Physical abuse
- Developmental delays
- Bruises, welts
- Sprains, dislocations, fractures
- Cigarette burns
- Scalding or burns, especially those resembling a stocking or glove from immersion of extremity into any hot liquid
- Internal injuries
- Injuries in various stages of healing
- Shaken baby syndrome (intracranial and intraocular bleeding without obvious head trauma)
- Dirt, fleas, lice on child

Sexual abuse
- Enuresis
- Red and swollen labia and rectum
- Vaginal tears
- Sexually transmitted diseases
- Chronic urinary tract infections
- Hyperactive gag reflex

Battered woman
- Injuries of head, neck, and shoulders
- Black eyes
- Injuries during pregnancy
- Sprains, dislocations, broken bones
- Bruises, welts
- Patterns left by objects used to inflict injury
- Repeated visits to health care facilities, especially emergency departments
- Complaints of pain without tissue injury
- Multiple injuries in various stages of healing

Elder victim
- Malnourishment or dehydration
- Fecal or urine smell on person
- Dirt, fleas, lice on person
- Pressure ulcers, sores, rashes
- Bruises, abrasions, fractures
- Hematomas, grip marks on arms
- Multiple injuries in various stages of healing

3. All states have laws and services in place to detect domestic elder abuse; the detection and handling of abuse incidents vary greatly from state to state.

D. Family violence

1. Violent acts in families do not occur randomly, but constitute a predictable, three-phase cycle.

   a. **Tension building:** the abuser blames the victim for problems in the abuser's life.

   b. **Serious abusive incident:** the tension in the abuser is relieved by the abusive incident.

   c. **Honeymoon:** the abuser becomes remorseful and promises an abusive incident will not happen again.

2. Victims of violence commonly have physical signs of abuse and, over time, behavioral and psychological signs are noted. (See *Table 9-1, Physical signs of abuse*, and *Table 9-2, Behavioral and psychological characteristics in victims of abuse*.)

3. Families in which violence occurs share certain characteristics.

   a. One or more members of the family become the focal point for family anxiety and are often blamed for problems.

TABLE 9-2

Behavioral and psychological characteristics in victims of abuse

Although behavioral and psychological signs of abuse are more difficult to assess than physical signs, nurses may use the information below as a guide to identify common characteristics of abuse victims.

Child victim

Physical abuse
- Fearful of caregiver
- Seeks affection from others
- May not cry when approached by an examiner or during a painful procedure
- Behavioral extremes (child is either very aggressive or very submissive)
- Poor academic performance
- Regressive behaviors and hyperactivity
- Self-injurious behaviors
- Runs away, abuses drugs or alcohol
- Lack of peer relationships

Sexual abuse
- Unusual interest in, or avoidance of, all things of a sexual nature
- Sleep problems, nightmares
- Seductiveness
- Statements that their bodies are dirty or damaged, or fear that there is something wrong with their genital area
- Aspects of sexual molestation in drawings, games, or fantasies

Battered woman

- Rationalizes abuse
- Fears leaving due to threats by partner
- Relationship with partner is male-dominant
- Isolates from friends and family
- Feels inadequate, accepts self-blame
- Acts so as not to provoke partner
- Emotionally and financially dependent on partner
- Feels powerless
- Uses alcohol or drugs
- Depression, suicidal thoughts
- Anxiety, recurrent nightmares

Elder victim

- Possible physical or mental impairment
- Aggressive or very submissive behavior
- Fearful of reporting abuse
- Dependency on caregiver
- Feelings of low self-esteem
- Feelings of hopelessness

b. The family roles are stereotypic, with rigid traditional sex roles and a strong power differential between parents (one parent, usually the man, is the sole authority in the family; the other parent is treated as one of the children rather than an equal partner).

c. Relationships in the family emphasize control over others.

d. The family may be secretive and isolated from others outside the family.

e. The communication patterns are dysfunctional and often involve denial, conflict avoidance, double-bind patterns, conditional loving, and rationalization of abuse.

4. Battered women often choose to remain in an abusive relationship; some of the reasons include:

a. Fear of physical reprisal if they leave

b. Feelings of self-blame, guilt, and depression, which can immobilize the victim

c. Emotional dependence and low self-esteem, and the belief that they do not deserve better treatment

d. Feeling that they have no choice and no control

e. Fear of being shunned by family and friends

f. Ties (emotional, financial) to the abuser, or religious or cultural beliefs that prevent leaving.

II. CAUSES OF ABUSE AND VIOLENCE

A. Key concepts

1. No single factor accounts for family violence; multiple factors exist in any situation of family violence or abuse.

2. Certain theories have attempted to explain the causative factors of abuse and violence.

B. Genetic theory

1. Theorists propose that genes and neurotransmitters may contribute to violent behavior.

2. Serotonin (5-HT) inhibits aggression; abnormally low levels of 5-HT result in a lack of control, loss of temper, and explosive rage.

C. Psychobiologic theory

1. Research has demonstrated that stimulation of the limbic system produces hostile and aggressive responses in humans.

2. Neurotransmitters, especially norepinephrine, dopamine, and serotonin, all play important roles in facilitating and inhibiting aggression; dysregulation of these substances is thought to be associated with violence.

3. Brain disorders, especially tumors in the limbic system and temporal lobe, can predispose a person to violent behavior.

D. Psychosocial and environmental theories

1. According to family theorists, violence occurs in dysfunctional families with problems involving unclear boundaries, enmeshment of individuals and roles, poor coping measures to handle stress, and multigenerational history of abuse.

2. Research based on cognitive-behavioral theory suggests that violence is learned from parents who use abuse as a method of discipline; the abuser acquires the belief that violence and aggression are acceptable and effective responses to real or imagined threats.
3. According to sociocultural theory, aggressive behavior is a product of one's culture and social structure.
   a. The United States has a long history of violence by one group of people over another.
   b. Current cultural glorification of violence as portrayed in movies, TV shows, video games, and the Internet have all been implicated as contributing factors to aggressive behaviors.
4. Based on interpersonal theory, issues of emotional deprivation in early childhood, along with growing up in an abusive environment, contribute to abusive behavior.
   a. As many as 80% of male abusers were raised in homes in which they were abused or observed their mothers being abused.
   b. Early emotional deprivation contributes to the development of an adult who needs much nurturance and support.
   c. Low self-esteem and fear of abandonment contribute to the abuser's attempt to isolate his partner, his increased jealousy, and his need to control.

III. MANAGING ABUSE AND VIOLENCE

A. Key concepts
1. Treatment of abuse victims depends on factors affecting the individual client, such as the type of abuse suffered, presence of physical injuries, age and physical condition of the victim, and the victim's unique family circumstances.
2. Types of treatment include visits to the emergency department, crisis intervention, counseling and therapy, and preventive measures.

B. Emergency care
1. Since 1991, institutions accredited by the Joint Commission on Accreditation of Healthcare Organizations (JCAHO) have been required to adopt the JCAHO's domestic violence standards into their emergency department protocols.
2. Emergency department standards include such protocols as:
   a. Routine screening of all adult and teenage women for intimate partner violence. Trained health care personnel ask simple and direct questions regarding abuse and sexual assault.
   b. When an acute incidence of violence and sexual assault has been established, proper documentation must include detailed, accurate, and nonjudgmental recording of injuries.
   c. Once abuse is identified and documented, an appropriate intervention/referral process should begin according to specific agency protocols as well as legal guidelines.

C. Crisis intervention

1. Crisis intervention may be used to respond to the immediate, short-term problems resulting from abuse; it requires careful collaboration with various health team members to ensure continuity of care.

2. **Public child welfare agencies** are charged with protecting children from harm and cruelty; the legal system can intervene by awarding temporary or permanent custody of children to individuals (relatives or foster parents) who will provide safe care.

3. Battered women may be referred to a **safe house** or **emergency shelter** to ensure protection for themselves and their children.

4. **Community social service agencies,** including special agencies for elderly clients, can provide various services to ensure safety and support for victims of violence.

D. Mental health services

1. **Therapeutic support** by means of individual or group counseling for victims of violence is available; group therapy for the abuser is thought to be the best method of treatment because it allows for vicarious learning, reduces client-therapist deadlock, and encourages breakthrough of denial.

2. **Individual counseling** for the abuser or violent perpetrator is also available.

3. **Family therapy** to break the cycle of abuse may be used.

E. Prevention

1. **Primary prevention** can take place in the community by identifying families at high risk for violence and by promoting educational programs and services that enhance family functioning.

2. **Secondary prevention** involves early detection and treatment for interpersonal violence.

NURSING PROCESS OVERVIEW

 ## IV. CARE OF THE CLIENT INVOLVED WITH FAMILY VIOLENCE

A. Assessment

1. Assess data for indications of possible abuse.
   a. Conduct a thorough examination to determine the nature and extent of the victim's physical injuries. (See *Table 9-1, Physical signs of abuse*, page 168.)
   b. Assess the victim for behavioral and psychological characteristics of abuse. (See *Table 9-2, Behavioral and psychological characteristics in victims of abuse*, page 169.)

2. Interview the victim to verify that abuse has occurred; use specific agency protocols for assessment, ensuring the following factors:
   a. Ensure privacy for assessment by questioning the client away from the suspected abuser; this will promote client trust.
   b. Use appropriate language for the client's age and developmental level.
   c. Ask questions that are simple, direct, and as nonthreatening as possible. (See *Key questions 9-1, Assessing clients who are victims of abuse*.)

KEY QUESTIONS 9-1
Assessing clients who are victims of abuse

Questions	Information gathered
Child victim	
Do you know why you were brought to the hospital?	Child's perception
How do you feel about being here?	Child's fears and other feelings
Can you tell me what happened to you?	Child's description of incident
Have you ever been hit with an object?	Past history of abuse
How do your parents (caregivers) discipline you?	Parenting behaviors
Battered woman	
Are you being threatened or hurt by your partner?	Willingness to acknowledge abuse
What's the worst episode you remember?	Past history of abuse
Have children been present when you were abused?	Escalation of violence
Have they ever been injured?	Child abuse
Elder victim	
I notice you have a number of bruises (or other injuries). Could you tell me what happened?	Willingness to acknowledge abuse
You seem frightened by your caregiver. Are you?	Validation of observation of relationship
Many patients tell me they have been hurt by someone close to them. Could this be happening to you?	Client's past history
When you disagree with your caregiver, what happens?	Family dynamics

   d. If possible, take meticulous notes (including exact quotes) to record conversations with the client and family.
   3. Identify the aspects of family behavior associated with family violence.
   a. Is there a lack of concern about the child or the elder person who is suspected of being abused?
   b. Are there inconsistencies between the nature and extent of injuries and the family or victim's explanation of what happened?
   c. Was there a delay in seeking help for injuries?
   d. Do the interactions between the client and family indicate conflict? Is there screaming or blaming of the victim for the injury?
   e. Is there a history of abusive behavior or substance abuse surrounding a family member?
   f. Are there descriptions (by the family) of children as aggressive, antisocial, and prone to injuries?
   g. Is there evidence of increased stress on the family system?

4. If the client is a victim of rape, take the following additional steps:
   a. Collect assessment data required by law from victims of rape.
   b. Follow agency protocol as well as legal guidelines to ensure an **unbroken chain of evidence.**
5. Be aware of personal (nurse's) feelings and responses to family violence and abuse.
   a. The nurse's personal memories may be reactivated by issues of violence and abuse.
   b. Negative feelings may emerge, including anger, blame, feeling overwhelmed, frustration, avoidance, fear, and disgust.
   c. Positive feelings may emerge, including hope, support, caring, helpfulness, commitment, and understanding.
   d. The nurse should seek support for self-responses and feelings that interfere with her ability to be therapeutic.

B. Nursing diagnoses

1. Analyze the collected data to determine the presence of abuse.
   a. Analyze the family functioning, including evidence of characteristics common in abusers and current stressors affecting the family.
   b. Analyze the family's coping resources and abilities, including use of community resources.
2. Establish individualized nursing diagnoses for the **abuse victim,** as needed.
   a. *Anxiety*
   b. *Delayed growth and development*
   c. *Fear*
   d. *Hopelessness*
   e. *Impaired skin integrity*
   f. *Ineffective coping*
   g. *Ineffective denial*
   h. *Pain*
   i. *Post-trauma syndrome*
   j. *Rape-trauma syndrome*
   k. *Risk for injury*
   l. *Risk for trauma*
   m. *Situational low self-esteem*
   n. *Spiritual distress*
   o. *Unilateral neglect*
3. Establish nursing diagnoses for the **family,** as needed.
   a. *Disabled family coping*
   b. *Impaired parenting*
   c. *Ineffective role performance*
   d. *Interrupted family processes*
   e. *Readiness for enhanced parenting*
   f. *Risk for self-directed or other-directed violence*
4. Establish nursing diagnoses for the **abuser,** as needed.
   a. *Chronic low self-esteem*
   b. *Deficient knowledge (specify)*

    c. Impaired social interaction

    d. Ineffective coping

    e. Ineffective role performance

    f. Noncompliance

    g. Risk for self-directed or other-directed violence

    h. Spiritual distress

C. Planning and outcome identification

1. Work with the client, family members, health team members, and community resource representatives in setting realistic goals.
2. Establish desired outcome criteria for the **victim of abuse.**
   a. The client will maintain safety.
   b. The client will receive treatment for physical and psychological injuries.
   c. The client will ventilate feelings by discussing the abusive situation.
   d. The client will develop behaviors of a functioning survivor.
3. Establish desired outcome criteria for the **family.**
   a. The family will identify interfamily violence or abuse.
   b. The family will remain free of violence.
   c. The family will accept assistance and follow through with community referrals.
   d. The family will implement appropriate coping measures to prevent further violence.
   e. The family will promote healthy growth and development of members.
4. Establish desired outcome criteria for the **abuser.**
   a. The abuser will demonstrate acceptance of responsibility for his own behavior.
   b. The abuser will establish and maintain impulse controls and coping strategies.
   c. The abuser will cope with the legal ramifications of abusive behavior, accepting court-determined punishment.
   d. The abuser will cooperate with the recommended treatment program.
   e. The abuser will refrain from violence against others.

D. Implementation

1. For the **abuse victim,** take the following measures:
   a. Provide first aid or medical treatment as needed.
   b. If violence or abuse is imminent, separate the victim from the perpetrator.
   c. Provide reports to state protective services for child and elder abuse as required by law; in the case of battered women, reporting is required when injury is from a gun, a knife, or other weapon.
   d. In cases of suspected sexual abuse, follow agency and legal protocols for collection and preservation of evidence in a recognized chain of custody procedure.
   e. Ensure sensitive, compassionate care of the victim.
   f. Support the victim for not tolerating abuse.
   g. Listen empathically to the victim's discussion of current and past abuse.
   h. Thoroughly document all injuries and the treatment provided.

      i. Collaborate with the health care team, including initiating interagency referrals and joint-case conferencing.

2. For the **child victim,** take the following measures:

      a. Ensure the child's comfort, using appropriate introductions and avoiding touching the child without permission during the interview.

      b. Use play activities, including drawings, to encourage disclosure (many children are hesitant or unable to verbalize trauma).

      c. Explain all medical tests and procedures in terms a child can understand prior to the procedures.

      d. Encourage the child's relationship with the parents; the nurse cannot become a substitute parent to the exclusion of the child's natural parents.

3. For the **abused woman,** take the following measures:

      a. Communicate acceptance, warmth, and a nonjudgmental attitude; avoid implying in any way that she is at fault for not leaving the abusive situation.

      b. Reinforce concern for her safety and her right to be free of abuse.

      c. Discuss available options, including shelters and legal protection by reporting abuse or seeking a court order.

      d. Respect the victim's decisions, including any decision to return to an abusive situation or a decision to not report the abuse; making decisions for the victim will further erode her self-esteem and reinforce her sense of powerlessness.

      e. Help the victim to develop a plan to ensure safety, including hiding an extra set of house and car keys; requesting a neighbor to call police if violence begins; having important documents (birth certificate, bank account numbers, social security numbers, and receipts for rent and utilities) available; having a list of phone numbers for emergency shelter, legal aid, police, counselor, and support groups.

4. For the **elder victim,** take the following measures:

      a. Be patient and allow the client enough time to discuss the situation.

      b. Respect the client's dignity and avoid being judgmental.

      c. Discuss options for ensuring the client's safety, such as temporary hospital admission, placement in a safe home, or a court order of protection.

      d. Provide a list of resources and support services, including adult protective services, public legal services, victim resource agency, local unit on aging, and 24-hour elder abuse hotline.

      e. If the elderly client is not competent to make decisions, guardianship arrangements need to be made.

5. For the **abuser,** take the following measures:

      a. If the perpetrator is threatening or under the influence of drugs or alcohol, call security or the police to ensure the safety of the family and staff.

      b. Inform the abuser of your duty to report the abuse to the appropriate agency.

      c. Enlist the aid of experienced health team personnel (clinical nurse specialist, social worker, protective agency representative, mental health crisis worker) to initiate intervention.

    d. Keep in mind that, in situations of child abuse, it may be more therapeutic for the nurse to view the abusive parent as a client and the child as a victim of abuse.

    e. Encourage the perpetrator to accept responsibility for the violent behaviors if he has acknowledged the abuse.

    f. Communicate the belief that violent behaviors can be controlled and that more appropriate functioning is possible.

    g. Encourage and refer the abuser to community resources, such as mental health services, parent education classes, self-help groups (Parents Anonymous), and respite care services for elders.

  6. For the **family,** take the following measures:

    a. Educate the family about the importance of individuals accepting responsibility for their own behavior.

    b. Teach them to acknowledge stressful situations.

    c. Advise them to develop problem-solving and coping strategies.

    d. Teach the parents effective parenting skills.

    e. Encourage the use of community resources and professional assistance in improving family functioning.

  7. For the **community,** take the following measures:

    a. Be a responsible professional member of the community by promoting social changes that enhances family functioning.

    b. Work to alleviate conditions associated with violence (poverty, inadequate housing, dysfunctional social attitude toward violence, substance abuse); for example, join community volunteer organizations (Victim's Resources) or lobby local, state, and federal legislators for changes helpful to families below the poverty level.

    c. Work to develop and maintain resources for families (child-care services, respite care for elders, educational programs, support groups); for example, join community volunteer organizations, such as parent-teacher groups or youth athletic leagues.

    d. Support and promote legal and legislative efforts to eliminate family violence.

E. Outcome evaluation

  1. The victim of violence achieves and maintains safety.

  2. The victim of violence demonstrates improved self-esteem and self-empowerment.

  3. The family uses community resources to achieve improved coping.

  4. The abuser accepts responsibility for violent behavior and follows through with any court-ordered punishment.

  5. The abuser refrains from violence against others.

Study questions

1. An 11-year-old child complains to the school nurse about nausea and dizziness. While assessing the child, the nurse notices a black eye that looks like a new injury. This is the third time in 1 month that the child has visited the nurse. Each time, the child provides vague explanations for various injuries. Which of the following is the school nurse's priority intervention?
1. Contact the child's parents and ask about the child's injury.
2. Encourage the child to be truthful with her.
3. Question the teacher about the parent's behavior.
4. Report suspicion of abuse to the proper authorities.

2. A community nurse is making a home visit to a family of three: a mother, a father, and their child. The mother tells the nurse that the father (who is not present) has hit the child on several occasions when he was drinking. The mother further explains that she has talked her husband into going to Alcoholics Anonymous and asks the nurse not to interfere, so her husband won't get angry and refuse treatment. Which of the following is the best response by the nurse?
1. The nurse agrees not to interfere if the husband attends an Alcoholics Anonymous meeting that evening.
2. The nurse commends the mother's efforts and agrees to let her handle things.
3. The nurse commends the mother's efforts and also contacts protective services.
4. The nurse confronts the mother's failure to protect the child.

3. During a well-child checkup, a mother tells the nurse about a recent situation in which her child needed to be disciplined by her husband. The child was slapped in the face for not getting her husband breakfast on Saturday, despite being told on Thursday never to prepare food for him. The nurse analyzes the family system and concludes it is dysfunctional. All of the following factors contribute to this dysfunction except:
1. conflictual relationships of parents.
2. inconsistent communication patterns.
3. rigid, authoritarian roles.
4. use of violence to establish control.

4. Which of the following statements about family violence is true?
1. Family violence affects every socioeconomic level.
2. Family violence is caused by drug and alcohol abuse.
3. Family violence predominantly occurs in lower socioeconomic levels.
4. Family violence rarely occurs during pregnancy.

5. The nurse is assessing a parent who abused her child. Which of the following risk factors would the nurse expect to find in this case?
1. Flexible role functioning between parents
2. History of the parent having been abused as a child
3. Single-parent home situation
4. Presence of parental mental illness

6. A woman is admitted to the emergency department with a fractured arm. She explains to the nurse that her injury resulted when she provoked her drunken husband, who then pushed her. Which of the following best describes the nurse's understanding of the wife's explanation?

1. The wife's explanation is appropriate acceptance of her responsibility.
2. The wife's explanation is an atypical reaction of an abused woman.
3. The wife's explanation is evidence that the woman may be an abuser as well as a victim.
4. The wife's explanation is a typical response of a victim accepting blame for the abuser.

7. A community nurse conducts a primary prevention, home-visit assessment for a newborn and mother. The mother has three other children, the oldest of whom is age 12. The mother tells the nurse that her 12-year-old daughter is expected to prepare family meals, to look after the younger children, and to clean the house once a week. Which of the following is the most appropriate nursing diagnosis for this family situation?

1. *Delayed growth and development, related to performance expectations of child*
2. *Anxiety (moderate), related to difficulty managing home situation*
3. *Impaired parenting, related to role reversal of mother and child*
4. *Social isolation, related to lack of extended family assistance*

8. What is the priority nursing intervention for a child or elder victim of abuse?

1. Assess the scope of the abuse problem.
2. Analyze family dynamics.
3. Implement measures to ensure the victim's safety.
4. Teach appropriate coping skills.

9. A nurse working in the emergency department is conducting an interview with a victim of spousal abuse. Which step should the nurse take first?

1. Contact the appropriate legal services.
2. Ensure privacy for interviewing the victim away from the abuser.
3. Establish a rapport with the victim and the abuser.
4. Request the presence of a security guard.

10. Which of the following assessment findings would lead the nurse to suspect that an 8-year-old child is the victim of sexual abuse?

1. The child is fearful of the caregiver and other adults.
2. The child has a lack of peer relationships.
3. The child has self-injurious behavior.
4. The child has interest in things of a sexual nature.

11. Which situation would the nurse identify as placing a client at high risk for caregiver abuse?

1. An adult child quits her job to move in and care for a parent with severe dementia.
2. An elderly man with severe heart disease resides in a personal care home and is visited frequently by his adult child.
3. An elderly parent with limited mobility lives alone and receives help from several adult children.
4. A wife cares for her husband who is in the early stages of Alzheimer's disease and has a network of available support persons.

12. While performing a prenatal assessment, the clinic nurse suspects that her client has been abused. Which of the following questions would be most appropriate?
1. Are you being threatened or hurt by your partner?"
2. "Are you frightened of your partner?"
3. "Is something bothering you?"
4. "What happens when you and your partner argue?"

13. Which nursing assessment findings are physical signs of sexual abuse of a female child? Select all that apply.
1. Enuresis
2. Red and swollen labia and rectum
3. Vaginal tears
4. Injuries in different stages of healing
5. Cigarette burns
6. Lice infestation

14. A client tells the community health nurse that her boyfriend has been abusive and she is afraid of him, but she doesn't want to leave. The client asks the nurse for assistance. Which nursing interventions are appropriate in this situation? Select all that apply.
1. Help the client to develop a plan to ensure safety, including phone numbers for emergency help.
2. Help the client to get her boyfriend into an appropriate treatment program.
3. Communicate acceptance, avoiding any implication that the client is at fault for not leaving.
4. Help the client to explore available options, including shelters and legal protection.
5. Tell the client that she should leave because things will not improve.
6. Reinforce concern for the client's safety and her right to be free of abuse.

Answer key

1. The answer is 4.

The nurse is obligated to report suspicion of child abuse to the appropriate protective services. Failure to do so can risk further endangerment of the child, and failure to report is a misdemeanor violation on the part of the nurse. The parents will be contacted and an investigation will proceed under the legal authority of the child protective service agency. Although the nurse would expect to establish rapport with the child, encouraging the child to be truthful would send the message that the nurse believes the child is lying; therefore, this intervention would be inappropriate. Questioning the teacher may or may not provide validation of the nurse's suspicions; regardless, this intervention does not ensure the child's safety, which is the priority.

2. The answer is 3.

The nurse would validate and reinforce the mother's efforts to seek help; however, the nurse must also report the abuse to the appropriate protective services. The priority is to maintain the child's safety. The responses in options 1 and 2 are inappropriate; the nurse is failing to provide for the child's safety and is not following legal guidelines. In option 4, the nurse is alienating the mother, as well as failing to follow legal guidelines and ensure the child's safety.

3. The answer is 1.

There is no evidence in this situation that the parents are in conflict; in fact, the mother is describing that the child "needed to be disciplined." Often, in dysfunctional families, one child is singled out to be the victim and is the recipient of blame for problems. The inconsistent communication pattern is that the child received conflicting messages regarding preparation of food. The rigid authoritarian roles demonstrated by the mother's indicate that the child needs discipline from the father. This is an example of a rigid role expectation of the father as disciplinarian. Also, the father used violence to retain the position of control.

4. The answer is 1.

Family violence occurs in all socioeconomic levels, races, religions, and cultural groups. Although violence is associated with substance abuse, it is not the singular cause. The statement that family violence predominantly occurs in lower socioeconomic levels is false. Abuse often occurs during pregnancy; about 23% of all pregnant women seeking prenatal care are victims of abuse.

5. The answer is 2.

One of the most important risk factors is a history of childhood abuse in the parent who abuses. Family violence follows a multigenerational pattern. Parents who are flexible in their roles are characteristic of healthy functioning, not abuse. Single-parent households and a history of mental illness are not established risk factors for child abuse by a parent.

6. The answer is 4.

Self-blame is a common psychological response for a woman who is a victim of abuse. In this situation, the message that

violence occurred because the woman provoked the abuser is accepted and owned by the victim; however, the victim is not responsible for the violence. The statements in options 2 and 3 are not true.

7. The answer is 3.

The role of a 12-year-old child in a family should not be that of the parent. In this situation, the child and mother have reversed roles. There is no evidence that the child has delayed growth or development, the mother in this situation is not demonstrating signs of anxiety, and there is no evidence in this situation that the family is socially isolated.

8. The answer is 3.

The priority intervention when a child or elderly person is involved in a situation of abuse is establishing the safety of the victim. Legislation in most states mandates the reporting of such abuse to ensure prompt intervention and safety. The question is asking about implementing a specific nursing action, not assessing the problem or analyzing the family dynamics. Teaching coping skills is important; however, the priority action involves ensuring safety.

9. The answer is 2.

Privacy, away from the abuser, is important. This allows the victim to discuss the problem freely, without fear of reprisal from the abuser (especially if she decides to return to the abusive situation). In this situation, it is not the nurse's responsibility to contact legal services; it is up to the woman to make the decision to report the abuse. However, whenever injury is inflicted with a gun, knife, or other weapon, the nurse is obligated to report the abuse. Although the nurse would want to establish rapport with the victim, her initial concern would not be to establish rapport with the abuser. The situation does not describe the abuser as currently violent or under the influence of substances; therefore, requesting a security presence is inappropriate at this time.

10. The answer is 4.

An 8-year-old child is in the latency phase of development; in this stage, the child's interest in peers, activities, and school is priority. Interest in sex and things of a sexual nature would occur appropriately during the age of puberty, not at this time. A child who is the victim of sexual abuse, however, may show unusual interest in sex. The assessments in the other answer choices may indicate abuse, but not necessarily sexual abuse.

11. The answer is 1.

In this situation, the adult child has given up her usual role as well as moved her place of residence to care for her parent. Caring for someone with severe dementia is very stressful, requiring almost 24-hour vigilance to ensure safety and meet needs. This situation places the caregiver at high risk for stress and abuse. The caregivers in option 2 are the staff working in the personal care home; the adult child does not have primary responsibility and, therefore, would not be at high risk for severe stress and

abuse. In options 3 and 4, the caregivers are receiving support and no one person has primary responsibility. This will decrease the risk for severe caregiver stress.

12. The answer is 1.

The use of a simple, direct question, asked in an empathic manner, is best to validate the presence of an abusive situation. The other questions are indirect and may not lead to the discussion of an abusive situation.

13. The answer is 1, 2, 3.

These are all indications that a female child has been the victim of sexual abuse. Options 4, 5, and 6 are signs of physical abuse of a child, not sexual abuse.

14. The answer is 1, 3, 4, 6.

These are all appropriate nursing interventions for the victim of domestic violence. The client is not responsible for seeking help for the abuser, and encouraging her to do so may reinforce the client's feeling responsible for the abuse. Advising the client to leave is inappropriate; the client must decide for herself whether to leave, and the nurse must respect any decision the client makes. Making the decision for the client will erode her self-esteem and reinforce her sense of powerlessness.

10

Childhood and Adolescent Psychiatric Disorders

I. OVERVIEW OF CHILDHOOD AND ADOLESCENT PSYCHIATRIC DISORDERS

A. Key concepts

1. Mental disorders in children are common, but are generally underdiagnosed and undertreated.

   a. Mental health problems occur in 15% to 22% of children and adolescents.

   b. Less than 20% of children and adolescents with a mental health problem receive treatment.

2. Attention deficit-hyperactivity disorder (ADHD) is the most common mental health disorder effecting children; its incidence is estimated at 6% to 9%.

B. Diagnosis

1. The diagnosis of mental disorders in children and adolescents depends on behavior that is inappropriate for the child's age and deviant when compared to cultural norms; the deviant behavior must also create deficits or impairments in adaptive functioning.

2. Knowledge of developmental theory is crucial to understanding infant, childhood, and adolescent disorders because deviation from developmental norms is an important warning sign of a problem. (See *Table 2-2, Comparing developmental theories*, page 27.)

3. Certain mental disorders characteristically develop during childhood; the most common of these include mental retardation, developmental disorders, elimination disorders, disruptive behavior disorders, and anxiety disorders.

4. Disorders that occur in children but also have a typical adult onset include mood disorders and psychotic disorders.

5. It is important to remember that children are not miniature adults, and symptoms of mental disorders may be different in a child or adolescent than in an adult with the same disorder. (See *Table 10-1, Comparing symptoms of mental illness at different developmental ages*.)

II. TYPES OF CHILDHOOD AND ADOLESCENT PSYCHIATRIC DISORDERS

A. Pervasive developmental disorders

1. These disorders are characterized by severe and pervasive impairment in several areas of development: reciprocal social interaction skills, communication skills, or the presence of stereotyped behavior, interests, and activities.

2. **Mental retardation** is characterized by substandard limitations in functioning, manifested by significantly subaverage intellectual functioning (an IQ less than 70) and related limitations in two or more adaptive skill areas.

   a. Adaptive skill areas include communication, self-care, activities of daily living, social skills, functioning in a community, self-direction, health and safety, functional academics, and leisure and work.

   b. Mental retardation manifests before age 18.

TABLE 10-1

Comparing symptoms of mental illness at different developmental ages

Symptoms of mental illness manifest differently in children, adolescents, and adults, as noted in the chart below.

Disorder	Child and adolescent	Adult
Major depressive disorder	■ Negativism, acting out ■ Physical complaints, weight loss ■ Delays or regression in developmental tasks ■ Sadness, apathy, clinging behavior ■ Nightmares ■ Academic difficulties ■ Intense mood swings ■ Self-loathing, low self-esteem ■ Suicidal thoughts	■ Depressed mood, sadness, crying ■ Decreased interest in previously enjoyable activities ■ Weight loss or gain ■ Insomnia or hypersomnia ■ Fatigue, loss of energy ■ Decreased ability to concentrate ■ Recurrent thoughts of death, suicide
Anxiety disorders	**Separation anxiety disorder** ■ Difficulty separating from mother (or other significant caregiver) ■ Worry, increased anxiety about possible harm coming to mother or caregiver ■ Anticipation of separation resulting in tantrums, crying, screaming, clinging behaviors ■ Refusal to attend school ■ Refusal to sleep at a friend or relative's house	**Generalized anxiety disorder** ■ Excessive worry, apprehension ■ Restlessness, irritability ■ Decreased ability to concentrate ■ Sleep disturbances

3. **Autistic disorder** (also called **infantile autism** and **childhood autism**) is characterized by markedly abnormal development in social interaction and communication as well as markedly restricted involvement in activities and interests.

  a. Symptoms of this disorder include such behaviors as impaired nonverbal communication; lack of interest in shared activities; delay or lack of spoken language; stereotyped, repetitive, or idiosyncratic language and motor mannerisms; and preoccupation with parts of objects.

  b. In the past, autism was often confused with childhood schizophrenia; however, recent genetic advances have made diagnosis easier. (See *Table 10-2, Comparing autism and childhood schizophrenia*, page 186.)

4. **Asperger's disorder** is a pervasive disorder with essential features that include severe and sustained development of restricted, repetitive patterns of behavior, interests, and activities.

  a. In contrast to autistic disorder, there are no delays in early language, and communication difficulties are usually related to social dysfunction.

  b. Mental retardation is not usually present.

5. **Pervasive developmental disorder not otherwise specified** is characterized by severely impaired social interaction and limited verbal communication; this is considered by many clinicians to be a milder form of autism.

TABLE 10-2

Comparing autism and childhood schizophrenia

Because autism and childhood schizophrenia are both characterized by profound problems with cognitive and behavioral functioning, these disorders were often previously misdiagnosed. However, recent genetic research and better understanding of disease development has made differentiating the two easier.

	Autism	Childhood schizophrenia
Incidence	■ 5 out of 10,000 births (boys affected 4 to 5 times more often than girls)	■ Rare
Age of onset	■ Before age 3	■ Between ages 5 and 10
Etiologic factors	■ Genetics, neurotransmitter abnormality, structural brain abnormality	■ Genetics, pregnancy and birth complications, structural brain abnormalities
Symptoms	■ Aversion to being held ■ Repetitive routines ■ Hand flapping and head banging ■ Clinging to inanimate objects ■ Language and speech difficulties ■ Mental retardation (in many cases)	■ Delusions and hallucinations ■ Regressive behaviors (can mimic those of autism) ■ Cognitive problems
Treatment	■ Medication to reduce repetitive movements and behaviors (antidepressants, such as fluvoxamine [Luvox] and clomipramine [Anafranil]) ■ Behavioral therapy ■ Special education ■ Family education	■ Medication to reduce psychotic symptoms (typical antipsychotics, such as chlorpromazine [Thorazine], and atypical agents, such as olanzapine [Zyprexa]) ■ Behavioral therapy ■ Individual psychotherapy ■ Family therapy and education

B. **Attention deficit and disruptive behavior disorders**

1. **Attention deficit hyperactivity disorder (ADHD)** is characterized by the appearance of at least six symptoms of inattention and/or six symptoms of hyperactivity-impulsivity that have persisted at least 6 months. (See *Display 10-1, Characteristics of ADHD.*)

   a. Impairment resulting from the symptoms must occur in two or more settings (school, work, home).

   b. Symptoms of this disorder are present before age 7.

2. **Conduct disorder** is marked by repetitive, persistent behavior in which the basic rights of others or major age-appropriate societal norms or rules are violated.

   a. Behaviors involve aggressive conduct that causes or threatens physical harm to people and/or animals; nonaggressive conduct that causes property loss or damage; deceitfulness or theft; and serious violations of rules.

   b. A significant number of children with this disorder develop antisocial personality disorder after age 18; substance abuse disorders are also common to this population.

DISPLAY 10-1
Characteristics of ADHD

Children with attention deficit hyperactivity disorder (ADHD) typically share some of these common characteristics, which are often identified by teachers, parents, and others in close contact with the client:
- difficulty paying attention to details
- careless mistakes in schoolwork
- difficulty concentrating on one activity at a time
- talking constantly, even at inappropriate times

- running around in a disruptive way when required to be seated or quiet
- fidgeting and squirming constantly
- trouble waiting for a turn
- easy distraction by things going on around them
- impulsively blurting out answers to questions
- misplacement of schoolbooks or toys
- inattention, even when directly addressed.

---

    3. Oppositional defiant disorder is characterized by a recurrent pattern of negativistic, defiant, disobedient, and hostile behavior toward authority figures that persists for at least 6 months.

        a. Typical behaviors include loss of temper, arguing with adults, actively defying or refusing to comply with rules of adults, deliberately annoying others, blaming others for own mistakes, being easily annoyed by others, and being angry and resentful.

        b. The diagnosis is made if the behaviors occur more frequently than typical for children of a comparable age and developmental level and if there is significant impairment in social, academic, or occupational functioning.

C. Anxiety disorders

    1. Anxiety disorders often begin in childhood or adolescence and continue into adulthood.

    2. Obsessive-compulsive disorder, generalized anxiety disorder, and **phobias** are common in children and adolescents, with symptoms similar to those seen in adults.

    3. Separation anxiety disorder is a childhood disorder characterized by the fear of being separated from the person to whom the child is most attached; symptoms include refusal to attend school, somatic complaints, severe anxiety about separation, and worry about harm coming to a significant caretaker. (See *Table 10-1, Comparing symptoms of mental illness at different developmental ages*, page 185.)

D. Schizophrenia

    1. Childhood schizophrenia is rare, and diagnosis is difficult; symptoms can mimic pervasive development disorders such as autism. (See *Table 10-2, Comparing autism and childhood schizophrenia.*)

    2. Although little research has been conducted on childhood schizophrenia, some characteristic behaviors have been noted, including:

        a. Severe cognitive and behavioral disturbances

        b. Social withdrawal

        c. Impaired communication.

    3. Schizophrenia in adolescents is more common.

        a. Incidence during late adolescence is high.

b. Symptoms are similar to those of adults; initial symptoms may include an extreme change in usual behaviors, social isolation, peculiar mannerisms, decreased academic performance, and acting-out behaviors.

E. Mood disorders

1. Mood disorders are less common in children and adolescents than in adults.

    a. The prevalence in children and adolescents ranges from 1% to 5% for **depressive disorders.**

    b. The existence of **bipolar disorder (manic type)** in young children is a matter of some controversy.

    c. Prevalence of bipolar illness in adolescents is estimated at about 1%; symptoms of depression in children are similar to those observed in adults. (See *Table 10-1, Comparing symptoms of mental illness at different developmental ages*, page 185.)

2. Children with mood disorders, especially adolescents, must be carefully assessed for an increased risk of **suicide**—the third leading cause of death in individuals ages 15 to 24. (See *Display 10-2, Warning signs of suicide in adolescents*.)

F. Substance abuse disorders

1. The symptoms and behaviors of substance abuse in children are similar to those in adults. (See Chapter 8, page 141, for a full discussion of specific substances and symptoms.)

2. About 32% of all adolescents have a substance abuse disorder.

    a. Rates of alcohol or illicit drug use are higher in boys than in girls.

    b. The greatest risk for developing a substance use disorder occurs between ages 15 and 24.

    c. Substance use can progress to addiction faster in adolescence; for example, substance use can progress to addiction in 2 years in adolescents compared with 15 to 20 years in adults.

3. Risk factors include a family history of substance abuse, dysfunctional family system, peer pressure, attempt at rebellion, conflicting societal messages about appropriate use and value of substances, poor self-esteem, and lack of or pressure to achieve academic success.

DISPLAY 10-2
Warning signs of suicide in adolescents

Suicide is the third leading cause of death during adolescence, and those with mood disorders are at serious risk. Nurses and other clinicians should be alert to the following warning signs:

- sudden withdrawal from friends, family, and regular activities
- violent or highly rebellious behaviors
- drug or alcohol abuse
- unusual neglect of personal appearance
- decline in quality of schoolwork; truancy
- running away
- excessive fatigue and somatic complaints
- poor response to praise or rewards
- verbal hints, overt threats about suicide
- giving away prized possessions

   4. Comorbidity with other psychiatric disorders (mood disorders, anxiety disorders, and disruptive behavior disorders) is common.

   5. Warning signs of adolescent substance abuse include the following:

      a. Decline in social and academic functioning

      b. Change from previous functioning, such as developing aggressive behaviors or withdrawing from family interaction

      c. Personality changes and low frustration tolerance

      d. Associations with other adolescents using substances

      e. Hiding or lying about use.

III. CAUSES OF CHILDHOOD AND ADOLESCENT PSYCHIATRIC DISORDERS

A. Key concepts

   1. There is no single cause of psychiatric disorders in children and adolescents.

   2. Multiple circumstances, including psychobiologic factors, family dynamics, and environmental influences, combine in a complex manner to cause mental illness.

B. Psychobiologic factors

   1. Genetics and family history have been implicated in such disorders as mental retardation, autism, childhood schizophrenia, conduct disorders, bipolar disorders, and anxiety disorders.

   2. Research has revealed the presence of structural brain abnormalities and neurotransmitter alterations in patients with autism, childhood schizophrenia, and ADHD.

   3. Prenatal influences, such as maternal infections, lack of prenatal care, and substance abuse by the mother, may all contribute to neurodevelopmental abnormalities associated with mental disorders.

   4. Birth trauma associated with a decreased oxygen supply to the fetus is significant in the development of mental retardation and other neurodevelopmental disorders.

   5. Chronic physical illness or disability may lead to coping difficulties for the child.

C. Family dynamics

   1. Child abuse has been closely linked to mental illness.

      a. Children subjected to ongoing abuse in early childhood have less developed brains.

      b. Abuse and its subsequent effect on the developing brain are associated with psychological problems, such as depression, memory problems, learning difficulties, impulsivity, and difficulties in relationships.

   2. A dysfunctional family system may also lead to mental illness in children.

      a. Relationships characterized by lack of nurturing, poor communication, lack of boundaries between generations, and enmeshment are all implicated in the development of mental disorders. (See page 246.)

      b. Inadequate coping skills in resolving conflict issues among family members also affect the child's mental health and development.

3. The lack of adequate parental role models can influence children to adopt dysfunctional behaviors.

D. Environmental factors

1. The effects of poverty—inadequate prenatal care, poor nutrition, and lack of necessities associated with insufficient income—adversely affect normal growth and development.
2. Homelessness among families is increasing at an alarming rate.
   a. Homeless children have multiple health needs that affect their emotional and psychological development.
   b. Studies have indicated an increased rate of minor childhood illnesses, developmental delays, and psychological problems among homeless children when compared with control samples.
3. Family culture, especially parental behaviors that are dramatically atypical from the surrounding culture, can lead to lack of peer group acceptance of the child and psychological difficulties.

IV. MANAGING CHILDHOOD AND ADOLESCENT PSYCHIATRIC DISORDERS

A. Key concepts

1. Management of childhood mental illness and psychiatric disorders is largely community-based, given today's managed care environment; however, hospital-based treatment may be used as well.
2. Medications are sometimes prescribed, depending on the specific disorder.

B. Community-based treatment

1. **Primary prevention** involves a variety of social programs directed at creating an environment that is health enhancing for children and supportive to parents; examples include:
   a. Early prenatal care
   b. Early intervention programs for parents with known risk factors for child-rearing problems
   c. Head Start programs.
2. **Secondary prevention** includes early case finding of children with problems in school systems so that prompt treatment may be initiated.
   a. Methods include individual counseling with school guidance programs and community mental health referrals, crisis intervention services for families in traumatic situations, group counseling in the school, and peer counseling programs.
   b. School nurses, community health nurses, and nurses employed in primary practice settings may all contribute to early case finding and initiation of prompt treatment.
3. Therapeutic support for children is provided through individual psychotherapy, play therapy, and special education programs for children who are unable to par-

ticipate in the normal school system; behavioral methods of treatment are commonly used to assist the child in developing more adaptive coping methods.

4. Family therapy and family education are important to assist families in acquiring necessary skills and support for making changes that enhance functioning of all family members.

C. Hospital-based treatment

1. Specialized units treating children and adolescents are established in psychiatric hospitals; treatment in these units is usually reserved for clients who have not benefited from less restrictive alternative methods, or for clients at high risk for violence to themselves or others.

2. Partial hospitalization programs are also available, providing on-site school programs directed toward the special needs of the child with a mental illness.

3. The use of seclusion and restraint for control of disruptive behavior is controversial.

   a. Research indicates that this method can be traumatic for the child and is not effective for learning adaptive responses.

   b. Least-restrictive measures include time-out, therapeutic holding, avoiding power struggles, and intervening early to prevent escalating behaviors.

D. Pharmacotherapy

1. Medications are used as one method of treatment.

2. Psychotropic medications are used cautiously in children and adolescent clients because multiple side effects are associated with these drugs. (See *Drug chart 10-1, Selected medications for treating childhood and adolescent psychiatric disorders*, page 192.)

   a. The physiologic differences of children and adolescents affect the dose, clinical response, and side effects of psychotropic medications.

   b. The developmental differences in neurotransmitters in children may affect the therapeutic effect of psychotropic medications, leading to inconsistent results, especially with tricyclic antidepressants.

NURSING PROCESS OVERVIEW

V. CARE OF THE CHILD OR ADOLESCENT WITH A PSYCHIATRIC DISORDER

A. Assessment

1. Review the client's history for precipitating stressors and significant data, including genetic-biologic vulnerability (family history), stressful family and life events, results of mental status exam, history of physical and psychological problems and their treatment, and medication history. (See *Key questions 10-1, Assessing children and adolescents with psychiatric disorders*, page 193.)

2. Note the child's growth and development patterns and compare them to standard instruments, such as the Denver Developmental Screening Test.

3. Note evidence of appropriate developmental task achievement for the child or adolescent. (See *Table 2-2, Comparing developmental theories*, page 27.)

DRUG CHART 10-1
Selected medications for treating childhood and adolescent psychiatric disorders

Drug ‹	Disorder or specific behaviors	Rationale for use
Typical antipsychotics chlorpromazine (Thorazine) haloperidol (Haldol) risperidone (Risperdal) *Atypical antipsychotics* olanzapine (Zyprexa)	▪ Childhood schizophrenia ▪ Other psychotic disorders ▪ Acute agitation ▪ Motor hyperactivity and impulsiveness	▪ Typical and atypical antipsychotics block dopamine receptor sites and thus decrease psychotic symptoms. Sedative effects of these drugs are useful for hyperactive states. The advantage of atypical antipsychotics is that they have fewer extrapyramidal side effects.
Tricyclic antidepressants clomipramine (Anafranil) imipramine (Tofranil) *Selective serotonin reuptake inhibitors (SSRIs)* fluoxetine (Prozac) fluvoxamine (Luvox) sertraline (Zoloft)	▪ Depression ▪ Attention deficit hyperactivity disorder (ADHD) ▪ Separation anxiety disorder ▪ Obsessive-compulsive disorder	▪ Tricyclic antidepressants are used to alter serotonin and norepinephrine and thus cause mood elevation. They also decrease repetitive behaviors. ▪ SSRIs selectively increase serotonin at the synapse and elevate mood.
Psychostimulants methylphenidate (Ritalin) pemoline (Cylert) *Nonstimulants* atomoxetine (Strattera)	▪ ADHD	▪ Psychostimulants alter neurotransmitters and thus increase attention span and the ability to concentrate. ▪ Nonstimulants block presynaptic norepinephrine transport in the brain, improving core symptoms of ADHD.

4. Perform a physical examination of the child or adolescent, noting normal and abnormal data.

5. Assess the client's behavioral responses for indications of an **attention disorder** or a **behavioral disorder**; be sure to assess direct interaction, observation of play, and interaction with family and peers.

   a. Is the client displaying aggressive or destructive behaviors?

   b. Does the client have academic problems? Truancy?

   c. Does the client have discipline or conduct problems?

   d. Does the client have problems with peers?

   e. Does the client demonstrate poor impulse control, rebellion, and defiance?

   f. Does the client demonstrate restlessness or hyperactivity?

   g. Does the client demonstrate sexual acting out?

   h. Does the client use or abuse substances, such as alcohol or illicit drugs?

   i. Does the client demonstrate withdrawal or social isolation?

KEY QUESTIONS 10-1
Assessing children and adolescents with psychiatric disorders

Questions	Information gathered
Who are the members of your family? *Who do you live with?*	Family system
Which people in your life do you think are supportive and helpful to you?	Quality of relationships with support persons
How do your parents or caregivers discipline you?	Family discipline patterns
What type of activities do you enjoy doing with your friends?	Positive and negative influences of peer group
Have you experienced any of the following? *– Parent-child conflict* *– School problems* *– Problems with peers* *– Running away* *– Trouble with legal system* *– Mood swings* *– Feelings of sadness, lack of interest* *– Suspicious or unusual thoughts*	Behavior, thoughts, and feelings indicative of specific disorders
What is your experience with alcohol, other drugs, or both?	Drug or alcohol use
What do you think are your strengths? What do you like about yourself?	Self-esteem

6. Observe for evidence of a **cognitive disorder.**
   a. Does the client have a lack of reality base or misperception of reality?
   b. Does the client have hallucinations or delusions?
   c. Does the client have language or speech problems?
   d. Does the client have poor attention span or learning difficulties?
   e. Does the client have unusual thought patterns or suspicion of others?
7. Observe for evidence of a **mood disorder.**
   a. Does the client have mood swings?
   b. Does the client have intense emotions (rage, devastation)?
   c. Does the client have a lack of affect?
   d. Does the client have feelings of sadness? Crying? Sense of hopelessness?
   e. Does the client have thoughts of suicide?
8. Assess the strengths and weaknesses of the client's **family system.**
   a. What are the anxiety levels of the family? What coping measures are used?
   b. What is the quality of the relationships in the family? Is there evidence of overt conflict?
   c. Are generational boundaries appropriate or blurred?

    d. Is communication open or poor?

    e. Is the family involved in a larger social system, such as extended family, friends, or community activities? *(Note:* The more isolated the family is from others, the more severe the pathology.)

    f. Does the family have basic knowledge of growth and development?

    g. What are the parenting skills? What are the methods of discipline?

B. Nursing diagnoses

  1. Analyze the situation to determine appropriate diagnoses for the client and family.

    a. Compare the client's growth and developmental level to norms appropriate for the age group.

    b. Prioritize the client's physical, behavioral, cognitive, and mood symptoms.

    c. Analyze the relationship of the client's symptoms to family system strengths and weaknesses.

    d. Analyze the client's level of self-esteem.

    e. Determine the client or family's view of the current problem.

  2. Establish individualized nursing diagnoses for client and family, as needed.

    a. Compromised family coping

    b. Delayed growth and development

    c. Disturbed thought processes

    d. Impaired social interaction

    e. Impaired verbal communication

    f. Ineffective coping

    g. Interrupted family processes

    h. Readiness for enhanced parenting

    i. Risk for impaired parent/infant/child attachment

    j. Risk for impaired parenting

    k. Risk for self-directed or other-directed violence

    l. Situational low self-esteem

C. Planning and outcome identification

  1. Work with the client and the family in setting realistic goals.

  2. Establish desired outcome criteria for the client and family.

    a. The client will demonstrate decreased anxiety levels and increased coping skills.

    b. The client will control impulsive or acting-out behaviors.

    c. The client will state improvement in mood.

    d. The client will demonstrate improved attention and the ability to participate in learning activities.

    e. The client will participate in the recommended treatment program and follow through with specific referrals.

    f. The client will interact with peers and establish friendships.

    g. The family will demonstrate improved ability to handle specific problematic child behaviors.

    h. The parents will actively participate in an ongoing treatment program.

D. Implementation

1. For **all clients,** take the following measures:

   a. Establish trust.

   b. Listen actively, demonstrating concern and support.

   c. Promote clear, honest, straightforward communication.

   d. Establish a position of neutrality; do not take sides of either the parent or child.

   e. Support the strengths of the client and the family.

   f. Use the cognitive model to explain the relationship among thoughts, feelings, and behavior (thoughts lead to feelings and behavior, but a person does not have to act on feelings or thoughts).

   g. Participate in the client's inpatient treatment plan; construct a safe, structured environment with the opportunity for the client to increase self-functioning and self-esteem.

   h. Positively reinforce acceptable behavior.

   i. Participate in play therapy, allowing the child to express himself through imaginative play.

   j. Collaborate with the client's family, school, and mental health team.

   k. Encourage the use of community support groups for the client and family.

   l. Teach the client and family information about the client's specific disorder and its treatment.

   m. Teach the family how to nurture the child's emotional health. (See *Client and family teaching 10-1, Guidelines for children and adolescents with psychiatric disorders.*)

CLIENT AND FAMILY TEACHING 10-1
Guidelines for children and adolescents with psychiatric disorders

Provide information about mental illness and the client's specific psychiatric disorder.
- Psychiatric disorders in children and adolescents occur because of a complex interaction among many factors; there is no single cause.
- Children and adolescents with a psychiatric disorder may respond to treatment, such as therapy for the child, family therapy and education, and medication.
- Prescribed medication, taken as directed, can help stabilize moods and bring about more normal behavior.

Teach the parents ways to nurture their child's emotional well-being.
- Focus on the "positives" in the child, providing praise when behavior is acceptable.
- When behavior escalates, decrease stimulation in the immediate environment and provide a time-out.

- Encourage the child's interests, and accept his limitations.
- Foster the child's self-worth and appropriate independence for age and developmental level.
- Set clear, consistent limits, and follow them.
- Seek help when overwhelmed by the child's feelings or behaviors, or when you cannot control your own anger and frustration.
- Maintain a parental role; children respond to parents who act as parents, not as friends.
- Strengthen spousal relationships; if separation or divorce occurs, negotiate and collaborate in areas involving the child.
- Maintain your own interests; overfocusing on the child's problems is not helpful.
- Seek help from community support groups, which focus on the experiences of children and families dealing with issues and problems concerning the child's diagnosis.

2. For the child or adolescent with a **pervasive developmental disorder,** take the following measures:
   a. Create a safe environment, and help the parents to do so at home.
   b. Help the parents to decrease their feelings of guilt and blame.
   c. Ensure the consistency of caregivers for the child in the hospital, in school, and at home.
   d. Help the parents and siblings identify and discuss their feelings, issues, and problems associated with living with a child with a severe disorder.
   e. Use diversion if the child has increased anxiety or acting-out behaviors; for example, engage the child in a physical activity (riding a bike, playing with a ball) or pleasurable activity (drawing, painting, playing a favorite game).
   f. Provide the child with familiar objects.
3. For the child or adolescent with **ADHD,** take the following measures:
   a. Administer a stimulant medication in the morning to maximize effectiveness for daytime activities.
   b. Assist the family with environmental manipulation to decrease stimuli for behavior control.
   c. Help the family to establish regularly scheduled times for eating, sleeping, playing, and doing homework.
   d. Collaborate with the client's school, family, and mental health team to ensure proper classroom placement.
4. For the child or adolescent with **conduct disorder** or **oppositional defiant disorder,** take the following measures:
   a. Establish firm, consistent limits, describing clearly the consequences of unacceptable behaviors.
   b. Assist the parents in defining and maintaining limits.
   c. Provide positive feedback for appropriate behaviors.
   d. Encourage the client to express anger in an appropriate verbal manner.
   e. Encourage the child to use exercise and activity to expend excess energy from increased anxiety or anger.
   f. Notice cues that behavior is escalating, and intervene early.
5. For the child or adolescent with an **anxiety disorder,** take the following measures (also see pages 45 and 46):
   a. Maintain a calm manner when the client and parents experience increased anxiety.
   b. Teach the client coping measures for handling anxiety.
   c. Use cognitive strategies in discussing the client's fears, pointing out reality issues.
   d. Assist the client to return to school immediately with family support, if separation anxiety is present.
6. For the child or adolescent with a **mood disorder,** take the following measures (also see pages 113 and 114):
   a. Teach the client and family about the client's mood disorder and its causes, symptoms, and treatment.
   b. Use appropriate measures to promote the client's self-esteem.
   c. Use cognitive measures in dealing with negative thoughts and feelings.

      d. Maintain an attitude of hopefulness.

      e. Initiate suicide precautions for the client at risk for suicide.

  7. For the child or adolescent with a **substance abuse disorder,** take the following measures (also see pages 158 and 159):

      a. Teach the client and family about abusive substances and their effects on physical and psychological well-being.

      b. Encourage the client and family to attend self-help groups (Alcoholics Anonymous, Narcotics Anonymous, Alateen, Alanon).

      c. Foster an attitude of hope that the client can achieve and maintain abstinence.

      d. Teach coping measures to handle uncomfortable feelings and situations.

E. Outcome evaluation

  1. The client controls impulsive behaviors.

  2. The client demonstrates normal mood stabilization.

  3. The client participates in an educational program at his appropriate level of ability.

  4. The client interacts socially with peer group.

  5. The client and family demonstrate improved coping skills.

  6. The client and family participate in the recommended treatment program and accept community referrals.

Study questions

1. A 9-year-old child is admitted to a psychiatric treatment unit accompanied by both parents. To establish trust and a position of neutrality, which action would the nurse take?

  1. Encourage the parents to leave while interviewing the child alone.

  2. Interview the child and parents together, observing their interaction.

  3. Provide diversion for the child, and interview the parents alone.

  4. Review the clinical record prior to interviewing the parents.

2. A community nurse is practicing primary prevention for psychiatric disorders in children. On which of the following risk factors would the nurse focus?

  1. Being raised in a single-parent home

  2. Family history of mental illness

  3. Lack of peer friendships

  4. Family culture

3. The school nurse is meeting with the school and health treatment team about a child who has been receiving methylphenidate (Ritalin) for 2 months. The meeting is to evaluate the results of the child's medication use. Which behavior change noted by the teacher will help determine the medication's effectiveness?

  1. Decreased repetitive behaviors

  2. Decreased signs of anxiety

  3. Increased depressed mood

  4. Increased ability to concentrate on tasks

4. Which behavioral assessment in a child is most consistent with a diagnosis of conduct disorder?

  1. Arguing with adults

  2. Gross impairment in communication

  3. Physical aggression toward others

  4. Refusal to separate from caretaker

5. A child with separation anxiety disorder has not attended school for 3 weeks, and she cries and exhibits clinging behaviors when her mother encourages attendance. The priority nursing action by the home-care psychiatric nurse would be to:
    1. assist the child to return to school immediately with family support.
    2. arrange for a home-school teacher to visit for 2 weeks.
    3. encourage family discussion of various problem areas.
    4. use play therapy to help the child express her feelings.

6. An adolescent hospitalized in a psychiatric unit initiates frequent fights with peers. Which implementation is most appropriate?
    1. Anticipate and neutralize potentially explosive situations.
    2. Ignore minor infractions of rules against fighting.
    3. Isolate the adolescent from contact with peers.
    4. Talk to the adolescent each time fighting occurs.

7. The community nurse visits the home of a child recently diagnosed with autism. The parents express feelings of shame and guilt about having somehow caused this problem. Which statement by the nurse would best help alleviate parental guilt?
    1. "Autism is a rare disorder. Your other children shouldn't be affected."
    2. "The specific cause of autism is unknown. However, it is known to be associated with problems in the structure of and chemicals in the brain."
    3. "Sometimes a lack of prenatal care can be the cause of autism."

    4. "Although autism is genetically inherited, if you didn't have testing you could not have known this would happen."

8. An adolescent with a depressive disorder is more likely than an adult with the same disorder to exhibit:
    1. negativism and acting out.
    2. sadness and crying.
    3. suicidal thoughts.
    4. weight gain.

9. The parents of a child with attention deficit hyperactivity disorder tell the nurse they have tried everything to calm their child and nothing has worked. Which action by the nurse is most appropriate initially?
    1. Actively listen to the parents' concern before planning interventions.
    2. Encourage the parents to discuss these issues with the mental health team.
    3. Provide literature regarding the disorder and its management.
    4. Tell the parents they are overreacting to the problem.

10. The nurse questions the parents of a child with oppositional defiant disorder about the roles of each parent in setting rules of behavior. The purpose for this type of questioning is to assess which element of the family system?
    1. Anxiety levels
    2. Generational boundaries
    3. Knowledge of growth and development
    4. Quality of communication

11. The nurse reinforces the behavioral contract for a child having difficulty controlling aggressive behaviors on the psychiatric unit. Which of the following is

the best rationale for this method of treatment?

1. It will assist the child to develop more adaptive coping methods.
2. It will avoid having the nurse be responsible for setting the rules.
3. It will maintain the nurse's role in controlling the child's behavior.
4. It will prevent the child from manipulating the nurse.

12. The nurse is teaching the parents of a child with a pervasive developmental disorder about how to deal with the child when his behavior escalates and he begins throwing things and screaming. Which guideline would be most helpful for the parents to deal with the situation?

1. Accept the child's limitations, and ignore this behavior.
2. Decrease stimulation in the environment, and provide a time-out.
3. Seek help when feeling overwhelmed by the child's behavior.
4. Tell the child to calm down, and encourage quiet activity.

13. The school nurse assesses a child newly diagnosed with attention deficit hyper-activity disorder (ADHD). Which of the following symptoms are characteristic of the disorder? Select all that apply.

1. Constant fidgeting and squirming
2. Excessive fatigue and somatic complaints
3. Difficulty paying attention to details
4. Easily distracted
5. Running away
6. Talking constantly, even when inappropriate

14. The psychiatric nurse is alert to warning signs of suicide in the adolescent population. From the following list, select those behaviors that are indicative of adolescent suicidal thinking. Select all that apply.

1. Giving away prized possessions
2. Associating with friends who are substance abusers
3. Sudden withdrawal from friends and family
4. Having difficulty concentrating on one thing at a time
5. Being easily distracted by environmental events
6. Verbal hints or threats about suicide

Answer key

1. The answer is **2**.

It is important for the nurse to be seen as a neutral person who is interested in the family as an adaptive functioning unit. By conducting the admission interview with the parents and child together, the nurse establishes this neutral role from the beginning. The responses in options 1 and 3 separate the parents and the child, and thus the nurse does not have an opportunity to establish a position of neutrality. Although the nurse would review the clinical record, this does not demonstrate to the family that she is an advocate for both the parents and the child.

2. The answer is **2**.

Abnormal genes and family history of mental illness have been implicated in many psychiatric disorders occurring in children and adolescents. There is no evidence that being raised in a single-parent home will increase a child's risk of developing a psychiatric disorder. Children who have problems with peers and withdraw from social interaction may have a psychiatric disorder; however, the nurse noting this problem would be practicing secondary, not primary, prevention. Family culture is not a risk factor unless parental behavior is dramatically atypical from surrounding culture.

3. The answer is **4.**
Methylphenidate (Ritalin) is used as a method of treatment for ADHD. Evidence of increased ability to concentrate on tasks while taking this medication would establish the drug's effectiveness. This medication will not decrease repetitive behaviors or signs of anxiety. Although it is a psychostimulant, this drug is not used for depression; consequently, mood elevation is not a measure of the drug's effectiveness in this situation.

4. The answer is **3.**
Physical aggression toward others is a significant criterion consistent with the diagnoses of conduct disorder. Arguing with adults may indicate a lesser disorder, oppositional defiant disorder. Conduct disorder is a problem that involves violation of social rules. Gross impairment in communication and refusal to separate from a caretaker are behaviors that are more consistent with other mental disorders that can affect children.

5. The answer is **1.**
When a child refuses to attend school as part of separation anxiety disorder, it is important to avoid reinforcing this behavior. The nurse's priority would be to assist the child to return to school immediately with support from the family. Arranging for a home-school teacher would reinforce the behavior of not attending school. Although encouraging family discussion of problem areas and the use of play therapy are appropriate

treatment interventions, the priority is returning the child to school.

6. The answer is **1.**
The nurse is responsible for maintaining a safe environment; therefore, it would be appropriate to observe for signs that an explosive situation is developing and to intervene to neutralize the situation, thereby preventing a fight. Ignoring minor infractions of rules against fighting would be incorrect, because fighting on a psychiatric unit would not be a minor infraction and should not be ignored. This could lead to unsafe situations that could escalate out of control. Isolation and seclusion are methods of intervention that can be used as a last resort after less restrictive means are employed. Talking to the adolescent each time a fight occurs does not indicate that the nurse is setting and enforcing clear, consistent rules. The nurse needs to maintain safety and would not allow fighting to occur if it could be avoided.

7. The answer is **2.**
This statement is factual and does not cast blame on anything the parents did or did not do. The parents are not questioning whether other children will be affected; their concern is directed to the current situation and their feelings about it. The statement in option 3 is not true: Lack of prenatal care may be a risk factor in pervasive developmental disorders, but it is not the cause of autism. Although it is thought that there is a genetic component in autism, research has not identified specific genes and there is no diagnostic test for this. The statement in option 4 is misleading and would not alleviate guilt.

8. The answer is **1.**
Adolescents sometimes demonstrate be-

havior that is uncharacteristic of an adult with a psychiatric disorder. In a depressive disorder, an adolescent's negativism and acting out could be signs of depression. Sadness, crying, and suicidal thoughts are behaviors of both adolescents and adults. An adult may experience either weight loss or weigh gain while depressed, whereas an adolescent may experience weight loss.

9. The answer is 1.
The nurse would encourage parents to fully discuss and describe their perception of the problem in order to assess the family system before determining appropriate interventions. In option 2, the nurse has not explored the problem and is deciding before adequately assessing the situation that the mental health team should be consulted. Providing literature regarding the disorder and its management may be a useful intervention; however, the initial action needs to involve a more thorough exploration of the parents' concerns. Telling the parents they are overreacting to the problem is inappropriate because it dismisses the parents' legitimate concerns and belittles their feelings.

10. The answer is 2.
An important element in assessing the family system is determining if the parents establish and maintain appropriate generational boundaries, establishing clear rules and expectations as part of the parental role. Although the parents may have anxiety regarding the role of parental rule setting, the nurse's question is not adequate to assess the anxiety levels. The question concerns the roles of the parents and the child in rule setting. It does not provide data regarding knowledge of growth and development or communication quality.

11. The answer is 1.
Behavioral therapy is employed for the purpose of developing adaptive behavior that will improve coping. The nurse does not avoid setting rules; it is the responsibility of the nurse to establish and maintain appropriate limits. The nurse works to enhance the child's self-functioning and responsibility for his own behavior using appropriate behavioral means to develop better coping. Although reinforcing behavioral contracts will help prevent manipulative behavior by the child, this is not the best rationale for using behavioral treatment, which aims to improve client behavior.

12. The answer is 2.
A child with a pervasive developmental disorder can have bizarre responses to environmental stimuli. By decreasing that stimulating effect and providing a time-out, the child can more readily de-escalate the behaviors. Escalating behaviors, such as those described, require intervention to promote safety. It is inappropriate to ignore this. The situation requires immediate intervention. The parents should seek help when overwhelmed, but they must intervene when safety is an issue. The response in option 4 is inadequate; the child will not be able to calm down without assistance.

13. The answer is 1, 3, 4, 6.
These behaviors are all characteristic of ADHD and indicate that the child is inattentive, hyperactive, and impulsive. Options 2 and 5 are signs of emotional distress in a child and could be associated with a number of different psychiatric diagnoses.

14. The answer is 1, 3, 6.
These are all warning signs that an ado-

lescent is having suicidal thoughts. The nurse should directly question any adolescent about suicide intent when these indicators are noted. Option 2 may indicate that the adolescent has a problem with substance use, but not necessarily suicide. Options 4 and 5 are signs of attention deficit hyperactivity disorder, not suicide.

11 Cognitive Impairment Disorders

I. OVERVIEW OF COGNITIVE IMPAIRMENT DISORDERS

A. Key concepts

1. **Cognitive impairment disorders** are a group of disorders characterized by deficits in cognition (the manner in which the brain processes information) and memory that represents a significant change from the client's previous level of functioning.

   a. The higher brain functions (such as reasoning, orientation, judgment, perception and attention) can all be affected.

   b. Personality and behavioral changes are also common in these disorders.

2. **Delirium** is an acute disorder characterized by cognitive impairment, attention deficit, and a reduced level of orientation (the ability to relate to time, place, and person).

3. **Dementia** is a chronic, progressive disorder characterized by severe impairments in cognitive processes and dysfunctions in personality and behavior.

4. **Amnestic disorders** are characterized by memory impairments in the absence of other significant cognitive impairments.

B. Diagnosing cognitive impairment disorders

1. Medical diagnosis of these disorders is made by careful screening to rule out other possible causes of symptoms.

2. Workup should include:

   a. Mental status examination and neuropsychological testing

   b. Comprehensive blood work, including complete blood count (CBC), blood chemistry panel, vitamin B_{12} and folate levels, thyroid panel, and liver and renal function tests

   c. Brain imaging studies, including computed tomography (CT), positron emission tomography (PET), and magnetic resonance imaging (MRI).

3. Depressive disorders in elderly clients may manifest with symptoms similar to those of cognitive impairment disorders; therefore, depressive disorder should be ruled out.

II. DELIRIUM

A. Key concepts

1. Delirium is characterized by a disturbed consciousness and change in cognition that develops over a short period of time; onset is acute and symptoms occur rapidly.

2. Evidence from the client's history, physical examination, or diagnostic testing indicates that the delirium is a direct physiologic consequence of a general medical condition, substance intoxication or withdrawal, use of medication, or toxin exposure or a combination of these factors.

3. Common symptoms of delirium include:

   a. Impaired consciousness and attention, disorientation

   b. Disorganized thinking and rambling speech

    c. Disturbance in the sleep-wake cycle, such as daytime sleepiness and night-time agitation

    d. Psychomotor changes (hyperactivity and agitation, or hypoactivity and somnolence)

    e. Misinterpretation of situations and reality, illusions, and hallucinations

    f. Labile mood (rapid, unpredictable shifts from one emotional state to another).

B. Types of delirium

    1. In **delirium due to a general medical condition,** multiple medical conditions can be associated with delirium; acute or chronic illnesses, hormonal and nutritional factors, sensory impairments, and various medications as well as surgical procedures can all contribute.

    2. In **substance-induced delirium** and **substance withdrawal delirium,** the client's history, physical examination, and diagnostic study findings indicate the delirium is associated with substance use.

    3. In **delirium due to multiple etiologies,** several medical conditions or a combination of substance use and medical conditions is evident.

    4. **Delirium not otherwise specified** is the *DSM-IV TR* classification applied when insufficient evidence exists to establish a definitive etiology.

C. Causes of delirium

    1. Delirium is complex and usually multifactored.

    2. The following risk factors are associated with delirium:

        a. Advanced age

        b. Preexisting illness

        c. Infection and/or electrolyte and metabolic imbalance

        d. Bone fractures

        e. Brain damage or dementia.

D. Managing delirium

    1. Treatment usually occurs in an acute care medical-surgical setting.

    2. The client typically undergoes a comprehensive diagnostic assessment, and physiologic symptoms are readily treated.

    3. Objectives of treatment include:

        a. Identification of the immediate cause

        b. Correction of the underlying cause

        c. Symptom management

        d. Supportive and safety measures.

III. DEMENTIA

A. Key concepts

    1. Dementia is characterized by multiple cognitive deficits that include memory impairment and at least one of the following cognitive disturbances: aphasia, apraxia, agnosia, or a disturbance in executive functioning.

2. The deficits must be severe enough to cause impairment in occupational or social functioning and must represent a decline in the client's previous level of functioning.

3. Common symptoms include:
   a. **Aphasia:** the loss of language ability; speech is often impoverished, and the client may have difficulty "finding" the right words
   b. **Apraxia:** an impaired ability to carry out motor activities despite intact sensory function
   c. **Confabulation:** filling in memory gaps with detailed fantasy believed by the affected individual
   d. **Sundown syndrome:** increased disorientation and confusion at night
   e. **Perseveration phenomenon:** repetitive behaviors, including pacing and echoing others' words
   f. Memory losses (initially, loss of recent memory; eventually, remote memory impairment)
   g. Disorientation to time, place, and person
   h. Decreased ability to concentrate or to learn new material
   i. Difficulty making decisions
   j. Poor judgment (for example, the client may not be aware of environmental considerations of safety and security).

B. Types of dementia

1. **Dementia of the Alzheimer's type,** the most common of all dementias, accounts for about two-thirds of all dementias involving those over age 65. (See *Table 11-1, Dementia of the Alzheimer's type.*)

2. **Vascular (multi-infarct) dementia,** the second-leading cause of dementia in elderly clients, occurs when blood clots block small blood vessels in the brain and destroy brain tissue.

3. Other types of dementia are associated with general medical conditions, such as Parkinson's disease, Pick's disease, Huntington's chorea, Creutzfeldt-Jakob disease, and HIV.

C. Causes of dementia

1. Dementia can develop as a result of chronic delirium caused by an untreated or untreatable acute condition.

2. Vascular disease may occur with such disorders as hypertension, arteriosclerosis, and atherosclerosis, resulting in cerebrovascular accident and ensuing dementia. (*Note:* Treating hypertension can decrease the client's risk of developing dementia of the Alzheimer's type.)

3. About 40% of those with Parkinson's disease develop dementia.

4. Certain genetic disorders, including Huntington's chorea and Pick's disease, cause dementia.

5. HIV infection can affect the central nervous system, causing HIV encephalopathy or AIDS dementia complex.

6. Structural disorders of brain tissue, such as normal pressure hydrocephalus and injury resulting from a head trauma, can lead to dementia.

TABLE 11-1
Dementia of the Alzheimer's type

The most common form of dementia affecting elderly clients, dementia of the Alzheimer's type may be categorized according to its stage and related symptoms. Although clients do not necessarily pass through the specific sequence of deterioration as outlined below, the stages are helpful in determining the client's current cognitive state.

Stage	Behavior	Affect	Cognitive changes
Mild	• Difficulty completing tasks • Decline in goal-directed activity • Lack of attention to personal appearance and activities of daily living • Withdrawal from usual social activities • Frequent searching for misplaced objects; may accuse others of stealing	• Anxious • Depressed • Frustrated • Suspicious • Fearful	• Recent memory losses (forgets appointments and conversations) • Time disorientation • Decreased ability to concentrate • Difficulty making decisions • Poor judgment
Moderate	• Socially inappropriate behavior • Self-care deficits (bathing, toileting, dressing, grooming) • Wandering and pacing • Hoarding objects • Hyperorality • Disturbance in sleep-wake cycle	• Labile mood • Flat, apathetic • Catastrophic agitation • Paranoia	• Recent and remote memory losses (amnesia) • Confabulation • Disorientation to time, place, and person • Some degree of agnosia, apraxia, and aphasia
Severe	• Decreased ability to ambulate or engage in other motor activities • Decreased swallowing ability • Complete self-care deficits (requires constant care) • Inability to recognize caregiver	• Flat, apathetic • Occasional catastrophic reactions may continue	• Progression of cognitive changes, with increased severity of amnesia, agnosia, apraxia, and aphasia

D. Alzheimer's disease

1. Onset of dementia of the Alzheimer's type is typically slow and progressive. (See *Table 11-1, Dementia of the Alzheimer's type*.)
2. Although no single cause has been implicated in the development of Alzheimer's disease, advancing age is the chief risk factor; incidence is as follows:
    a. Age 65 to 75—5% to 8%
    b. Age 75 to 85—15% to 20%
    c. Age 85 years and older—25% to 50%.
3. Other possible causes point to genetic factors and organic and inorganic etiologies.
    a. Family history and genetic mutations or sequencing may also play a role in its development.
       – Familial Alzheimer's disease has an early onset (age 30 to 40) and accounts for less than 5% of all Alzheimer's cases.
       – Genetic mutations on chromosomes 1, 14, and 21 have been identified as increasing the risk of this disorder.

DRUG CHART 11-1
Medications for treating symptoms of dementia

Classification	Drug	Rationale for use
Anticholinesterase drugs	donepezil (Aricept) galantamine hydrobromide (Reminyl) rivastigmine tartrate (Exelon)	Interfere with the enzyme acetylcholinesterase, which acts to break down acetylcholine, allowing acetylcholine to remain longer at synapses.
Antioxidants	vitamin E	Combats the oxidation process that synthesizes cytotoxic free radicals. There is some evidence that this will delay symptoms.
N-methyl-D-aspartate (NMDA) receptor antagonists	memantine	Prevents the release of glutamate, which is thought to be a factor in the degeneration of neurons.

- The e-4 allele of the lipid-carrying plasma protein apolipoprotein E is associated with increased risk of Alzheimer's disease.

  b. Nearly all individuals with Down syndrome develop the neuropathologic changes of Alzheimer's disease by the fifth decade of life.

  c. Other contributing factors may include low education level, female gender, presence of depression, and brain injury.

4. The pathophysiology of Alzheimer's disease follows a specific course, which is evident at autopsy (still the gold standard diagnosis) and, in some cases, identified through imaging studies before death occurs.

  a. Autopsy usually reveals reduced brain weight, cortical atrophy, and enlarged ventricles.

  b. Accumulated amyloid protein material (plaque) distributed throughout the gray matter of the cortex is commonly found.

  c. Neurofibrillary tangles, intracellular collections of abnormal filaments, contribute to the death of neurons.

  d. Neurochemical and neurotransmitter changes, including the loss of acetylcholine (major cholinergic neurotransmitter), are associated with the loss of cognitive functions of attention and memory.

  e. Inflammation in the brain has been identified as an early change; however, it is not known if this is a cause or a result of Alzheimer's disease.

E.   Managing dementia

1. Treatment of this progressive, degenerative disorder is directed toward a long-term outcome and maintaining the client's quality of life.

2. A multidisciplinary team approach that includes the collaborative efforts of nurses, doctors, dietitians, psychiatrists and psychologists, social workers, pharmacists, and rehabilitative specialists (occupational, physical, and activity therapists) is commonly used.

3. Statistics indicate that 7 out of 10 people with Alzheimer's disease live at home, and family and friends care for 75% of them; thus, a family focus on treatment and management is vital.

4. Community-focused management varies, depending on the client's needs and level of functioning.

    a. Community nurses provide home health visits.

    b. Adult day-care services provide therapeutic activities, rehabilitative services, recreation, and respite services for caregivers.

    c. Residential (personal care) facilities provide assisted living for some clients.

    d. About half of all skilled nursing facility residents reportedly have Alzheimer's disease.

    e. The Alzheimer's Association is a national organization that provides family and caregiver support groups, educates the community, funds research, and lobbies for legislative action.

5. Pharmacologic intervention may include the use of commonly prescribed medications or experimental therapies.

    a. Certain medications may be used to slow the client's rate of decline (by increasing acetylcholine levels and helping to maintain neuronal functioning) or to manage the client's behavior and distressing symptoms. (See *Drug chart 11-1, Medications for treating symptoms of dementia,* and *Drug chart 11-2, Medications for behavior modification in dementia.*)

    b. Experimental therapies include the use of nonsteroidal anti-inflammatory drugs (NSAIDs) to reduce the risk of Alzheimer's disease and antioxidant (vitamin E) therapy to protect neurons.

DRUG CHART 11-2
Medications for behavior modification in dementia

Classification	Drug	Behavior treated
Benzodiazepines (BZAs)	lorazepam (Ativan)	Anxiety and agitation
Non-BZA antianxiety agents	buspirone (BuSpar)	
Anticonvulsants	carbamazepine (Tegretol) valproic acid (Depakote)	
Antipsychotics Typical	haloperidol (Haldol)	Hallucinations and combative behavior
Atypical	risperidone (Risperdal)	
Antidepressants (selective serotonin reuptake inhibitors)	nefazodone (Serzone)	Depression

IV. AMNESTIC DISORDERS

A. Key concepts

1. **Amnestic disorders** are characterized by a disturbance in memory that is due to either the direct physiologic effects of a general medical condition or the persisting effects of a substance (drug of abuse, medication, or toxin exposure).

2. Common symptoms include:
   a. Impaired ability to learn new information or an inability to recall previously learned information or past events
   b. Confabulation (making up information to fill memory gaps)
   c. Profound amnesia resulting in disorientation to place and time
   d. Apathy, lack of initiative, and emotional blandness
   e. Lack of insight into memory deficits
   f. Disorientation to self (rarely occurs; more common in dementia).

3. Onset may be acute (such as from a traumatic brain injury, stroke, or other cerebrovascular event) or insidious and slow (such as from prolonged substance abuse, chronic neurotoxic exposure, or sustained nutritional deficiency).

B. Types of amnestic disorders

1. In **amnestic disorder due to a general medical condition,** the client's condition stems from a specific medical disorder (such as a cerebrovascular accident, traumatic brain injury, or encephalitis).

2. **Substance-induced persisting amnestic disorder** is characterized by impaired learning that directly results from the use of a substance (such as alcohol, sedatives, hypnotics, or opiates) as evidenced by the client's history, physical examination, and laboratory findings.

3. The label **amnestic disorder not otherwise specified** may be applied when no other cause has been identified.

C. Causes of amnestic disorders

1. Common causes of amnestic disorder include head trauma, hypoxia, and acute CNS infections.

2. Chronic thiamine deficiency associated with alcoholism (Korsakoff's syndrome) also causes this disorder.

D. Management of amnestic disorders

1. Treatment is similar to that of delirium if the amnestic disorder is an acute problem.

2. When the disorder is chronic, treatment is similar to that of dementia.

V. CARE OF THE CLIENT WITH A COGNITIVE IMPAIRMENT DISORDER

A. Assessment

1. Review the client's history and physical examination for characteristic signs and symptoms associated with the diagnosed disorder.
2. Assess for dementia using standardized tools.
   a. The Mini-Mental Status Exam (MMSE) is a well-studied and established screening test for dementia.
   b. The Short Portable Mental Status Questionnaire, the Clock-Drawing Test, the Modified MMSE, and the Seven-Minute Screen may also be used, although these tests have not been evaluated as extensively as the MMSE.
   c. The Functional Activities Questionnaire (FAQ) is a test that detects functional limitations rather than cognitive deficits.
3. Assess for depression because clients with cognitive impairments commonly have a depressed mood; about 40% to 50% of all clients with Alzheimer's disease have depressive symptoms, which are more common in early stages and treatable with antidepressant medications. (See *Table 11-2, Comparing delirium, dementia, and depression in the elderly client*, page 212.)
4. Ask the client pertinent questions to determine the degree of cognitive impairment. (See *Key questions 11-1, Assessing clients with cognitive impairment disorders*, page 213.)
   a. "What is today's date (day, month and year)?"
   b. "Where are you now?"
5. Interview the client, caregiver, and family members, making direct observations about the client's status in the following areas:
   a. **Behavior:** What are the client's capabilities for performing self-care and activities of daily living? Does the client exhibit socially unacceptable behaviors? Does he wander and pace? Are sundown or perseveration phenomena present?
   b. **Affect:** Does the client demonstrate anxiety? Emotional lability? Depression or apathy? Irritability? Suspiciousness? Helplessness? Frustration?
   c. **Cognitive responses:** What is the client's orientation level? Does he have recent or remote memory loss? Difficulty in problem solving, organizing, or abstracting? Deficits in judgment? Evidence of aphasia, agnosia, or apraxia?
6. Spend time with the caregiver or family to elicit the following information:
   a. **Primary caregiver:** Who is the client's primary caregiver, and how long has care been provided? *(Note:* Late stages of dementia of the Alzheimer's type can be especially difficult because family resources may be exhausted.)
   b. **Available support systems:** Who do the caregiver and other family members rely on for respite and support?
   c. **Knowledge base:** What do the caregiver and family members know about available client care and community resources? (Note any areas requiring further teaching.)

TABLE 11-2

Comparing delirium, dementia, and depression in the elderly client

Use the information in this chart to help differentiate the symptoms of delirium, dementia, and depression in the elderly client with a cognitive impairment disorder.

	Delirium	Dementia	Depression
Onset	■ Acute (develops in hours to days)	■ Gradual, insidious (developing within months to years)	■ Can be gradual (developing within weeks to months); obvious symptoms apparent at least for 2 weeks
Initial symptoms	■ Acute confusion ■ Disorientation (time, place, and person)	■ Difficulty planning, organizing, and completing complex tasks (balancing checkbook, meal planning) ■ Recent memory loss (forgetting appointments, misplacing objects)	■ Depressed mood ■ Lack of interest in usual activities
Continuing symptoms	■ Sensory alterations (illusions, hallucinations) ■ Alteration in the sleep-wake cycle ■ Motor changes (increased or decreased agitation and somnolence)	■ Disorientation (time, place) ■ Anxiety, agitation, paranoia (blaming people for stealing misplaced objects) ■ Depressed mood, apathy, loss of spontaneity ■ Lack of attention to grooming, hygiene ■ Lack of regard to safety (leaving stove on, going outside dressed inappropriately) ■ Pacing, wandering ■ Remote memory losses ■ Disorientation to time, place, and person	■ Complaints of memory loss, poor concentration ■ Feelings of helplessness, hopelessness ■ Sleep problems (hypersomnia, insomnia) ■ Appetite loss, weight loss ■ Physical complaints (headache, muscle aches, GI symptoms) ■ Self-neglect, poor hygiene ■ Thoughts of suicide

    d. **Spiritual support system:** Does the family belong to a spiritual group that can provide support?

    e. **Specific concerns:** Does the client or caregiver have any specific concerns that need further discussion and attention?

B. Analysis

    1. After analyzing the data, differentiate client priorities.

    2. Evaluate the client and family's coping abilities as well as the client's level of anxiety and potential for acting out.

    3. Analyze the degree of impairment related to the client's specific cognitive disorder.

    4. Analyze resources available to the client, caregiver, and family.

KEY QUESTIONS 11-1
Assessing clients with cognitive impairment disorders

Questions	Information gathered
Ask the client to state his name, address, and current location as well as the time, season, and year.	Orientation status
Ask the client to repeat six to seven digits in a forward sequence.	Attention span
Have the client name three objects (such as a watch, glass, and clock), and then have him repeat naming them. Ask him to repeat them again after 5 minutes.	Recent memory
Ask the client to state his mother's maiden name, brothers' and sisters' names, and children and grandchildren's names.	Remote memory
Ask the client about any changes in eating or sleeping habits, somatic complaints, or lack of interest in usually pleasurable things.	Presence of depression
Ask the client about his usual activities of daily living.	Ability to plan and complete activities of daily living

C. Nursing diagnoses

1. Establish appropriate nursing diagnoses for the client as needed.
    a. Acute confusion
    b. Anxiety
    c. Chronic confusion
    d. Disturbed sensory perception (specify: visual, auditory, kinesthetic, gustatory, tactile, olfactory)
    e. Disturbed sleep pattern
    f. Disturbed thought processes
    g. Imbalanced nutrition: Less than body requirements
    h. Impaired home maintenance
    i. Impaired verbal communication
    j. Ineffective coping
    k. Ineffective role performance
    l. Self-care deficit (specify: feeding, bathing or hygiene, dressing or grooming, toileting)
    m. Social isolation
    n. Risk for self-directed or other-directed violence
2. Establish appropriate nursing diagnoses for the caregiver and family as needed.
    a. Caregiver role strain
    b. Disabled family coping
    c. Interrupted family processes

D. Planning and outcome identification

1. Work with the client, caregiver, and family in setting realistic goals.
2. Establish desired outcome criteria for the client.
   a. The client will remain safe and free from injury.
   b. The client will demonstrate decreased anxiety levels.
   c. The client will remain oriented at level of ability; if orientation is not possible, the client will feel validated and accepted.
   d. The client will maintain existing ability to perform activities of daily living with cues as necessary.
   e. The client will maintain adequate fluid and nutritional levels.
   f. The client will pose no harm to himself or others.
   g. The client will follow a schedule of activity and rest.
   h. The client will experience minimal catastrophic reactions.
3. Establish desired outcome criteria for the caregiver and family.
   a. The caregiver and family will identify and use available support systems.
   b. The caregiver and family will demonstrate effective use of measures to prevent burnout.
   c. The caregiver and family will verbalize confidence in ability to provide client care.

E. Implementation

1. Take the following measures to maintain the client's **safety:**
   a. Provide emergency measures (for aspiration, injury, seizures) as necessary.
   b. Anticipate environmental safety hazards, and remove objects that pose a risk to the client; keep surroundings clutter-free.
   c. Minimize the risk of cardiovascular problems (anemia, hypertension, angina) by promoting proper diet, medications, exercise, and rest.
   d. Monitor drugs and drug interactions, ensuring safe doses for elderly clients; pay special attention to medications with anticholinergic properties as well as to medications that may cause drowsiness or postural hypotension.
2. Use the following responses to address the client's **cognitive deficits:**
   a. Call the client by name, and introduce yourself; use short, clear messages; and give directions one at a time.
   b. Support the client's memory by using calendars, orientation boards, seasonal reminders, signs, and labels, as needed.
   c. Avoid stressful demands, and limit client decision-making.
   d. Offer activities within the client's ability.
   e. Avoid or limit socially embarrassing situations; support and maintain the client's dignity.
   f. Do not reinforce or agree with hallucinations, illusions, or delusions; respond to and focus on the client's feelings.
   g. Use reminiscence techniques to encourage the client to capitalize on more intact remote memories.
      - Encourage the client to talk about past events; use a tape recorder to tape reminiscences, then play them back for the client.
      - Use family photo albums to stimulate reminiscence.

TABLE 11-3

Comparing reality orientation and validation therapy techniques

Both reality orientation and validation therapy are useful for clients with cognitive impairments. However, reality orientation attempts to refocus the client's awareness on the current environment, whereas validation therapy acknowledges the client's feelings and memories in an attempt to redirect her awareness and attention.

	Reality orientation	Validation therapy
Purpose	■ To establish or maintain the client's awareness of her current environment	■ To establish a connection between the nurse and client by validating emotional memories
Appropriate use	■ Useful as a first attempt to help the client regain awareness of the current environment, especially when she is suffering from a temporary loss of awareness	■ Useful when reality orientation is resisted or ineffective; may be helpful as a calming method when the client misperceives her environment
Specific techniques	■ Establish eye contact with the client, introduce yourself, and state the client's name; smile. ■ Use short, simple sentences when providing orienting information. ■ Structure the environment using clocks, calendars, orientation boards, seasonal decorations, and family pictures.	■ Establish eye contact with the client, introduce yourself, and state the client's name; smile. ■ Validate the client's feelings. ("You seem upset.") ■ Repeat part of what the client said. ("You need to fix dinner for your husband...") ■ Reflect what seems to be the client's underlying feelings. ("You miss your husband.") ■ Continue to talk with the client about the topic (husband). ■ As the client becomes calmer, redirect her to the appropriate current activity.

    h. Use validation therapy when the client no longer responds to reality orientation techniques. (See *Table 11-3, Comparing reality orientation and validation therapy techniques.*)

3. Take the following measures to maintain the client's **level of functioning** for performing activities of daily living:

    a. Promote a balance of rest and activity.

    b. Support the client in self-sufficiency; use cues and positive reinforcement.

    c. Assist with toileting on a structured schedule; use disposable pants as needed to preserve the client's dignity.

    d. Maintain a balanced diet, and ensure adequate fluids; offer finger foods if the client has difficulty with utensils.

4. Take the following measures to avoid and minimize **catastrophic reactions:**

    a. Maintain consistent structure and routines.

    b. Decrease environmental stimuli when the client is anxious.

    c. Avoid rapidly approaching or touching the client when he is irritable, agitated, or suspicious.

CLIENT AND FAMILY TEACHING 11-1

Guidelines for clients with dementia

Provide information about dementia (including its symptoms and the progressive nature of the disease):
- Dementia is a chronic, progressive disease that alters the client's thinking, personality, and behavior.
- The client may be depressed, anxious, fearful, or suspicious at times; medications can help relieve some of these symptoms, especially in the early stages of illness.
- The client's memory will be impaired, and he will require frequent reminders to perform daily tasks.
- The client may be prone to wandering and pacing and will require supervision; appropriate exercise may help reduce these activities.

Provide the caregiver and family with helpful home care measures:
- Use memory aids (clocks, labels, calendars, lists), and structure the client's daily routine (regular times for sleeping and awakening, meals, activities, and rest periods).
- Maintain good nutrition (frequent, small meals are better for the client with a poor appetite).
- Respond to the client's memory impairment and losses by attempting to gently reorient him as long as this is not upsetting.
- Maintain a regular bedtime routine to promote sleep: eliminate caffeine after 2 p.m., provide a quiet environment, use a nightlight, perform toileting prior to bed.
- Provide directions and instructions with simple words, using gestures when helpful and needed.
- Institute safety measures: remove or lock up objects or cleaning agents that can harm the client; remove throw rugs and extension cords; paint hot water faucets red; secure all doors and windows.
- Keep in mind that wandering is expected. Prepare for this by having the client wear an identification bracelet and registering him with the police (the Safe Return Program is a joint effort of the Alzheimer's Association and local police departments).
- Remove the client from upsetting situations to prevent catastrophic reactions (avoid crowds, strangers, confusion, and noise).

Help the caregiver and family to plan for the terminal stage of dementia:
- The client will gradually experience a loss of ambulation, caregiver recognition, and conversation; eventually, his disease will progress to a vegetative state.
- A hospice-type approach may be used in the late stage (palliative measures, comfort, limited medications and medical interventions).

---

    d. When the client is agitated, remain with him and maintain a calm, supportive manner.

    e. Use nightlights and calm interaction to decrease sundowning.

  5. Provide appropriate information to the caregiver and family caring for the client with a cognitive impairment disorder. (See *Client and family teaching 11-1, Guidelines for clients with dementia*, and *Client and family teaching 11-2, Guidelines for preventing caregiver burnout.*)

F. Outcome evaluation

  1. The client demonstrates decreased anxiety and increased feelings of security within a structured environment.

  2. The client maintains a maximum degree of orientation within his level of ability.

  3. The client maintains the ability to perform activities of daily living within a structured environment.

  4. The client refrains from acting out.

  5. Family members use all available support services and community resources.

CLIENT AND FAMILY TEACHING 11-2
Guidelines for preventing caregiver burnout

When caring for a client with an impaired cognitive disorder, such as delirium or dementia, remember that it's important to take time for yourself to prevent burnout.

- Get enough rest.
- Maintain proper nutrition.
- Maintain a sense of humor.
- Ask for help from other family members, community agencies, and support groups (Alzheimer's Association).

- Take breaks and vacations; use respite and day-care services.
- Make time for enjoyable activities and hobbies.
- Expect feelings of anger, grief, and loss as the client's illness progresses.
- Openly talk about your feelings, frustrations, and difficulties with supportive persons (family members, friends, health care professionals, and support group members).

Study questions

1. The nurse enters the room of a client with a cognitive impairment disorder and asks what day of the week it is; what the date, month, and year are; and where the client is. The nurse is attempting to assess:
1. confabulation.
2. delirium.
3. orientation.
4. perseveration.

2. Which of the following best describes dementia?
1. Memory loss occurring as part of the natural consequence of aging
2. Difficulty coping with physical and psychological change
3. Severe cognitive impairment that occurs rapidly
4. Loss of cognitive abilities, impairing ability to perform activities of daily living

3. Which of the following will the nurse use when communicating with a client who has a cognitive impairment?
1. Complete explanations with multiple details
2. Pictures or gestures instead of words
3. Stimulating words and phrases to capture the client's attention
4. Short words and simple sentences

4. A 75-year-old client has dementia of the Alzheimer's type and confabulates. The nurse understands that this client:
1. denies confusion by being jovial.
2. pretends to be someone else.
3. rationalizes various behaviors.
4. fills in memory gaps with fantasy.

5. Which ability should a nurse expect from a client in the mild stage of dementia of the Alzheimer's type?
1. Remembering the daily schedule
2. Recalling past events
3. Coping with anxiety
4. Solving problems of daily living

6. An 82-year-old man is admitted to the medical-surgical unit for diagnostic confirmation and management of probable delirium. Which statement by the client's daughter best supports the diagnosis?
1. "Maybe it's just caused by aging. This usually happens by age 82."
2. "The changes in his behavior came

on so quickly! I wasn't sure what was happening."

3. "Dad just didn't seem to know what he was doing. He would forget what he had for breakfast."

4. "Dad has always been so independent. He's lived alone for years since Mom died."

7. An elderly client with Alzheimer's disease becomes agitated and combative when a nurse approaches to help with morning care. The most appropriate nursing intervention in this situation would be to:

1. tell the client firmly that it is time to get dressed.

2. obtain assistance to restrain the client for safety.

3. remain calm and talk quietly to the client.

4. call the doctor and request an order for sedation.

8. Which goal is a priority for a client with a *DSM-IV TR* diagnosis of delirium and the nursing diagnosis *Acute confusion related to recent surgery secondary to traumatic hip fracture*?

1. The client will complete activities of daily living.

2. The client will maintain safety.

3. The client will remain oriented.

4. The client will understand communication.

9. Which of the following is *not* included in the care plan of a client with a moderate cognitive impairment involving dementia of the Alzheimer's type?

1. Daily structured schedule

2. Positive reinforcement for performing activities of daily living

3. Stimulating environment

4. Use of validation techniques

10. In clients with a cognitive impairment disorder, the phenomenon of increased confusion in the early evening hours is called:

1. aphasia.

2. agnosia.

3. sundowning.

4. confabulation.

11. An 80-year-old man is accompanied to the clinic by his son, who tells the nurse that the client's constant confusion, incontinence, and tendency to wander are intolerable. The client was diagnosed with chronic cognitive impairment disorder. Which nursing diagnosis is most appropriate for the client's son?

1. *Risk for other-directed violence*

2. *Disturbed sleep pattern*

3. *Caregiver role strain*

4. *Social isolation*

12. Which of the following outcome criteria is appropriate for the client with dementia?

1. The client will return to an adequate level of self-functioning.

2. The client will learn new coping mechanisms to handle anxiety.

3. The client will seek out resources in the community for support.

4. The client will follow an established schedule for activities of daily living.

13. A family member expresses concern to a nurse about behavioral changes in an elderly aunt. Which would cause the nurse to suspect a cognitive impairment disorder?

1. Decreased interest in activities that she once enjoyed

2. Fearfulness of being alone at night

3. Increased complaints of physical ailments

4. Problems with preparing a meal or balancing her checkbook

14. During the home visit of a client with dementia, the nurse notes that an adult daughter persistently corrects her father's misperceptions of reality, even when her father becomes upset and anxious. Which intervention should the nurse teach the caregiver?
1. Anxiety-reducing measures
2. Positive reinforcement
3. Reality orientation techniques
4. Validation techniques

15. A client with moderate dementia has frequent catastrophic reactions during shower time. Which of the following interventions should be implemented in the plan of care? Select all that apply.
1. Assign consistent staff members to assist the client.
2. Accomplish the task quickly, with several staff members assisting.
3. Schedule the client's shower at the same time of day.
4. Sedate the client 30 minutes prior to showering.
5. Tell the client to remain calm while showering.
6. Use a calm, supportive, quiet manner when assisting the client.

Answer key

1. The answer is **3**.
The initial, most basic assessment of a client with cognitive impairment involves determining his level of orientation (awareness of time, place, and person). The nurse may also assess for confabulation and perseveration in a client with cognitive impairment; but the questions in this situation would not elicit the symptom response. Delirium is a type of cognitive impairment; however, other symptoms are necessary to establish this diagnosis.

2. The answer is **4**.
The impaired ability to perform self-care is an important measure of a client's dementia progression and loss of cognitive abilities. Difficulty or impaired ability to perform normal activities of daily living, such as maintaining hygiene and grooming, toileting, making meals, and maintaining a household, are significant indications of dementia. Slowing of process-

es necessary for information retrieval is a normal consequence of aging. However, the global statement that memory loss occurs as part of natural aging is not true. Dementia is not normal; it is a disease. Difficulty coping with changes can be experienced by any client, not just one with dementia. The rapid occurrence of cognitive impairment refers to delirium.

3. The answer is **4**.
Short words and simple sentences minimize client confusion and enhance communication. Complete explanations with multiple details and stimulating words and phrases would increase confusion in a client with short attention span and difficulty with comprehension. Although pictures and gestures may be helpful, they would not substitute for verbal communication.

4. The answer is **4**.
Confabulation is a communication device

used by patients with dementia to compensate for memory gaps. The remaining answer choices are incorrect.

5. The answer is 2.
Recent memory loss is the characteristic sign of cognitive difficulty in early Alzheimer's disease. The ability to recall past events is usually retained until the later stages of this disorder. Remembering daily schedules, coping with anxiety, and solving problems of daily living are areas that would pose difficulty in the early phase of Alzheimer's disease.

6. The answer is 2.
Delirium is an acute process characterized by abrupt, spontaneous cognitive dysfunction. Cognitive impairment disorders (dementia or delirium) are not normal consequences of aging. Option 3 would be characteristic of someone with dementia. Although option 4 provides background data about the client, it is unrelated to the current problem of delirium.

7. The answer is 3.
Maintaining a calm approach when intervening with an agitated client is extremely important. Telling the client firmly that it is time to get dressed may increase his agitation, especially if the nurse touches him. Restraints are a last resort to ensure client safety and are inappropriate in this situation. Sedation should be avoided, if possible, because it will interfere with CNS functioning and may contribute to the client's confusion.

8. The answer is 2.
Maintaining safety is the priority goal for an acutely confused client who recently had surgery. All measures to promote physiologic safety and psychosocial well-being would be implemented. This client

would not be capable of completing activities of daily living, and safety is a priority over these tasks. The goals of remaining oriented and understanding communication would be appropriate only after the client's acute confusion has resolved.

9. The answer is 3.
A stimulating environment is a source of confusion and anxiety for a client with a moderate level of impairment and, therefore, would not be included in the plan of care. The remaining options are all appropriate interventions for this client.

10. The answer is 3.
Sundowning is a common phenomenon that occurs after daylight hours in a client with a cognitive impairment disorder. The other options are incorrect responses, although all may be seen in this client.

11. The answer is 3.
The son's description exemplifies some of the problems commonly encountered by a primary caregiver who is caring for someone with a cognitive impairment disorder. Although the other nursing diagnoses are possibilities, the scenario does not provide enough information to validate any of these.

12. The answer is 4.
Following established activity schedules is a realistic expectation for clients with dementia. All of the remaining outcome statements require a higher level of cognitive ability than can be realistically expected of clients with this disorder.

13. The answer is 4.
Making a meal and balancing a checkbook are higher level cognitive functions that, when unable to be performed, may signal onset of a cognitive disorder.

Although the remaining behaviors may occur, they are not associated only with cognitive impairment and may indicate depression or other problems.

14. The answer is 4.

Validation techniques are useful measures for making emotional connections with a client who can no longer maintain reality orientation. These measures are also helpful in decreasing anxiety. Anxiety-reducing measures and positive reinforcements will also be appropriate, but validation techniques will provide both anxiety reduction and positive reinforcement for the client. Reality orientation techniques are not useful when the client can no longer maintain reality contact and becomes upset when misperceptions are corrected.

15. The answer is 1, 3, 6.

Maintaining a consistent routine with the same staff members will help decrease the client's anxiety that occurs whenever changes are made. A calm, quiet manner will be reassuring to the client, also helping to minimize anxiety. Moving quickly with several staff will increase the client's anxiety and may precipitate a catastrophic reaction. The use of sedation is not indicated and may increase the risk of client injury from side effect of drowsiness. Telling the client to remain calm is inappropriate because a client with dementia cannot respond to such a direction.

12 *Crisis Intervention*

I. OVERVIEW OF CRISES

A. Key concepts

1. A **crisis** is an overwhelming reaction to a threatening situation in which an individual's usual problem-solving skills and coping responses are inadequate for maintaining psychological equilibrium.

   a. All individuals experience problems and crises at one time or another.

   b. Because each person responds uniquely to problems, a crisis is determined by the individual's perception of the problem.

   c. Crises are not necessarily pathological; they can stimulate growth and learning.

2. A crisis is a time-limited event and usually resolves, either successfully or unsuccessfully, within a brief period (typically 4 to 6 weeks).

   a. Crisis resolution is considered successful when the individual's functioning is restored or enhanced through new learning.

   b. When crisis resolution is unsuccessful, the individual's functioning diminishes and fails to achieve the precrisis level.

3. **Balancing factors,** when available, increase the chance of a successful resolution to a crisis; the presence of three important factors may serve as predictors of a good outcome:

   a. A realistic, rather than distorted, perception of the precipitating event

   b. Situational supports (family, friends) to help through the crisis

   c. Effective coping mechanisms to alleviate anxiety.

4. **Crisis intervention** is a method of providing assistance to those affected by a crisis in which the immediate problem is resolved and psychological equilibrium is restored.

B. Types of crises

1. Crises are generally grouped into three major categories. (See *Table 12-1, Categorizing crises.*)

TABLE 12-1
Categorizing crises

Crises are grouped into three major categories as shown below.

Developmental (maturational)	Situational	Adventitious
■ Beginning school	■ Divorce	■ Floods
■ Puberty	■ Death	■ Earthquakes
■ Graduation	■ Job loss	■ Wars
■ Marriage	■ Academic failure	■ Violence
■ Birth of a child	■ Diagnosis of a serious illness	■ Rape
■ Children leaving home		■ Murder
■ Retirement		■ Kidnapping
		■ Terrorist acts

> *a.* A **developmental crisis** occurs in response to a transition from one stage of maturation to another in the life cycle (such as the transition from adolescence to adulthood).
>
> *b.* A **situational crisis** occurs in response to a sudden, unexpected event in an individual's life; these events generally revolve around experiences of loss (such as the death of a loved one).
>
> *c.* An **adventitious crisis** occurs in response to a severe trauma or natural disaster; these crises can affect individuals, communities, and even nations.

2. Recent acts of violence and terrorism in the United States have affected the feelings of safety and security of many Americans.

   a. Bombing of the Oklahoma City federal office building (April 19, 1995)

   b. Massacre at Columbine High School (April 20, 1999)

   c. Terroristic attacks involving the World Trade Center and Pentagon building (September 11, 2001)

3. Consequently, mental health services now play an important part in the emergency planning of federal, state, and local agencies.

   a. Victims, if they survive, may suffer severe physical injuries as well as post-traumatic stress syndrome, depression, or other symptoms. (See *Table 12-2, Symptoms associated with crises.*)

   b. Rescuers often suffer psychological stress as a result of witnessing the effects of terror.

TABLE 12-2
Symptoms associated with crises

During crises, individuals commonly experience a range of symptoms indicative of their inability to cope with an overwhelming situation or event.

Physical symptoms	▪ Somatic complaints (headaches, gastrointestinal symptoms, pain) ▪ Appetite disturbances (significant weight loss or gain) ▪ Sleep disturbances (insomnia, nightmares) ▪ Restlessness, tearfulness, irritability
Cognitive symptoms	▪ Confusion, difficulty concentrating ▪ Racing thoughts ▪ Inability to make decisions
Behavioral symptoms	▪ Disorganization ▪ Impulsive, angry outbursts ▪ Difficulty carrying out usual role responsibilities ▪ Withdrawal from social interaction
Emotional symptoms	▪ Anxiety, anger, guilt ▪ Sadness, depression ▪ Paranoia, suspicion ▪ Helplessness, powerlessness

c. Even those not directly involved in such events (witnesses, television viewers) may be affected by the experience and manifest symptoms common to those experiencing the actual crisis.

C. Sequence of crisis development

1. The **precrisis period** is characterized by a state of emotional equilibrium.
2. During the **crisis period,** the client's usual coping mechanisms fail and symptoms begin to manifest. (See *Table 12-2, Symptoms associated with crises.*)
3. The **postcrisis period** marks the resolution of the crisis and is characterized by a return to the client's baseline state of physical and mental health.

II. MANAGING CRISES

A. Key concepts

1. Crisis management (intervention) aims to provide timely assistance to an individual or a group of people during a crisis.
   a. For an individual, assistance is typically provided through telephone counseling, hotlines, and brief crisis counseling (1 to 6 sessions).
   b. Assistance for groups or communities usually involves a team approach.
      - **Mobile crisis teams** are interdisciplinary and provide services to groups or communities affected by particular crisis events.
      - **Disaster response teams** follow an organized plan to provide help to large population segments affected by natural disasters.
2. **Critical incident stress debriefing** is directed at groups of professionals (hospital personnel, police, firefighters) who have been involved in a crisis situation.

B. Nursing's role in crisis intervention

1. Nurses provide direct services to people in crisis and serve as members of crisis intervention teams.
   a. Nurses working in acute- and chronic-care hospital settings assist individuals and families who are responding to the crisis of a serious illness, hospitalization, or death.
   b. Nurses in community settings (doctors' offices, clinics, schools, businesses) provide assistance to individuals and families involved in developmental and situational crises.
2. Nurses working with a particular group of clients should anticipate situations in which crises may occur.
   a. **Maternal-child nursing:** Anticipated crises may include the birth of a premature or stillborn child, miscarriage, and birth anomalies.
   b. **Pediatric nursing:** Crises may include the onset of serious illness, chronic or debilitating illnesses, traumatic injuries, or a dying child.
   c. **Medical-surgical nursing:** Various crises, including the diagnosis of a serious illness, debilitating illness, hospitalization for acute or chronic problems, loss of a body part or function, and death and dying, are commonly encountered.

      d. **Gerontologic nursing:** The nurse should anticipate such crises as cumulative losses, debilitating illness, dependency, and nursing home placement.

      e. **Emergency nursing:** Crises in the emergency department may include physical trauma, acute illness, treatment of rape victims, and death.

      f. **Psychiatric nursing:** Common crises include hospitalization for mental illness, life stressors for the seriously mentally ill, and suicide.

3. The psychiatric mental health nurse specialist (APRN or CNS) may assume the role of a crisis intervention worker by:

      a. Establishing rapport and communicating hope and optimism

      b. Assuming an active, directive role, if necessary

      c. Making suggestions and offering alternatives (including referrals to appropriate agencies, such as a child welfare agency or medical clinics)

      d. Supporting the client in choosing alternatives

      e. Collaborating with other professionals to obtain necessary services and resources for the client.

C. Principles of crisis intervention

1. The goal of crisis intervention is to return the individual to the precrisis level of functioning, with an emphasis on strengthening and supporting healthy aspects of functioning.

2. Crisis intervention involves a systematic, problem-solving approach (similar to the nursing process) that involves:

      a. **Assessing** the individual's perception of the problem, as well as the strengths and weaknesses of the individual and family support systems

      b. **Planning specific outcomes** or goals based on priorities

      c. **Providing direct intervention,** such as providing shelter for a client who has been evicted from his home or referring a client to a "safe house" when spousal abuse has occurred

      d. **Evaluating outcomes and results of the intervention.**

3. Maslow's *Hierarchy of Needs* provides a working framework to help determine the priorities for specific interventions:

      a. **Physical resources** necessary for survival (food, shelter, safety)

      b. **Social resources** necessary for regaining a sense of belonging (family support, social network, community support)

      c. **Psychological resources** necessary for regaining self-esteem (positive reinforcement, goal accomplishment).

4. Individuals involved in major traumatic events (terrorism, violence, natural disasters) require a multidisciplinary approach and early intervention.

      a. Research indicates that multiple-session, early intervention is beneficial, especially for individuals exhibiting crisis symptoms.

      b. Mass disasters require preplanned, well-coordinated, and multidisciplinary intervention efforts.

      c. Medications are not routinely indicated after traumatic events.

NURSING PROCESS OVERVIEW

 III. CARE OF THE CLIENT REQUIRING CRISIS INTERVENTION

A. Assessment

1. Identify the precipitating event and the circumstances of the crisis. (See *Key questions 12-1: Assessing clients experiencing crises.*)
2. Determine the client's perception of the crisis, including the underlying needs that the crisis threatens, the degree of life disruption, and the client's symptoms. (See *Table 12-2, Symptoms associated with crises*, page 224.)
3. Determine the presence of balancing factors, including whether the client has a realistic perception of the crisis events, situational supports (family, friends, financial resources, spiritual resources, community supports), and the use of coping mechanisms.
4. Identify the client's strengths.

B. Nursing diagnoses

1. Analyze the client's unique perception of the crisis and the events precipitating it.
   a. Evaluate the adequacy of the client's balancing factors and degree of personal, social, and environmental supports.

KEY QUESTIONS 12-1
Assessing clients experiencing crises

Question	Information gathered
What happened to you?	Client's perception of events (realistic or distorted)
What are your thoughts and feelings about what happened?	Cognitive and emotional symptoms
Are you experiencing any physical symptoms or changes in your usual behaviors?	Physical, behavioral symptoms
Have you ever experienced anything similar to this in your life? If so, how did you cope at that time?	Previous experience with crises, coping measures used in the past
What do you think are your personal strengths?	Client's recognition of strengths
Who do you feel is supportive or helpful to you in your life?	Support systems available
What have you tried to do so far to resolve the crisis?	Use of coping measures in the present situation

    b. Determine the degree to which others (the client's family, social network, community) are affected by the crisis.

  2. Establish individualized nursing diagnoses for the client, family, and/or community, including the following as needed:

    a. *Caregiver role strain*

    b. *Disturbed body image*

    c. *Dysfunctional grieving*

    d. *Ineffective community coping*

    e. *Ineffective coping*

    f. *Ineffective denial*

    g. *Ineffective role performance*

    h. *Posttrauma syndrome*

    i. *Powerlessness*

    j. *Rape-trauma syndrome*

    k. *Readiness for enhanced family coping*

    l. *Risk for self-directed or other-directed violence*

    m. *Spiritual distress*

C. Planning and outcome identification

  1. Assist the client, family, and/or community in setting realistic short-term goals based on a return to a precrisis level of functioning.

  2. Establish desired outcome criteria for the client, family, and/or community.

    a. The client will verbalize the meaning of the crisis situation.

    b. The client will discuss options for resolution.

    c. The client will identify resources available for assistance.

    d. The client will choose a strategy for coping with the crisis.

    e. The client will implement necessary measures to bring about crisis resolution.

    f. The client will maintain safety when the situation escalates.

D. Implementation

  1. For a client experiencing a **general crisis,** take the following measures:

    a. Establish rapport by active listening and use of empathic responses.

    b. Encourage the client to fully discuss the crisis situation, and help him to verbalize his thoughts and feelings.

    c. Support the client's strengths and use of coping measures.

    d. Use a problem-solving approach.

    e. Intervene to deter any plans for self-harm or suicide.

      – Recognize warning signs of self-violence, such as the client's direct statements about suicidal threats, hinting that others will be better off when she is gone, or the presence of depression. (See *Display 6-1, Quick assessment of suicide risk factors*, page 112.)

      – Perform a suicide lethality assessment.

      – Remove dangerous objects from the client's immediate environment.

      – Collaborate with mental health team members to determine whether hospitalization is necessary.

    f. Provide crisis intervention, as needed, depending on the specific situation (such as working as a team member in post-terrorism crisis intervention).

2. For an **angry** or **violent** client in crisis, take the following measures:
   a. Intervene early to prevent the client from acting violently toward others.
      - Recognize verbal signs of escalating anger (shouting, rapid speech, demanding attention, making aggressive statements).
      - Recognize nonverbal signs of escalating anger (tightened jaw, tense posture, clenched fists, pacing).
   b. Use appropriate measures to deescalate the client's anger.
      - Answer the client's angry questions and demands by providing factual information in a supportive and reassuring manner.
      - Respond to underlying feelings of anxiety, fear, and frustration (such as by saying, "It seems to me that you're feeling frustrated about not going home when you expected.").
      - Allow the client to vent anger verbally, recognizing that the nurse may receive displaced anger.
      - Avoid defending or justifying personal behavior or the behavior of others (treatment team members, hospital policies).
      - Monitor personal body language, using a relaxed posture with arms hanging loosely at sides.
      - Allow the client to assume control over the problem by offering alternative solutions for resolution.
   c. Respond to the client's violent behavior.
      - Protect yourself by standing between the client and the exit door, so escape is possible.
      - Protect others by instructing them to leave the area.
      - Follow agency protocol, initiating a violence code if necessary (such as when a client threatens to hurt another client or a staff member, or if the client is throwing objects or breaking furniture).
   d. Follow violence code guidelines, ensuring that the least restrictive measures are implemented before seclusion or restraint is attempted (personnel responding to a violence code, including nurses, must first receive appropriate training).
      - The team should include at least five staff to ensure a show of force.
      - One team member acts as the leader, who will interact with the client and direct the team response.
      - The team leader is positioned at the head of the group, with the other members behind in rows of two to three.
      - If physical restraint is necessary, the team leader decides who will take each limb and who will take the head (to prevent biting).
      - The team acts as one and accomplishes a smooth, face-down takedown.
      - Holding regular drills in which these techniques are practiced can ensure safety and avoidance of client and staff injury.

E. **Outcome evaluation**
1. The client identifies a relationship between stressors and symptoms experienced during a crisis.
2. The client evaluates possible solutions to the crisis.
3. The client selects appropriate solutions to his problems.
4. The client returns to a precrisis state or improves the situation or his behavior.
5. The client, family, and community remain safe as a result of appropriate interventions when acting-out behavior occurs.

Study questions

1. The school nurse receives a referral from a teacher about a sudden behavior change in a 13-year-old girl who has become increasingly withdrawn and uninterested in her schoolwork. Upon interviewing the girl and her teacher, the nurse notes that the girl's behavioral changes correspond with a rapid onset of puberty. Which type of crisis is the girl experiencing?
   1. Adventitious crisis
   2. Developmental crisis
   3. Situational crisis
   4. Natural crisis

2. The nurse is intervening with a client who experienced a crisis following the sudden death of a loved one. Which of the following actions should the nurse take after establishing initial rapport?
   1. Ask the client to describe his social support system.
   2. Call the client's family to discuss the problem.
   3. Encourage the client to describe in detail what happened.
   4. Refer the client to a bereavement support group.

3. The nurse assesses balancing factors to predict a client's response to a crisis and eventual outcome. Which of the following is the best example of a balancing factor?
   1. Age
   2. Physical health status
   3. Situational supports available
   4. Type of crisis event

4. Which approach by the nurse is best when responding to a client in crisis?
   1. Behavioral approach
   2. Nondirective approach
   3. Problem-solving approach
   4. Supportive approach

5. Which of the following best describes the role of the nurse as a member of a crisis intervention team?
   1. Assistive role
   2. Collaborative role
   3. Educational role
   4. Managerial role

6. Which outcome is most appropriate following nursing intervention for a client in crisis?
   1. The client will analyze problems with lifestyle choices.
   2. The client will improve weaknesses in personal development.
   3. The client will learn new adaptive measures to decrease anxiety.
   4. The client will return to a level of precrisis functioning.

7. A client who has been raped tells the emergency department nurse that the rape was her fault because she walked down an alley on her way to school. Which response by the nurse would be best in this situation?
1. Accept the client's statement that this was risk-taking behavior.
2. Ask the client what other behaviors may have been risky.
3. Emphasize that the rapist, not the client, is responsible.
4. Suggest that the client discuss this issue later.

8. A client angrily shouts to the clinic nurse, "You'd better get me in to see the doctor now, or I'll see that you regret it." Which of the following is the best initial response by the nurse to deescalate this situation?
1. Call for assistance from security.
2. Explain to the client the reason why the doctor is busy.
3. Firmly tell the client not to shout, but to be patient.
4. Respond empathically to the client's underlying frustration.

9. A homeless client with a history of mental illness tells the clinic nurse that someone has taken all of the blood pressure pills she received at her last visit to the clinic. The nurse notes that the client is dirty and unkempt and appears to have lost weight since her last visit. Upon questioning, the nurse learns that the client has not been eating regularly because of her fear that the person taking the pills works at the local soup kitchen. Which nursing intervention is the priority in this situation?
1. Call the local mental health center and make a referral.
2. Make immediate provisions for the client to eat.

3. Provide the client with a new supply of medication.
4. Suggest that the client wash up in the clinic bathroom.

10. Which of the common symptoms should the nurse anticipate during assessment of a client experiencing a crisis?
1. Feelings of depersonalization, loose associations, flat affect
2. Lack of regard to social norms, apathy, hallucinations
3. Mood swings, feeling of boundless energy, grandiose beliefs
4. Somatic complaints, difficulty performing life roles, poor concentration

11. What is the best rationale for identifying client strengths when evaluating someone experiencing a crisis?
1. It allows the nurse to better determine the nursing diagnosis.
2. It helps the nurse understand the client's unique personality.
3. The nurse can better educate the client about his strengths.
4. Reinforcing the client's strengths will aid in coping.

12. The psychiatric nurse hears shouting in the day room and finds a client threatening to kick the television because the other clients in the room have refused to change the channel. The nurse intervenes by instructing other clients to leave the area. Which intervention is most appropriate to protect the nurse while using deescalating measures?
1. Position herself between the exit door and the client
2. Stand within an arm's length of the client
3. Stand next to the client with hands at her side
4. Sit in a chair next to the client

13. The medical-surgical nurse assesses a client who suffered a broken leg while attempting to leave her home, which was demolished by a fire. Which of the following questions are appropriate for the nurse to ask in this situation? Select all that apply.

1. "How did you feel about your parents while growing up?"

2. "What happened to you?"
3. "Who do you feel is supportive or helpful to you?"
4. "What have you done so far to try and resolve this crisis?"
5. "What kind of work do you do?"
6. "Do you have any hobbies that interest you?"

Answer key

1. The answer is 2.

A *developmental crisis* is one that occurs in response to a particular transition from one stage of maturation to another in the life cycle. Puberty marks the transition from childhood to adolescence. An *adventitious crisis* occurs in response to severe trauma or disaster. A *situational crisis* occurs in response to sudden, unexpected events in an individual's life. Puberty is neither sudden nor unexpected; it is a normal transition. A *natural crisis* is not a clinical type of crisis.

2. The answer is 3.

It is important for the nurse to assess the client's perception of the overwhelming problem and the events preceding the crisis situation because these are the factors that define the crisis. Determining the social support system is important; however, this assessment would follow the client's description of the problem (the first step in crisis intervention). Calling the family to discuss the problem or referring the client to a bereavement support group may or may not be appropriate, depending on the client's perception of the problem; but, again, these would occur later in the intervention.

3. The answer is 3.

Situational supports (family, friends, and others the client can rely on for help) are important balancing factors that will help predict a good outcome. Other balancing factors include the client's realistic (rather than distorted) perception of the crisis and the availability of effective coping mechanisms to alleviate anxiety. Although the client's age and physical health status may be influential in predicting outcome resolution, they are not considered balancing factors. Likewise, the type of crisis is not considered a balancing factor.

4. The answer is 3.

Crisis intervention employs a systematic, problem-solving approach in attempting to help clients deal with crises. A behavioral approach or a nondirective approach would not be used. Although a supportive approach (supporting the client's strengths) is part of crisis intervention, the overall method guiding the nurse is the problem-solving approach.

5. The answer is 2.

As an integral member of a health care team, the nurse must collaborate with other professionals to help clients resolve crises. The nurse may assist and teach clients during the process, but the chief role is one of a collaborative team member. The nurse may or may not assume a managerial role on the team.

6. The answer is 4.

Crisis intervention is designed to enable the individual, group, or community to return to a precrisis state of equilibrium as soon as possible by resolving immediate problems. Analyzing the client's lifestyle choices and improving weaknesses in personal development are goals more appropriate for a longer-term therapeutic intervention, in which the focus is on insight development. Although the client may learn new, adaptive measures as a result of crisis intervention, this is not the goal.

7. The answer is 3.

The client's feeling of self-blame is a common response to a rape-trauma crisis. However, this is not a realistic perception of the event, and the nurse should point out reality (telling the victim that the rapist is responsible). The responses in options 1 and 2 would only serve to reinforce the client's misperception that her own behavior caused the rape and, therefore, are incorrect. The response in option 4 is incorrect because it avoids addressing the client's distress and is unsupportive to the situation.

8. The answer is 4.

In this situation, the nurse can best respond to the client's anger by using empathy to address his underlying feelings (frustration). This approach will help to deescalate anger. Because the client's anger has not escalated to physical, acting-out behavior, calling security would be premature. Defending the doctor is inappropriate in this situation. Also, this might further escalate the client's anger. It is im-

portant to respond to the client's underlying feelings. If the nurse firmly tells the client not to shout and to be patient, the client is likely to see this as nonsupportive and authoritarian, which would only escalate his anger.

9. The answer is 2.

Following Maslow's *Hierarchy of Needs* to determine crisis intervention priorities, the nurse must make immediate provisions for the client to eat because this basic need is currently unmet. All of the remaining interventions would be appropriate during crisis intervention; however, providing nutrition is the first priority.

10. The answer is 4.

A client who is experiencing a crisis has difficulty performing usual life roles because of acute distress. He also typically has somatic symptoms and poor concentration resulting from the physiologic stress response. All of the remaining symptoms commonly occur with the onset of mental illness, but they are not characteristic of a crisis response.

11. The answer is 4.

An important principle of crisis intervention is the strengthening and support of healthy aspects of an individual's functioning. This is important because the client needs to resolve the crisis and identifying his individual strengths will enhance his ability to cope. Although the remaining responses are generally true and reflect good nursing practice, they are not the primary reason for assessing client strengths during a crisis.

12. The answer is 1.

Standing between the client and the exit door will allow the nurse to quickly exit the area if the client attempts physical aggression. Standing within an arm's length of the client would not afford enough protection. Standing or sitting next to the client could be misinterpreted as a threat, and the client may lash out.

13. The answer is 2, 3, 4.

These questions will help the nurse understand the client's perspective of the crisis events, the available support systems, and the coping measures attempted thus far. The remaining options are irrelevant to the client's current predicament and will not assist the nurse in analyzing the crisis experience.

13 *Group Therapy*

I. OVERVIEW OF GROUP THERAPY

A. Key concepts

1. A **group** is a collection of individuals whose association is based on a shared purpose or common interests, values, and goals.

2. **Group dynamics** are the underlying forces working to produce behavior patterns in groups; these forces include group roles, stages of group development, and group norms.

3. A **group process** is the combined verbal and nonverbal interactions occurring within the group and the meanings they convey; it includes:

   a. Communication content (what is said verbally)

   b. Relationships among members

   c. Seating arrangements

   d. Speaking patterns or tones

   e. Body language and gestures

   f. Group themes, which may be overtly or covertly expressed.

4. There are three general types of group therapy: psychotherapy groups, therapeutic groups, and self-help groups.

II. GROUP DYNAMICS

A. Key concepts

1. Groups can be **curative.**

   a. Working in a group setting allows clients to develop better insight through shared information about common problems.

   b. Several factors associated with a group's interpersonal interactions may play a role in effecting a cure. (See *Display 13-1, Curative factors of group therapy.*)

2. **Group norms** are the implicit or explicit rules of conduct defining member behavior.

DISPLAY 13-1
Curative factors of group therapy

Group therapy provides a forum for support, shared information, and insight development that can lead to better coping, healthier behaviors and, ultimately, a cure. The following curative factors, outlined by Irvin D. Yalom in his **Theory and Practice of Group Psychotherapy**, play an important role in a group setting:

- Installation of hope (belief that problems can be solved)
- Universality of experience (support from others with a similar problem)
- Imparted information (shared knowledge)
- Altruism (concern and support for others)
- Corrective experience of primary family group (re-experiencing and resolving early conflicts)
- Socialization development (learning and developing new skills)
- Initiative behaviors (role modeling)
- Interpersonal learning (perceptions of self by members)
- Group cohesiveness (sense of belonging)
- Catharsis (sharing positive and negative feelings)
- Existential factors (self-direction of one's life)

TABLE 13-1
Leadership styles and group functioning

Leadership style can have a significant effect on group dynamics and functioning, as highlighted below.

Leadership style	Characteristics of leader	Effect on group members
Authoritarian	▪ Exerts total control ▪ Makes all decisions ▪ Discourages sharing among members ▪ Task-oriented	▪ Can lead to frustration and anger among members ▪ May encourage scapegoating ▪ May foster passive-aggressive behavior (such as absenteeism)
Democratic	▪ Encourages member involvement ▪ Fosters collaboration and cohesiveness ▪ Promotes open communication	▪ Promotes feeling that individual members are valued ▪ Fosters loyalty ▪ Encourages productivity
Laissez-faire	▪ Functions as resource/consultant ▪ Provides minimal direction ▪ Promotes minimal interpersonal interactions	▪ Can cause members to feel lost or without direction ▪ Promotes disorganization ▪ May lead to apathy

---

   a. **Productive norms** enhance the group's function (such as agreeing that all members' opinions are valued or allowing only one member to speak at a time).

   b. **Nonproductive norms** inhibit the group's function (for example, not allowing disagreements or accepting absenteeism and tardiness).

   3. Leadership of a group may be shared (by co-leaders or co-therapists), or the group may be led by one individual; common leadership includes authoritarian, democratic, and laissez-faire styles. (See *Table 13-1, Leadership styles and group functioning.*)

   4. Group therapy can occur in both inpatient and outpatient community settings; brief inpatient stays and managed care directives provide a financial incentive for using group methods of treatment.

B. Stages of group development

   1. Groups work through three typical stages of development.

   2. In the **orientation stage,** group expectations are established and group norms are specified.

   a. Anxiety levels may be high among members.

   b. Superficial sharing occurs.

   3. During the **working stage,** members work productively on the established goals and focus on the purpose of the group.

   a. Members increase their level of self-disclosure.

   b. A cohesiveness develops within the group.

   4. In the **termination stage,** summarization of the group experience (closure) occurs.

   a. Members share feelings of sadness or loss.

b. Some may reexperience anxiety felt during the orientation stage.

C. Group roles

1. Each member typically has a role within the group.
2. These roles can overlap and change among members, depending on the situation; they may also be helpful or impede the group.
3. Typical roles include:
    a. **Initiator:** suggests innovative ideas and starts interactions
    b. **Coordinator:** organizes and integrates the progress of the group
    c. **Evaluator:** appraises group performance
    d. **Information seeker:** elicits facts
    e. **Gatekeeper:** screens input and maintains open communication
    f. **Encourager:** offers praise and acceptance
    g. **Harmonizer:** maintains peace through compromise and alternatives
    h. **Commentator:** processes the group interactions
    i. **Blocker:** inhibits group advancement
    j. **Recognition seeker:** seeks self-praise
    k. **Monopolizer:** controls by endless talking
    l. **Self-confessor:** discloses personal information inappropriately.

D. Role of the nurse

1. In group therapy, the nurse's role depends on her educational level and experience, as outlined by the ANA *Standards of Psychiatric-Mental Health Clinical Nursing Practice.*
2. The **psychiatric-mental health generalist** or **registered nurse** works with groups on issues that pose immediate problems with clients' health or well-being (medication teaching groups, stress management groups).
3. The **psychiatric-mental health clinical specialist** or **nurse practitioner** works as a group therapist, using her knowledge of behavior at the interpersonal and group levels.

III. TYPES OF GROUPS

A. Psychotherapy groups

1. Psychotherapy focuses on encouraging members to analyze and improve interpersonal functioning.
2. Groups are designed around a specific theoretical framework. (See Chapter 2, page 21.)
3. The most common types of psychotherapy groups include:
    a. Psychoanalytic group therapy
    b. Interpersonal group therapy
    c. Cognitive-behavioral group therapy.

B. Therapeutic groups

1. Therapeutic groups focus on group relations, interactions among members, and immediate issues of living and behaving (relationship conflicts, job-related coping problems, health issues).

2. Several types of groups are available to clients on both an inpatient and outpatient basis.

   a. **Support groups** provide acceptance and empathy for members, reinforce existing strengths, and reduce anxiety; examples include posttraumatic stress groups, cancer support groups, and Recovery, Inc.

   b. **Activity groups** (art, music, and dance groups) facilitate communication and interaction by encouraging expression of feelings in nonverbal ways; they also enhance self-esteem.

   c. **Education groups** (medication management, stress management) provide information on topics of interest; they empower clients through self-management of behaviors.

   d. **Socialization groups** (clubs, hobby groups) help members to improve interaction skills and plan activities for mutual enjoyment.

   e. **Reality-orientation groups** (current events groups) assist clients with cognitive impairments by using a variety of environmental reminders (such as clocks, television, radio, newspapers, magazines).

   f. **Community meeting groups** (inpatient groups on a particular psychiatric unit) explore common concerns and focus on problems in group-living situations.

     – They discuss and clarify rules, requests, and privileges.

     – They also encourage clients to be self-directed.

C. Self-help groups

1. Members (rather than mental health professional leadership) run the group.
2. Members share the same problem (such as an addiction), which is the chief focus of the group's work, and offer strategies for coping.
3. Examples include:

   a. Alcoholics Anonymous (AA) and Narcotics Anonymous (NA)

   b. Al-Anon and Alateen, for families of alcoholics and substance abusers

   c. Recovery, Inc., for people with mental health problems

   d. Overeaters Anonymous, modeled after AA principles, for people with addictive eating behaviors.

NURSING PROCESS OVERVIEW

 ## IV. CARE OF THE CLIENT IN GROUP THERAPY

A. Assessment

1. Assess the individual client behaviors within the group.
2. Assess group processes, noting such factors as:

   a. Seating preferences

   b. Communication patterns (who talks, to whom communication is directed, how often an individual speaks)

   c. Nonverbal patterns of communication (tone of voice, body language)

   d. Response to group norms

   e. Roles assumed by individual members.

B. Nursing diagnoses

1. Recognize how the group's behavior and your own behavior affect individual group members (for example, group behavior may trigger an emotional response in some members).
2. Analyze group dynamics and group processes.
3. Establish individualized nursing diagnoses for clients within the group, as needed:
   a. *Anxiety*
   b. *Decisional conflict (specify)*
   c. *Deficient knowledge (specify)*
   d. *Impaired social interaction*
   e. *Impaired verbal communication*
   f. *Ineffective coping*
   g. *Ineffective health maintenance*
   h. *Posttrauma syndrome*
   i. *Readiness for enhanced management of therapeutic regimen*
   j. *Situational low self-esteem*

C. Planning and outcome identification

1. Work with group members in setting realistic goals.
2. Establish desired outcome criteria for the group and individual members.
   a. Members will participate in group activities.
   b. Members will demonstrate concern for individual members of the group.
   c. Members will focus on the identified purpose related to the specific group type and task.
   d. Members will improve communication and socialization skills.
   e. Members will learn effective ways to manage therapeutic regimens.
   f. Members will demonstrate improved individual coping behaviors.

D. Implementation

1. During the **orientation phase,** take the following measures:
   a. Provide directives and establish the contract for meeting schedules, purpose, and goals for the group.
   b. Encourage open communication and feedback from all members.
   c. Discuss and establish group norms of behavior.
2. During the **working phase,** take the following measures:
   a. Assume the appropriate role as leader, depending on the type of group.
   b. Listen, observe, and provide therapeutic feedback.
   c. Comment on behavior that enhances or hinders group progress.
   d. Recognize conflicts and discuss them in an open manner.
   e. Foster self-esteem among members.
   f. Focus on immediate issues and problems of members.
   g. Provide appropriate information in an educational group setting.
   h. Ensure the participation of all members.
3. During the **termination phase,** take the following measures:
   a. Assume a supportive role in assisting members to identify and discuss termination feelings.

    b. Encourage evaluation of group and individual members' progress.

    c. Refer those whose needs were not met by the group for further evaluation and treatment.

E. Outcome evaluation

1. The group exhibits shared allegiance and responsibility.
2. The group demonstrates active participation by all members.
3. The group accomplishes its goals or purpose.
4. The group communicates among all members, not just between leaders and members.
5. Individual members demonstrate use of communication skills.
6. Individual members apply problem-solving skills to their own life.
7. Individual members report improved coping and behavior.
8. Individual members state effective ways to manage their therapeutic regimen.

Study questions

1. During a support group meeting, one of the members continually interrupts when others are talking and offers solutions to problems addressed. Which of the following is the best way for the nurse leader to intervene?
1. Ask the group to address this behavior.
2. Ignore the interruption.
3. Tell the client who is speaking to proceed.
4. Review the established group norms.

2. The nurse group leader assesses communication and relationships among members, seating arrangements, and group themes. In doing this, which of the following is the nurse leader analyzing?
1. Group behavior
2. Group norms
3. Group process
4. Group roles

3. The nurse assesses that a number of parents in a child-care clinic have misconceptions about child development in relationship to discipline. In which type of group setting would the nurse address this issue?
1. Activity group
2. Education group
3. Self-help group
4. Support group

4. Clients involved in a psychotherapy group identify negative cognitions and work toward changing thoughts in order to influence behaviors. Which theoretical framework is the focus of this group psychotherapy?
1. Cognitive-behavioral framework
2. Interpersonal framework
3. Psychoanalytic framework
4. Self-help framework

5. The community nurse is working with a support group and notes a high rate of absenteeism and minimal participation by members. Which leadership style is the nurse most likely using in this situation?
1. Authoritarian
2. Democratic
3. Laissez-faire
4. Progressive

6. When working in the community with a caregiver support group, the nurse establishes group expectations and discusses norms of group behavior. Which stage is this group in?
1. Orientation
2. Reorganization
3. Working
4. Termination

7. The nurse must evaluate the effectiveness of a therapy group during the termination stage. Which of the following would be the best way to determine this?
1. Ask members to discuss effectiveness.
2. Elicit the leader's opinion.
3. Measure members' participation in problem solving.
4. Refer to the established group norms.

8. Community meetings are held as part of the therapeutic milieu on an inpatient psychiatric unit. The purpose of these meetings is to:
1. encourage expression of feelings in nonverbal ways.
2. provide information on topics of interest.
3. focus on issues arising from group living.
4. provide direction from the treatment team.

9. The nurse group leader of a support group in a partial hospitalization community program notes that the group atmosphere has become negative and nonaccepting of members. Which nursing intervention would be best?
1. Ask members to be more accepting.
2. Ignore this observation until the group decides to discuss it.
3. Select the most prominent offenders for private discussion.
4. Share this observation with the group.

10. The nurse initiates a medication management teaching group for clients who were recently prescribed antidepressant medications. Which nursing diagnosis would be the most appropriate for the individuals in this group?
1. *Anxiety*
2. *Decisional conflict (taking antidepressants)*
3. *Ineffective coping*
4. *Readiness for enhanced management of therapeutic regimen*

11. The psychiatric nurse-generalist is beginning a small group for the purpose of medication teaching. Which of the following nursing actions are appropriate during the orientation phase of this group? Select all that apply.
1. Provide medication teaching.
2. Foster self-esteem building.
3. Discuss norms for group behavior.
4. Comment on the behavior of individual members.
5. Encourage open communication among members.
6. Establish a group contract.

Answer key

1. The answer is 1.

Directing the group to look at this behavior helps members to explore and resolve disruptive interpersonal actions, and facilitates the group process. Ignoring this behavior would deny the group an opportunity to examine and resolve problems. Telling the client who is speaking to proceed or reviewing the established group norms would hinder group development because the nurse is taking control.

2. The answer is 3.

Group process encompasses the verbal and nonverbal interactions within the group, which are represented by communication, seating, and content of group themes. Group behavior is a part of the group process. Group norms refer to implicit or explicit rules of conduct defining members' behavior. Group roles are various aspects of behavior that individuals may assume within a group.

3. The answer is 2.

An education group is best designed to impart information on topics of common interest to a group, such as the child development information needed by the parents in this situation. Activity groups encourage nonverbal expression of feelings and would be inappropriate for this situation. Self-help groups are member-run rather than planned by mental health team members. Support groups are designed to provide acceptance and empathy for members, not to impart identified knowledge.

4. The answer is 1.

In this situation, the psychotherapy group is using a cognitive-behavioral framework.

An interpersonal framework would emphasize interpersonal sharing and fostering of communication between members to improve interpersonal functioning. A psychoanalytic framework would promote insight development into problem areas through examination of early developmental issues. A self-help framework would be member-run; it would focus on members' sharing specific problems that are common to all members and offering suggested solutions.

5. The answer is 1.

When the leader style is authoritarian, the group may demonstrate passive-aggressive behavior, such as absenteeism and minimal participation. Democratic leadership leads to loyalty and productive group work. Laissez-faire leadership may contribute to disorganized group functioning and apathy. Option 4 does not describe a leadership style.

6. The answer is 1.

The orientation phase of a group sets expectations of purpose or goals and specifies group norms. Reorganization does not describe a stage of group development. Working and termination are other phases of group development, consisting of productive work (working stage) and summarizing group experiences (termination stage).

7. The answer is 3.

Evaluation of a group's effectiveness would include determining the participation of members in the problem-solving process. Groups that are effective will have accomplished this goal. Asking the members to discuss effectiveness would be appropriate during the working phase of the group, but it would not provide evaluation data. Although eliciting the opinion of the leader is valuable, measuring participation would provide objective data. Adhering to group norms is a part of the group process that is best determined during the working phase.

8. The answer is 3.
Community encompasses both clients and staff, and meetings are held on a regular basis to provide a means of focusing on important issues related to living together in a group situation. Encouraging nonverbal expression of feelings describes the purpose of an activity group. Providing information on topics of interest describes the purpose of an educational group. Providing direction from the treatment team is not consistent with a community approach, in which self-direction is encouraged.

9. The answer is 4.
The nurse would facilitate the group process by commenting on behavior that hinders group functioning. Asking members to be more accepting or selecting the most prominent offenders for private discussion are incorrect because, in these cases, the nurse is assuming responsibility for directing a solution to the problem. Ignoring the negative, nonaccepting atmosphere until the group decides to discuss it avoids dealing with an important issue to group functioning.

10. The answer is 4.
Readiness for enhanced management of therapeutic regimen is the best nursing diagnosis for individuals who participate in group learning about treatment. *Anxiety, Decisional conflict,* and *Ineffective coping* do not apply to this situation because there is no evidence the clients are anxious, conflicted about taking antidepressants, or have difficulty coping at this time.

11. The answer is 3, 5, 6.
These actions by the nurse group leader are important during the orientation phase to set the stage for a working group. Options 1 and 4 are more appropriate in the actual working phase of the group. Self-esteem building is not the purpose of an educational group; however, as part of the working phase, it may be effective on the group process.

14 *Family Therapy*

I. OVERVIEW OF THE FAMILY SYSTEM

A. Key concepts

1. A **family** is a social system composed of two or more people who coexist and have strong emotional attachments, regular interaction, and shared concerns and responsibilities.

2. Families may be further defined as follows:

   a. A **nuclear family** is composed of a mother and a father (married or unmarried) and their child or children (by birth or adoption).

   b. An **extended family** is a broad group of people related by blood and marriage, including grandparents, uncles, aunts, and cousins.

   c. A **single-parent family** is composed of a parent and a child or children (by birth or adoption).

   d. A **blended family** is a married or unmarried couple, one or both of whom were married previously, and includes his, her, or their child or children.

   e. An **alternative family** is composed of persons with or without blood or marital ties who live together to achieve common goals.

3. A **system** is a set of elements that have reciprocal interactions or relationships; the family is considered a system.

   a. A **suprasystem** is a broad system composed of multiple smaller systems (neighborhood, community, cultural group, nation).

   b. A **subsystem** is composed of smaller subsets of the family (siblings, parents, parent-child, intergenerational relatives).

4. **Boundaries** are parameters defining who is inside and outside the system.

   a. Boundaries may be **open** (allowing free interchange), **closed** (restricting interaction), or **diffuse** (unclear).

   b. Diffuse boundaries may change the definition of who is inside or outside the system.

5. **Homeostasis** is the maintenance of system continuity, constancy, and equilibrium; all systems (including families) strive to maintain homeostasis.

B. Interdependent family systems

1. Change in any one part of a family system affects all other parts and the system as a whole.

2. Roles, behaviors, and relationships among family members are maintained in relative constancy.

3. **Coalitions** or **dyads**, formed among members of the system, may become problematic; for example, an intergenerational dyad may hinder intergenerational communication.

4. **Triangles** are emotional configurations involving three family members or two family members and an issue; for example, by pulling in a child to deflect attention away from the spousal conflict, a conflictual relationship between spouses can be calmed.

C. Levels of differentiation

1. **Differentiation,** the process of becoming an individual and developing autonomy, occurs within the family system.
2. Different family members may be at different differentiation levels.
   - *a.* A person with a **low** level of differentiation is characteristically governed by emotions, acts impulsively, and has difficulty with sharing and giving in a relationship.
   - *b.* Someone with a **moderate** level of differentiation has less emotional fluctuation, but may tend to view the world in "black/white" or "either/or" terms; relationships may be lasting, but in times of anxiety, fusion or loss of self-functioning may occur.
   - *c.* A person with a **high** level of differentiation typically maintains a balance between emotions and intellect.
     - The individual views the world in its contextual framework and has a capacity to understand multiple perspectives.
     - Relationships are characterized by mutual respect for the uniqueness and differences of others.

D. Family relationships and stages

1. Relationships among family members may be characterized or affected by:
   - *a.* **Mutual respect:** members value and encourage the differences and uniqueness of each individual
   - *b.* **Enmeshment (fusion):** overinvolvement among members with the expectation that the individuals in a family think and act alike
   - *c.* **Disengagement:** underinvolvement among members and estrangement of individuals in the family
   - *d.* **Schismatic parental relationship:** existence of an overt conflict between parents that forces a child or children to "take sides"
   - *e.* **Skewed parental relationship:** dysfunction of one spouse leads to an imbalance of roles and functioning within the family.
2. Families proceed through predictable developmental stages corresponding to the life cycle; each phase may be characterized by a particular set of adjustments that can be stressful for the family, including:
   - *a.* Coupling or marriage (relationship negotiation)
   - *b.* Childbearing (adjusting to parenting)
   - *c.* Preschool-age children (coping with toddlers)
   - *d.* School-age children (interacting with wider social system)
   - *e.* Teenage children (coping with independence)
   - *f.* Empty nest (spousal relationship renegotiation)
   - *g.* Retirement (redefining self)
   - *h.* Aging (handling losses).
3. Families can be classified as either functional or dysfunctional based on their ability to work effectively as a system. (See *Table 14-1, Comparing functional and dysfunctional family systems*, page 248.)

E. Family functioning in society

1. Families function within the larger societal system.

TABLE 14-1
Comparing functional and dysfunctional family systems

Families are classified as either functional or dysfunctional based on how successfully they measure up to characteristics commonly shared by all families. Any family may have functional and dysfunctional elements at any given time.

Characteristics	Functional family	Dysfunctional family
Role definitions	▪ Clearly defined as to who does what, when, where, and how ▪ Flexible in response to need; members can fill in or take over as necessary	▪ Unclear definitions resulting in unaccomplished important tasks ▪ Rigid in response to need; unable to fill in or take over when necessary
Boundaries	▪ Clearly defined among family subsystems as well as suprasystems ▪ Maintains open boundaries that encourage multiple exchanges from family to larger systems	▪ Unclear or diffuse; difficult to determine subsystems ▪ Closed boundaries that discourage interactions of family with larger social systems
Belief systems	▪ Beliefs supported by facts and reality ▪ Ability of family members to identify and discuss differences	▪ Beliefs based on stereotypes, myths, and biases ▪ May be unable to recognize or understand belief patterns; beliefs may not be open to discussion
Communication	▪ Clear, direct, congruent verbal and nonverbal communication	▪ Confusing, indirect communications; possible incongruency between verbal and nonverbal communication ▪ May have double-bind patterns; recipient is a victim and cannot win ("Do what I tell you—be more independent!")
Differentiation	▪ Encourages individuation of members ▪ Respects differences	▪ Discourages individuation of members ▪ Is threatened by differences
Resolution of problems	▪ Defines and names problems, explores alternative solutions, evaluates solutions ▪ Uses necessary resources for assistance	▪ Cannot define problems or generate alternative solutions ▪ Uses resources for assistance ineffectively

2. They perform the following tasks:
   a. **Physical maintenance of members:** provision of food, shelter, and clothing
   b. **Physical and emotional resource allocation:** allocation of expenses, goods, space, and emotional support
   c. **Division of labor:** division of duties involving financial responsibilities, household management, and child rearing
   d. **Socialization of members:** provision of physical, emotional, social, and spiritual guidance
   e. **Entry and release of members:** birth, adoption, moving out, visitation, living-in
   f. **Order:** conforming to family or societal rules, standards, and norms

g. **Interaction with larger systems:** interacting with church, school, neighborhood, community, and society

h. **Cultural transmission:** instillation of values, beliefs, roles and functioning, and traditions

II. FAMILY THERAPY IN NURSING

A. Key concepts

1. The goal of family therapy is to bring about beneficial change in individual members by focusing on the family as a whole.
2. This may be accomplished in several ways:
   a. Using the family's strengths to assist in identifying problems, setting goals for change, and solving problems
   b. Fostering open communication among family members
   c. Assisting one or more family members to differentiate.
3. Therapists use a historical view of family membership and functioning across generations to understand current problems; this may include:
   a. Taking a family history
   b. Constructing a family **genogram,** a pictorial representation of the family over time that includes births, deaths, marriages, and other significant events. (See *Figure 14-1, Constructing a family genogram*, page 250.)

B. Types of therapy

1. **Family systems therapy,** developed by Murray Bowen (1979), assists family members to avoid being dominated by emotional reactivity and to achieve a higher level of differentiation of self.
2. **Structural therapy,** which was developed by Salvador Minuchin (1974), encourages change within the family organization to modify each family member's position in the group.
3. **Interactional therapy,** developed by Virginia Satir (1964), identifies invisible, unspoken laws governing family relationships and uses communication theory to promote improvement in relationships.

C. Role of the nurse

1. The **psychiatric-mental health nurse specialist** (APRN or CNS) can function as a family therapist, using family theory to provide services (such as family diagnosis or psychotherapeutic intervention).
2. The **psychiatric-mental health nurse generalist** (RN, C) typically follows a nursing process approach in dealing with families; responsibilities may include:
   a. Assessment of family roles, functions, and needs as well as establishing standard North American Nursing Diagnosis Association (NANDA) nursing diagnoses
   b. Education of families regarding illnesses, resources, and treatment regimens as well as working with members to provide effective illness management
   c. Use of therapeutic communication to assist families to improve communication

FIGURE 14-1

Constructing a family genogram

A family genogram is a schematic diagram that traces a family over generations. It typically identifies genders of family members, relationships among members (marriages or liasons, children),
and significant events (births, deaths, and sometimes cause of death).

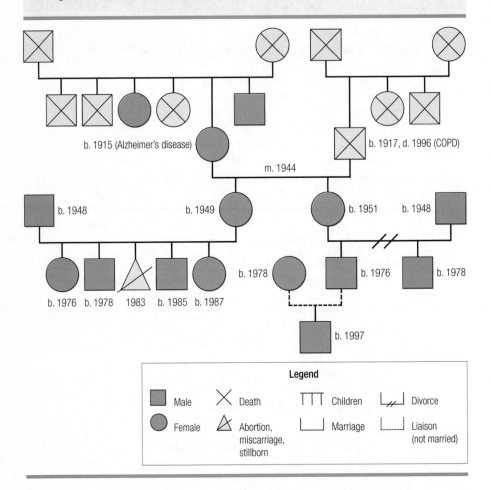

d. Collaboration with other health team members to enhance family functioning and improve the health of its members; this collaboration includes providing referrals and acting as a case manager.

NURSING PROCESS OVERVIEW

 III. CARE OF THE CLIENT IN FAMILY THERAPY

A. Assessment

1. Question the family about membership and other pertinent information. (See
   Key questions 14-1, Assessing families in therapy.)

KEY QUESTIONS 14-1
Assessing families in therapy

Questions	Information gathered
Who are the members of your family?	Family boundaries and genogram
Where do the family members live?	Shared and nonshared living arrangements
To what particular culture or ethnic group does your family belong? *Are there any health practices or customs that are important to your family?*	Cultural and ethnic identification and practices
Who provides significant support to the members of your family?	Internal and external resources
What would you say are your family's special strengths?	Family perception of strengths
Describe your family's usual communication patterns.	Communication patterns
Describe the current issues or problems affecting your family.	Family perception of problems

   a. Identify the family's developmental stage as well as the internal and external stressors affecting the family.
   b. Determine the family's ethnic and cultural beliefs and health practices.
   c. Review significant aspects of the family history.
  2. Collect data necessary to construct a family genogram.
  3. Identify family strengths, support systems, and communication patterns.
  4. Determine the family's perception of the problem.

B. Nursing diagnoses
  1. Analyze family characteristics to determine whether the family is functional or dysfunctional. (See *Table 14-1, Comparing functional and dysfunctional family systems*, page 248.)
  2. Analyze internal and external stressors on family functioning in relation to the current problem.
  3. Establish nursing diagnoses applicable to the family, as needed:
   a. Compromised family coping
   b. Disabled family coping
   c. Interrupted family processes
   d. Readiness for enhanced family coping

C. Planning and outcome identification
  1. Work with family members to establish realistic goals.
  2. Establish desired outcome criteria.
   a. Family members will use resources both within and outside the family to cope with problems.

b. Family members will communicate clearly, using congruent verbal and non-verbal messages.

c. Family members will assume clearly defined roles and responsibilities according to the situation.

d. Family members will encourage individual growth and autonomy of members.

D. Implementation

1. Develop an alliance with the family based on trust.
2. Remain neutral and objective; avoid taking sides.
3. Focus on immediate problems and relationships.
4. Model clear, congruent verbal and nonverbal communication.
5. Help the family to define who "owns" the problem and who is responsible for resolution.
6. Assist the family to develop effective communication skills, such as active listening and the use of "I" messages ("You" messages are generally accusatory and create conflict).

    a. An "I" message conveys exactly how behavior affected the well-being of the speaker; this type of message is less likely to cause anger and defensiveness because it encourages each person to be responsible for his own feelings.

    b. For example, rephrase "You should be more responsible about being on time" to say, "When I waited for an hour and you weren't home, I was really worried."

7. Support and enhance the family's existing coping skills.
8. Provide education regarding:

    a. The biological nature and signs and symptoms of mental illness

    b. Rationale for treatment recommendations

    c. Monitoring psychotropic medications

    d. Problem-solving techniques.

9. Refer the family to a qualified family therapist when problems are beyond the scope of nursing intervention at the generalist level.
10. Collaborate with the mental health team and family regarding recommendations for treatment and follow-up.
11. Encourage family members to take time for leisure pursuits and to maintain community involvements to prevent caregiver burnout.

E. Outcome evaluation

1. Family members successfully use available resources for coping with problems.
2. Family members demonstrate clear, congruent communication.
3. Family members fulfill roles and responsibilities.
4. Family members demonstrate autonomous, differentiated behaviors.

Study questions

1. The school guidance counselor refers a family with an 8-year-old child to the mental health clinic because of the child's frequent fighting in school and truancy. Which of the following data would be a priority to the nurse doing the initial family assessment?
1. The child's performance in school
2. Family education and work history
3. The family's perception of the current problem
4. The teacher's attempts to solve the problem

2. When interacting with a mother and father who are divorcing, the nurse notes that the major theme of parental disagreement is the behavior of their 13-year-old daughter. The father states that the daughter is irresponsible and lacks respect for his authority, whereas the mother cites the belief that a strict, authoritarian father rules the daughter. This situation is an example of which family systems concept?
1. Differentiation of child
2. Enmeshed relationship of parents
3. Skewed parental relationship
4. Triangulation of child

3. A 19-year-old client is admitted to a psychiatric inpatient facility for treatment of major depression. The nurse learns that the client's father has been on total disability for 3 months since an accident and that the mother has recently experienced relapse of a chronic alcohol problem. The nursing diagnosis established is *Ineffective coping related to situational stressors*. Which goal (outcome criteria) is most appropriate for intervention?
1. Establish the client's independence from the family system.

2. Ensure the mother's compliance with alcohol treatment.
3. Identify parental ownership of the problem.
4. Assist with use of family and external resources to cope with problems.

4. The parents of a young man with schizophrenia express feelings of responsibility and guilt for their son's problems. How can the nurse best educate the family?
1. Acknowledge the parents' responsibility.
2. Explain the biological nature of schizophrenia.
3. Refer the family to a support group.
4. Teach the parents various ways they must change.

5. The nurse collecting family assessment data asks, "Who is in your family and where do they live?" Which of the following is the nurse attempting to identify?
1. Boundaries
2. Ethnicity
3. Relationships
4. Triangles

6. The school nurse is conducting a class on parent-child relationships to encourage functional family development. Which statement should the nurse include when teaching the class about family resolution of conflict situations?
1. Children need to be encouraged to accept parental advice.
2. Conflict generally does not arise in functional families.
3. Discussion of conflict in a clear, direct way is important.
4. Solutions to conflicts should be provided by a neutral party.

7. According to the family systems theory, which of the following best describes the process of differentiation?
1. Cooperative action among members of a family
2. Development of autonomy within the family
3. Incongruent messages wherein the recipient is a victim
4. Maintenance of system continuity or equilibrium

8. The nurse is interacting with a family consisting of a mother, a father, and a hospitalized adolescent who has a diagnosis of alcohol abuse. The nurse analyzes the situation and agrees with the adolescent's view about family rules. Which intervention is most appropriate?
1. The nurse should align with the adolescent, who is the family scapegoat.
2. The nurse should encourage the parents to adopt more realistic rules.
3. The nurse should encourage the adolescent to comply with parental rules.
4. The nurse should remain objective and encourage mutual negotiation of issues.

9. A 16-year-old girl has returned home following hospitalization for treatment of anorexia nervosa. The parents tell the family nurse performing a home visit that their child has always done everything to please them and they cannot understand her current stubbornness about eating. The nurse analyzes the family situation and determines it is characteristic of which relationship style?
1. Differentiation
2. Disengagement
3. Enmeshment
4. Scapegoating

10. A family is in treatment with a family therapist for multiple problems. The nurse collaborating with the therapist learns that members of the family expect everyone to think alike about important issues and discourage disagreement. Which nursing action would be most appropriate during the implementation phase of the nursing process?
1. Assist each member to use "I" communication messages.
2. Tell the family they must comply with the therapist's recommendations to get the most out of therapy.
3. Determine how the family perceives the problems.
4. Provide literature on effective family functioning.

11. The staff nurse on an inpatient psychiatric unit meets with the family of a newly admitted first-time client. During the discussion, the nurse realizes that the family does not understand the client's care plan. In keeping with the nurse generalist role, which information should the nurse include in her family teaching? Select all that apply.
1. Signs and symptoms of the client's diagnosed illness
2. How invisible, unspoken laws govern family relationships
3. The nature of family triangles
4. Rationale for treatment recommendations
5. How to monitor for psychotropic medication side effects
6. The difference between skewed and schismatic relationships

Answer key

1. The answer is 3.

The family's perception of the problem is essential because change in any one part of a family system affects all other parts and the system as a whole. Each member of the family has been affected by the current problems related to the school system and the nurse would be interested in the data. The child's performance in school and the teacher's attempts to solve the problem are relevant and may be assessed; however, priority would be given to the family's perception of the problem. The family education and work history may be relevant, but are not a priority.

2. The answer is 4.

Triangulation in a family system refers to the emotional configuration involving three family members or two members and an issue. In this situation, the conflict between the spouses is handled by deflecting attention away from themselves and onto the child. Differentiation is the process of developing autonomy within the family system. An enmeshed relationship between parents refers to their overinvolvement, with the expectation that everyone in the family should think and act alike. A skewed parental relationship is characterized by having one spouse who is dysfunctional; therefore, the roles are imbalanced.

3. The answer is 4.

There are several problems currently facing this family, including the father's disability, the mother's relapse, and the child's hospitalization. Mobilizing and using resources from both inside the family (strengths) and outside the family (support systems) will constitute the most appropriate outcome for the nursing diagnosis. Autonomy or differentiation of self takes place within the family system and does not mean that independence from the family system occurs. Ensuring the mother's compliance with alcohol treatment and identifying ownership of the problem as belonging to the parents are incorrect responses, because each member of the family is involved in the current problems.

4. The answer is 2.

The parents are feeling responsible and this inappropriate self-blame can be limited by supplying them with the facts about the biologic basis of schizophrenia. Acknowledging the parents' responsibility is neither accurate nor helpful to the parents and would only reinforce their feelings of guilt. Support groups are useful; however, the nurse needs to handle the parents' self-blame directly instead of making a referral for this problem. Teaching the parents various ways to change would reinforce the parental assumption of blame; although parents can learn about schizophrenia and what is helpful and not helpful, the approach suggested in this option implies the parents' behavior is at fault.

5. The answer is 1.

Family boundaries are parameters that define who is inside and outside the system. The best method of obtaining this information is asking the family directly who they consider to be members. The question asked by the nurse would not elicit information about the family's ethnicity or culture, nor does it address the nature of the family relationship.

6. The answer is **3.**

A family's ability to discuss difficult issues openly among members reflects healthy behavior. Communication needs to be reciprocal between parents and children. Healthy, functional families are defined not by the absence of conflict, but by the manner in which it is handled. The family needs to work out solutions, not have solutions provided by another.

7. The answer is **2.**

Differentiation is the process of becoming an individual, developing autonomy while staying in contact with the family system. Cooperative action among family members does not refer to differentiation, although individuals who have a high level of differentiation would be able to accomplish cooperative action. Incongruent messages in which the recipient is a victim describe double-bind communication. Maintenance of system continuity or equilibrium is homeostasis.

8. The answer is **4.**

The nurse who wishes to be helpful to the entire family must remain neutral. Taking sides in a conflict situation in a family will not encourage negotiation, which is important for problem resolution. If the nurse aligned with the adolescent, then the nurse would be blaming the parents for the child's current problem; this would not help the family's situation. Learning to negotiate conflict is a function of a healthy family. Encouraging the parents to adopt more realistic rules or the adolescent to comply with parental rules does not give the family an opportunity to try to resolve problems on their own.

9. The answer is **3.**

Enmeshment is a fusion or overinvolvement among family members whereby the expectation exists that all members think and act alike. The child who always acts to please her parents is an example of how enmeshment affects development. In many cases, a child who develops anorexia nervosa exerts control only in the area of eating behavior. The remaining options are not appropriate to the situation described.

10. The answer is **1.**

Use of "I" communication messages will allow each member to begin to identify and discuss differences. This process is healthy and will encourage differentiation. The family therapist does not "tell" the family what to do; however, the therapist helps members find solutions to their own problems. Determining how the family perceives their problems is appropriate during the assessment phase and would have been part of the data collection done initially. Literature is helpful in educating the family; however, this situation calls for a nursing action that will stimulate differentiation of members.

11. The answer is **1, 4, 5.**

Teaching the family to recognize signs and symptoms, explaining the reason for treatment, and advising them how to monitor for side effects—all within the role of the nurse generalist—will help the family become active participants in the client's recovery. The remaining options are issues more appropriately handled by an advanced practice psychiatric nurse functioning in the role of a family therapist.

15 Somatic Therapies

I. OVERVIEW OF PSYCHOPHARMACOLOGY AND OTHER SOMATIC THERAPIES

A. Key concepts

1. Many mental illnesses (such as schizophrenia, depression, and anxiety disorder) once thought to be purely psychological are now known to be associated with chemical imbalances of neurotransmitters in the brain.

   a. **Neurotransmitters** are chemical messengers that carry inhibiting or stimulating messages from one neuron to another across the space **(synapse)** between them.

   b. **Receptor sites** are channels or specially tailored protein molecules located on presynaptic and postsynaptic cell membranes, where neurotransmitters are accepted.

2. **Psychotropic (psychoactive) drugs,** the mainstay of psychopharmacology, exert their effect in the brain; they are used to relieve behavioral and emotional symptoms of mental illness.

3. Psychotropic drugs work by altering the amount of neurotransmitters available at the synapse in the following ways:

   a. Preventing reuptake of the neurotransmitter at the presynaptic neuron

   b. Binding to receptor sites at the postsynaptic neuron (thus preventing the neurotransmitter from entering the receptor)

   c. Preventing enzymes present at the synapse from metabolizing neurotransmitters

   d. Affecting the ion channels of nerve cell membranes.

4. Selected neurotransmitters that can be altered by psychotropic drugs include:

   a. **Dopamine:** primarily affected by antipsychotics

   b. **Serotonin:** primarily affected by antidepressants and antipsychotics

   c. **Norepinephrine:** affected by mood-stabilizing agents, antidepressants, antipsychotics, and psychostimulants

   d. **Gamma-aminobutyric acid (GABA):** primarily affected by antianxiety agents

   e. **Acetylcholine:** affected by anticholinesterase agents, antipsychotics, and antidepressants.

5. Besides standard pharmacologic measures, somatic therapies for treating mental illness may include the use of medicinal herbs and other biological treatments.

B. Medicinal herbs

1. The use of **natural herbs** in treating emotional symptoms has grown tremendously over the last 10 years with the increased popularity of **complementary and alternative medicine (CAM).** (See *Table 4-2, Complementary and alternative medicine treatment*, page 66.)

2. Although herbs are currently not regulated in the United States, their safety and effectiveness can be validated by the U.S. Food and Drug Administration (www.fda.gov) and the National Center for Complementary and Alternative Medicine (www.ncam.nih.gov).

3. Some examples of herbal medicines commonly used include:

a. St. John's Wort and SAMe (S-adenosylmethionine): alleviate mild depression

b. Kava: decreases anxiety symptoms

c. Ginkgo leaf extract: improves memory

d. Melatonin: improves sleep and counteracts jet lag.

C. Other biological treatments

1. **Electroconvulsive therapy (ECT)** is used primarily for treating depression but has also been used to treat mania, catatonia, and schizophrenia that is unresponsive to medications; it requires a consent form and may be administered 2 to 3 times per week, for a total of 6 to 12 treatments.

   a. The procedure involves inducing unconsciousness, then passing an electric current through the brain; the client's vital signs, oxygenation, and cardiac functioning are carefully monitored before, during, and after ECT.

   – Short-acting anesthesia is used to induce unconsciousness.

   – An electric current (70 to 150 volts) is applied through the brain for 0.5 to 2 seconds, producing a seizure that lasts 30 to 60 seconds.

   b. Following ECT, the client is monitored according to routine postoperative protocols.

2. **Light therapy (phototherapy)** involves exposing the client to an artificial light source in the winter to relieve depression in seasonal affective disorder (SAD).

3. **Repetitive transcranial magnetic stimulation (TMS)** is an experimental treatment for depression; it involves sending an electric current through a wire coil on the client's head to generate a magnetic field, causing neurochemical changes in targeted brain areas.

4. **Eye movement desensitization reprocessing (EMDR)** is a controversial treatment for posttraumatic stress disorder; it involves asking the client to recall traumatic memories while making a series of rapid lateral eye movements.

II. ANTIPSYCHOTICS (NEUROLEPTICS)

A. General information

1. Antipsychotics are classified as either typical or atypical; for a list of commonly used antipsychotic drugs, see *Drug chart 15-1, Antipsychotic (neuroleptic) drugs*, page 260.

2. They are used to alleviate psychotic symptoms (hallucinations, delusions, paranoid thinking, poor reality contact) that may occur in clients with schizophrenia, bipolar disorders, and cognitive impairment disorders.

3. Antipsychotics may also be used to treat acute agitation, rage, and hyperactive states, which can occur in various mental disorders; additionally, they are used to treat intractable vomiting, hiccoughs, and vertigo.

4. Antipsychotics are prescribed for adults and children; however, caution is needed when administering these agents to elderly clients with decreased kidney and liver function because side effects are intensified (low doses are recommended for elderly clients).

5. These drugs are not recommended for use during pregnancy and lactation.

DRUG CHART 15-1
Antipsychotic (neuroleptic) drugs

Classification	Drug
*High-potency typical neuroleptics**	fluphenazine † (Prolixin) haloperidol † (Haldol) perphenazine (Trilafon) thiothixene (Navane) trifluoperazine (Stelazine)
Moderate-potency typical neuroleptics ‡	loxapine (Loxitane) mesoridazine (Serentil) molindone (Moban)
Low-potency typical neuroleptics §	chlorpromazine (Thorazine) chlorprothixene (Taractan) thioridazine (Mellaril)
Atypical neuroleptics	clozapine (Clozaril) olanzapine (Zyprexa) pimozide (Orap) quetiapine (Seroquel) risperidone (Risperdal) sertindole (Serlect) ziprasidone (Geodon)
Dopamine system stabilizer	aripiprazole (Abilify)

* Low-dose range; increased extrapyramidal symptom (EPS) response and seizure risk; low incidence of anticholinergic effects.

† These medications can be given in an oil suspension (decanoate) that is administered intramuscularly and has delayed onset and prolonged action. Administration may be 1 to 2 times weekly or up to 1 time per month.

‡ Mild-dose range; moderate EPS response; moderate hypotensive and anticholinergic effects.

§ High-dose range; low EPS response; increased sedative, hypotensive, and anticholinergic effects.

B. Typical antipsychotic agents

1. Typical antipsychotics block selected dopamine receptors in the striatal and limbic areas of the brain, an action believed to reduce psychotic symptoms.
   a. These antipsychotics also affect other receptors, including those for histamine, serotonin, norepinephrine, and acetylcholine.
   b. The effect on these receptors accounts for the multiple side effects.
2. **Pharmacokinetics** is as follows:
   a. Peak plasma levels occur 2 to 4 hours after administration, while serum half-life is 20 to 40 hours; the drug accumulates in fatty tissue, which accounts for the persistence of the drug's effect when it is stopped.
   b. The recommended dosage varies widely for these drugs; dosage titration is important for targeting specific changes in an individual client's symptoms.
   c. Tolerance does not develop with these drugs.

    d. Oral absorption is significantly affected by foods and stomach acidity level; consequently, these drugs should be taken at least 2 hours after eating and should not be used concurrently with antacids or histamine$_2$ (H$_2$) blocking agents (cimetidine).

    e. Asians require one-half to one-third the usual dose because they are more sensitive to drug side effects (related to p-450 genetic differences).

    f. Long-acting preparations are available for haloperidol (Haldol) and fluphenazine (Prolixin); they are administered I.M. via depot injection, and effects last 2 to 4 weeks.

3. Contraindications include:

    a. Known allergic response to any antipsychotics

    b. CNS depression

    c. Parkinson's disease

    d. Blood dyscrasias

    e. Hepatic disease

    f. Acute narrow-angle glaucoma

    g. Benign prostatic hypertrophy.

4. Interactions are as follows:

    a. Additive anticholinergic effects occur when antipsychotics are taken with antihistamines, antidepressants, antiparkinsonian agents, and other drugs with anticholinergic effects.

    b. Additive hypotensive effects are possible when antipsychotics are taken with other agents that lower blood pressure (beta blockers, calcium channel blockers, antianginal nitrate preparations).

    c. Because caffeine and nicotine interfere with therapeutic effects, intake of these substances should be minimized (no more than 10 cigarettes or 200 mg of caffeine daily).

    d. Antipsychotics potentiate the CNS depressant effects of alcohol and barbiturates.

5. Common side effects include the following (see *Table 15-1, Managing common side effects of psychotropic drugs*, pages 262 and 263):

    a. Anticholinergic effects, including dry mouth, blurred vision, urinary retention, and constipation

    b. Cardiovascular effects, including postural hypotension and tachycardia

    c. Sedation, drowsiness, and lack of alertness

    d. Photosensitivity, including sunburn and rash

    e. Weight gain

    f. Endocrine changes, including amenorrhea and gynecomastia

    g. Extrapyramidal effects. (See *Table 15-2, Treating extrapyramidal effects of psychotropic drugs*, page 264.)

6. Some **serious but uncommon side effects** can occur with use of antipsychotic agents (see *Table 15-3, Managing serious side effects of psychotropic drugs*, page 265):

    a. Agranulocytosis (white blood cell [WBC] level < 2,000 µl)

    b. Acute dystonic reaction, characterized by severe, sudden muscle spasms

TABLE 15-1

Managing common side effects of psychotropic drugs

Side effects	Nursing interventions
Anticholinergic effects	
Dry mouth	Suggest the use of sugarless gum or candy, rinsing the mouth frequently with water (advise avoiding commercial mouthwash, which will increase dryness).
Blurred vision	Caution the client to avoid driving or operating heavy machinery until vision problem subsides. Eye pain can indicate acute narrow-angle glaucoma; if this occurs, notify the doctor.
Urinary retention	Teach the client to report sensation of bladder fullness or incomplete emptying. Assess for bladder distention; clients with benign prostatic hypertrophy are susceptible to acute urinary retention, requiring catheterization.
Constipation	Encourage the client to drink 6 to 8 glasses of water daily, add fiber to his diet, and exercise regularly.
Cardiovascular effects	
Postural hypotension	Teach the client to change positions slowly, especially when moving from a lying to standing position. Assess the client's blood pressure (take lying, sitting, and standing pressures to validate postural changes, if necessary).
Arrhythmias	Teach the client to report sensations of racing pulse or heartbeat, feelings of light-headedness and dizziness. Assess the pulse (radial and apical).
CNS effects	
Headache	Advise the client that this effect may be temporary until he adjusts to the medication. Instruct him to check with his provider before taking any over-the-counter medications (acetaminophen and some nonsteroidal anti-inflammatory drugs may be contraindicated).
Drowsiness, fatigue, decreased mental alertness	Teach the client to take the prescribed dose at bedtime (for medications that decrease mental alertness and that are taken once daily). Advise him to use caution when driving or operating machinery while this effect persists.
Gastrointestinal effects	
Nausea, decreased appetite, diarrhea	Instruct the client to take medications with meals (suggest eating six small meals rather than three larger ones). Teach him to maintain normal fluid intake and to report continued diarrhea to his doctor.
Weight gain, increased appetite	Advise the client about the importance of consuming adequate calories to maintain normal weight. Encourage following a regular exercise program; discourage frequent snacking with high-calorie foods.

TABLE 15-1

Managing common side effects of psychotropic drugs *(continued)*

Side effects	Nursing interventions
Endocrine effects	
Amenorrhea (in women)	Instruct the client about continuing the use of appropriate birth-control measures because pregnancy can still occur.
Gynecomastia (in men)	Inform the client about the possibility of this effect; encourage him to discuss his feelings about body image changes.
Sexual dysfunction (anorgasmia in women, erectile dysfunction in men)	Teach the client to report any changes in sexual desire or functioning because dosage or medication may be decreased or changed.

    c. Tardive dyskinesia, characterized by involuntary mouth, tongue, and facial movements

    d. Seizures

    e. Hepatotoxicity, which may be characterized by jaundice, nausea, and abdominal pain

    f. Neuroleptic malignant syndrome, which is a severe reaction that can be fatal.

C. Atypical antipsychotic agents

    1. Atypical antipsychotics block dopamine receptors in the limbic system and affect serotonin receptors in the cortical areas of the brain.

    2. The indications, contraindications, and interactions are similar to those of typical antipsychotic agents; however, they offer the following advantages over typical antipsychotics:

        a. Atypical antipsychotic agents reduce positive symptoms of schizophrenia (hallucinations, delusions) as well as lessen the negative symptoms (blunted affect, apathy, and social withdrawal).

        b. These agents cause decreased (or no) extrapyramidal effects because they do not affect dopamine in striatal areas.

        c. Rapid-dissolving preparations of olanzapine (Zyprexa) and risperidone (Risperdal) are available; they begin to dissolve with saliva and can be swallowed without water.

    3. Common side effects are similar to those of typical antipsychotics and include the following:

        a. Seizures

        b. Agranulocytosis, which is associated primarily with clozapine (incidence of 1% to 2%)

          – The FDA currently mandates weekly testing of WBC counts for the first 6 months while taking these drugs.

          – Biweekly testing can then be instituted if counts are acceptable.

TABLE 15-2

Treating extrapyramidal effects of psychotropic drugs

Various involuntary movements known as extrapyramidal side effects are produced by many psychotropic drugs, which block dopamine at receptor sites. A standard assessment tool, such as the Abnormal Involuntary Movement Scale (AIMS), may be used to detect these symptoms. Common treatments and nursing interventions are included below.

Effect	Treatment	Nursing interventions
Pseudoparkinsonism drooling, lack of facial responsiveness, shuffling gait, and fine intention tremors	■ Administer an antiparkinson (anticholinergic) drug: – benztropine (Cogentin) – biperiden (Akineton) – trihexyphenidyl (Artane).	■ Assess for this effect; note that elderly clients are more susceptible. ■ Notify the doctor if this occurs.
Acute dystonic reaction muscle spasms of jaw, tongue, neck, or eyes; laryngeal spasms may occur	■ Stop drug and administer antidote: – benztropine (Cogentin) – diphenhydramine (Benadryl).	■ Treat as an emergency. ■ Withhold any further doses. ■ Administer the antidote if a standing order has been provided. If no order is available, alert the doctor immediately. ■ Reassure the client.
Akasthisia motor restlessness	■ Administer an antiparkinson drug: – benztropine (Cogentin) – biperiden (Akineton) – trihexyphenidyl (Artane). ■ May reduce antipsychotic dose if symptom persists.	■ Assess for this effect. ■ Administer an antiparkinson (anticholinergic) drug. ■ Reassure the client.
Tardive dyskinesia involuntary movements of mouth, tongue, and face; movements may extend to fingers, arms, and trunk	■ No antidote available. Stop drug or continue at a lower dose; if necessary, change to another medication.	■ Assess for this effect; note that elderly clients are more susceptible. ■ Notify the doctor if this occurs.

   D. Dopamine system stabilizer (DSS)
      1. Currently, only one drug is available in this class: aripiprazole (Abilify).
      2. DSS restores dopamine activity in cortical levels of the brain and reduces dopamine in limbic areas, thus decreasing psychotic symptoms.
      3. This drug is not metabolized by P-450 enzymes; therefore, few drug-drug interactions occur.
      4. **Common side effects** include headache, nausea, vomiting, constipation, insomnia, lightheadedness, and akathisia. (See *Table 15-1, Managing common side effects of psychotropic drugs*, pages 262 and 263 and *Table 15-3, Managing serious side effects of psychotropic drugs*, page 265.)

TABLE 15-3
Managing serious side effects of psychotropic drugs

Side effect and symptoms	Treatment	Nursing interventions
Agranulocytosis White blood cell (WBC) level < 2,000; sore throat, low-grade fever, malaise, mouth sores	▪ Stop drug. ▪ Initiate reverse isolation for client safety.	▪ Monitor complete blood count, paying particular attention to decreasing WBC. ▪ Notify the doctor. ▪ Withhold any further doses. ▪ If the client's WBC level decreases, institute infection precautions.
Seizures Tonic-clonic seizure activity	▪ Reduce dose or stop drug. ▪ Add an anticonvulsant medication to prevent further seizures.	▪ Ensure the client's safety during any seizure activity. ▪ Notify the doctor. ▪ Administer anticonvulsant medication as prescribed.
Hepatotoxicity Abnormal liver function series (elevated enzymes); fever, nausea, jaundice, abdominal pain	▪ Stop drug. ▪ Treat symptoms with bed rest, good nutrition, and adequate fluids.	▪ Monitor the client for any symptoms described. ▪ Monitor results of liver function studies. ▪ Notify the doctor if hepatotoxity is suspected. ▪ Ensure adequate rest, nutrition, and fluids.
Neuroleptic malignant syndrome Altered consciousness, severe hyperthermia (102° F [38.9° C] and higher), diaphoresis, tachycardia, and extrapyramidal effects resulting from massive dopamine blockade in the brain and CNS	▪ Stop drug. ▪ Administer a drug that stimulates dopamine receptors, such as bromocriptine (Parlodel). ▪ Administer I.V. fluids, hypothermia measures, and antiarrhythmic medication.	▪ Monitor for any symptoms described. ▪ Withhold any further doses. ▪ Notify the doctor. ▪ Prepare to transfer the client to the intensive care unit.
Serotonin syndrome Severe hypothermia, altered muscle tone (hyperreflexia), altered consciousness, tachycardia, and diaphoresis resulting from use of antidepressants (increase serotonin bioavailablilty)	▪ Stop drug. ▪ Administer a serotonin receptor antagonist, such as methysergide (Sansert) or cyproheptadine (Periactin). ▪ Administer I.V. fluids, hypothermia measures, and antiarrhythmic medication.	▪ Ensure selected serotonin reuptake inhibitors and monoamine oxidase inhibitors are not used concurrently; monitor for the appropriate "washout" period when switching between these groups. ▪ Monitor the client for any symptoms described. ▪ Withhold any further doses. ▪ Notify the doctor. ▪ Prepare to transfer the client to the intensive care unit.

III. ANTIDEPRESSANTS

A. General information

1. Antidepressants are a group of drugs generally used to treat depression, including symptoms of depressed mood, loss of interest in activities or pleasure, altered sleep patterns, and somatic complaints.

2. They are also used to treat anxiety disorders (especially panic attacks), phobic disorders, and obsessive-compulsive disorder; additionally, they are used to treat anxiety symptoms that occur with depressive disorder.

3. Antidepressants may be further classified based on their mechanism of action and general usage; see *Drug chart 15-2, Antidepressant drugs*, for a list of classifications and specific drugs.

DRUG CHART 15-2
Antidepressant drugs

Classification	Drug
Tricyclic antidepressants	amitriptyline (Elavil) amoxapine (Asendin) clomipramine (Anafranil) desipramine (Norpramin) doxepin (Sinequan) imipramine (Tofranil) maprotiline (Ludiomil) nortriptyline (Aventyl, Pamelor) protriptyline (Vivactil) trimipramine (Surmontil)
Monoamine oxidase inhibitors	isocarboxazid (Marplan) moclobemide (Manerix) phenelzine (Nardil) tranylcypromine (Parnate)
Selective serotonin reuptake inhibitors	citalopram (Celexa) escitalopram (Lexapro) fluoxetine (Prozac) fluvoxamine (Luvox) paroxetine (Paxil) sertraline (Zoloft)
Atypical antidepressants	bupropion (Wellbutrin) trazodone (Desyrel)
Serotonin-norepinephrine reuptake inhibitors	mirtazapine (Remeron) nefazodone (Serzone) reboxetine (Edronax, Vestra) venlafaxine (Effexor)

B. Tricyclic antidepressants (TCAs)

1. TCAs work by blocking the reuptake of several neurotransmitters (nonselective action) at presynaptic neurons; neurotransmitters affected include serotonin, norepinephrine, acetylcholine, and dopamine.

2. TCAs are prescribed for adults and elderly clients; however, they should be used with caution in elderly clients because of the potential cardiac effects.

   a. Selective serotonin reuptake inhibitors (SSRIs), such as setraline (Zoloft) and fluvoxamine (Luvox), are being prescribed for children and appear to be working well.

   b. TCAs are not recommended during pregnancy and lactation.

3. Pharmacokinetics of TCAs is as follows:

   a. Because the serum half-life is 20 to 126 hours, TCAs can be taken once daily.

   b. Therapeutic blood levels must be established to ensure optimal dosage.

   c. Although tolerance does not develop with these drugs, taking three times the maximum dose can be lethal; TCAs must be used with extreme caution in clients at risk for suicide.

   d. Therapeutic effectiveness takes 2 to 4 weeks; the client may become discouraged and discontinue taking the drug if not advised about this.

4. **Contraindications** include:

   a. Cardiovascular disease, which can be a serious problem (a baseline ECG is recommended prior to TCA treatment, especially in the elderly client)

   b. Glaucoma

   c. Benign prostatic hypertrophy

   d. Liver and renal diseases.

5. **Interactions** are as follows:

   a. Fatal interactions may occur with concurrent use of antiarrhythmics, monoamine oxidase inhibitors (MAOIs), or SSRIs.

   b. Additive anticholinergic effects may occur when TCAs are taken with antihistamines, antipsychotics, antiparkinsonian agents, and other drugs with anticholinergic effects.

   c. Additive serotonergic effects may occur when TCAs are combined with other categories of antidepressant drugs.

   d. Additive sympathomimetic effects may occur when TCAs are combined with drugs causing adrenergic stimulation; the combination may cause tachycardia and hypertension.

   e. Additive hypotensive effects may occur when TCAs are combined with drugs that lower blood pressure (beta blockers, calcium channel blockers, antianginal nitrate preparations).

   f. Bleeding may be increased when TCAs are combined with warfarin (Coumadin).

6. **Common side effects** include the following (see *Table 15-1, Managing common side effects of psychotropic drugs*, pages 262 and 263):

   a. Anticholinergic effects, including dry mouth, blurred vision, urinary retention, and constipation

   b. Cardiovascular effects, including hypotension, hypertension, arrhythmias, prolonged QRS complex, and heart failure

TABLE 15-4
Tricyclic antidepressant overdose

Tricyclic antidepressants produce various toxic effects, the most serious of which affect the cardiovascular system, central nervous system, and peripheral nervous system. An overdose can cause blockage of acetylcholine at receptor sites, resulting in anticholinergic toxicity and rapidly developing symptoms. Untreated, toxicity can be fatal.

Symptoms	Treatment
▪ Sedation	▪ Monitor the client's vital signs and ECG readings.
▪ Ataxia	▪ Maintain a patent airway.
▪ Agitation	▪ Administer cathartics or gastric lavage with activated charcoal.
▪ Stupor	
▪ Coma	▪ Administer cholinergic-stimulant medication, such
▪ Convulsions and respiratory depression	as physostigmine (Antilirium).

    c. Photosensitivity

    d. Gastrointestinal effects, including anorexia and nausea

    e. CNS effects, including sedation and fatigue.

  7. Serious side effects are possible with TCAs (see *Table 15-3, Managing serious side effects of psychotropic drugs*, page 265) and may include:

    a. Overdose (for specific symptoms, see *Table 15-4, Tricyclic antidepressant overdose*)

    b. Serotonin syndrome, which is characterized by hypothermia, hyperreflexia, tachycardia, diaphoresis, and decreased level of consciousness

    c. Agranulocytosis (WBC level < 2,000 µl)

    d. Seizures.

C. Monoamine oxidase inhibitors (MAOIs)

  1. MAOIs inhibit the enzyme monoamine oxidase, which is responsible for breaking down excess serotonin and norepinephrine at the synapse; when this enzyme is inhibited, the neurotransmitters remain active at the synapse. (See *Drug chart 15-2, Antidepressant drugs*, page 266, for a list of commonly used MAOIs.)

  2. Pharmacokinetics for this group is as follows:

    a. The serum half-life is unknown for these drugs.

    b. The enzyme monoamine oxidase is also normally active in the liver; consequently, use of these drugs inhibits the liver's activity, leading to elevated levels of other drugs that are normally metabolized in the liver.

    c. Therapeutic effectiveness is reached in 2 to 4 weeks.

  3. Contraindications include:

    a. Cardiovascular disease or history of stroke

    b. Hyperthyroidism

    c. Pheochromocytoma

    d. Elective surgery (MAOIs should be discontinued at least 2 weeks before surgery because MAOIs increase the risk of severe hypotension when anesthesia is given).

TABLE 15-5
Substances that interact with MAOIs

Certain substances interact with monoamine oxidase inhibitors (MAOIs) to produce a dangerous additive sympath-omimetic effect. MAOIs increase norepinephrine levels; combining an MAOI with drugs containing ephedrine, epi-nephrine, phenylephrine, or phenylpropanolamine further increases these levels. Foods and beverages containing tyramine can cause a hypertensive crisis when combined with an MAOI and should be avoided.

Drugs	Foods	Beverages
■ Over-the-counter cold and cough preparations	■ Products containing brewer's yeast	■ Beer
■ Over-the-counter allergy medications	■ Broad beans	■ Coffee
■ Prescribed drugs, such as psychostimulants	■ Pickles, sauerkraut	■ Tea
■ Substances of abuse, including cocaine and amphetamines	■ Bananas, figs, raisins	■ Chianti wine
	■ Cheddar or aged cheese, yogurt	
	■ Chicken liver, pickled herring	
	■ Smoked salmon, snails	
	■ Chocolate, licorice, soy sauce	

4. **Interactions** are as follows:
   a. Additive serotonergic effects may occur when an MAOI is combined with any other antidepressant. (See *Table 15-3, Managing serious side effects of psychotropic drugs*, page 265.)
   b. Additive anticholinergic effects are possible when the drug is combined with drugs having anticholinergic side effects.
   c. Additive sympathomimetic effects may occur when an MAOI is combined with drugs that stimulate the sympathetic nervous system (epinephrine, nor-epinephrine, amphetamines, over-the-counter cold preparations) or with foods containing tyramine. (See *Table 15-5, Substances that interact with MAOIs.*)
5. **Common side effects** include (see *Table 15-1, Managing common side effects of psychotropic drugs*, pages 262 and 263):
   a. Anticholinergic effects
   b. Cardiovascular effects
   c. CNS stimulation, resulting in anxiety, agitation, restlessness, and insomnia (clients should report this effect because drug may need to be discontinued).
6. **Serious side effects** include (see *Table 15-3, Managing serious side effects of psychotropic drugs*, page 265):
   a. Agranulocytosis
   b. Hepatic toxicity
   c. Hypertensive crisis, which is associated with tyramine-containing substances. (See *Table 15-5, Substances that interact with MAOIs.*)
      – Symptoms include severe occipital headache, nausea, vomiting, elevated blood pressure, photophobia, dilated pupils, and arrhythmia.
      – Treatment is directed at measures to decrease blood pressure, such as oral administration of nifedipine (Procardia) or I.V. phentolamine (Regitine).

TABLE 15-6

Common side effects of SSRIs

Side effect	Nursing interventions
Insomnia	▪ Instruct the client to take the dose early in the day. ▪ Teach the client to eliminate caffeine. ▪ Encourage the client to use relaxation techniques before bed.
Headache	▪ Instruct the client to use analgesics as prescribed and to check with the doctor before taking any over-the-counter drugs. ▪ If the client has severe headaches, check with the doctor about the possibility of discontinuing the drug.
Weight loss	▪ Encourage the client to consume adequate calories to maintain weight. Note that extreme caution is needed when the client has an eating disorder.
Sexual dysfunction Anorgasmia in women, ejaculatory dysfunction in men	▪ Advise the client that sexual dysfunction is possible with these drugs, and instruct him to speak with the doctor because another antidepressant may be prescribed.

D. Selective serotonin reuptake inhibitors (SSRIs)

1. SSRIs specifically affect the neurotransmitter serotonin by preventing its reuptake at the synapse. (See *Drug chart 15-2, Antidepressant drugs*, page 266, for a listing of specific drugs in this group.)

2. Because other neurotransmitters are not affected, these drugs do not have the same side effects as other antipsychotic agents. (See *Table 15-6, Common side effects of SSRIs.*)

3. **Pharmacokinetics** is as follows:

   a. The serum half-life is 20 to 168 hours; therefore, SSRIs can be given once daily.

   b. Tolerance does not develop, and these drugs have a low potential for overdose.

   c. Therapeutic effectiveness occurs in 2 to 4 weeks.

4. **Contraindications** include:

   a. Hypersensitivity reactions

   b. Severe hepatic or renal disease

   c. Seizures

   d. Diabetes mellitus.

5. **Interactions** include the following:

   a. Additive CNS depressive effects may occur when combining SSRIs with alcohol, antihistamines, and opioids.

   b. Additive serotonergic effects are possible when SSRIs are combined with other antidepressants (TCAs, MAOIs); allow a 5-week "washout" period when switching from an SSRI to an MAOI.

   c. SSRIs may increase the risk of toxicity from other drugs (digitoxin, phenytoin, lithium, warfarin).

E. Atypical antidepressants

1. These drugs do not have a well-explained mechanism of action, although they are thought to act similarly to TCAs. (See *Drug chart 15-2, Antidepressant drugs*, page 266, for a list of specific drugs in this category.)
2. Their main advantage over TCAs is fewer side effects, particularly fewer anticholinergic and cardiovascular effects.
3. **Pharmacokinetics** for each drug in this category is unique to the drug; consult a pharmacology text for greater details.
4. **Contraindications** and **interactions** include:
   a. Digoxin preparations (use with trazodone increases the risk of digitalis toxicity)
   b. Zyban, a smoking-cessation medication that contains buproprion (combined use can cause seizures).
5. **Common side effects** are as follows:
   a. Seizures, which are associated with buproprion
   b. Priapism (prolonged painful penile erection), which is associated with trazodone.

F. Serotonin-norepinephrine reuptake inhibitors (SNRIs)

1. A new generation of antidepressants, SNRIs selectively inhibit the reuptake of both serotonin and norepinephrine.
2. SNRIs have the same general uses and characteristics as other antidepressants.
3. **Common side effects** include GI upset, dose-related hypertension, insomnia, restlessness, headache, and irritability. (See *Table 15-1, Managing common side effects of psychotropic drugs*, pages 262 and 263.)
4. Caution should be used with nefazone because serious liver failure has been reported; it has been withdrawn from use in Europe.

IV. MOOD STABILIZERS

A. General information

1. Mood stabilizers are a class of drugs that include antimanics and anticonvulsants. (See *Drug chart 15-3, Mood stabilizer drugs*.)

DRUG CHART 15-3
Mood stabilizer drugs

Classification	Drug
Antimanics	lithium carbonate (Eskalith, Lithane)
Anticonvulsants	carbamazepine (Tegretol) gabapentin (Neurontin) lamotrigine (Lamactal) oxcarbazepine (Trileptal) topiramate (Topamax) valproic acid (Depakene, Depakote)

2. Specific uses include:

  a. Treatment of the manic cycle of bipolar disorder

  b. Prevention of recurrent episodes of mania and depression characteristic in bipolar disorder

  c. Treatment of schizoaffective disorder and episodes of acute hyperactivity associated with other mental disorders.

3. These drugs are prescribed for children and adults; however, elderly clients are particularly sensitive to toxicity because of decreased renal function.

4. They are not recommended for use during pregnancy and lactation.

B. Antimanics (lithium carbonate)

  1. Although its mechanism of action is poorly understood, lithium is thought to normalize reuptake of neurotransmitters, including serotonin, norepinephrine, dopamine, and acetylcholine.

  2. Unlike most of the psychotropic medications, lithium exerts its action intracellularly rather than at the synapse.

  3. Pharmacokinetics include the following:

  a. The serum half-life is about 24 hours.

  b. Lithium is metabolized by the kidneys and is similar in chemical structure to sodium, competing at various body receptor sites with sodium; if sodium intake is reduced or serum sodium levels are depleted, lithium will be reabsorbed rather than excreted by the kidney and may reach toxic levels in the body.

  c. The blood level of lithium has a narrow therapeutic range (0.6 to 1.2 mEq/L); blood levels greater than 1.5 mEq/L are considered toxic.

  d. Upon initiation of lithium, blood is drawn either daily or every 2 to 3 days until a therapeutic level is identified for the individual client.

  e. When the client's symptoms resolve, the lithium dose is decreased for maintenance treatment of one-half to two-thirds the acute dose; blood levels are then monitored every 2 to 3 months or when a problem is suspected.

  4. Contraindications include:

  a. Hypersensitivity response (to lithium)

  b. Renal disease

  c. Thyroid disease

  5. Interactions are as follows:

  a. Concurrent use with anesthetics, angiotensin-converting enzyme (ACE) inhibitors, nonsteroidal anti-inflammatory drugs (NSAIDs), tetracycline, or thiazide diuretics increases the risk of lithium toxicity.

  b. The risk of lithium toxicity also increases when sodium intake is less than 2 g/day; when fluids and sodium are lost due to excessive exercise, dehydration, or gastrointestinal illness; and when fluid intake is less than 6 to 8 glasses of water daily.

  c. Lithium levels may decrease if the drug is taken with acetazolamide, theophylline preparations, mannitol or other osmotic diuretics, sodium bicarbonate, or xanthines.

  6. Common side effects include (see *Table 15-1, Managing common side effects of psychotropic drugs*, pages 262 and 263):

TABLE 15-7
Preventing lithium toxicity

Lithium toxicity is a serious, potentially life-threatening condition. Clients receiving lithium should be advised of the following ways to prevent toxicity:
- Restrict caffeine intake.
- Maintain adequate water intake (6 to 8 glasses per day).
- Maintain adequate sodium intake (2 g daily).
- When exercising, drink fluids containing essential electrolytes (sports drinks).
- Contact the doctor if severe gastrointestinal symptoms develop.
- Inform all health care providers about lithium therapy, especially when surgical procedures are planned.
- Contact the doctor if symptoms indicating toxicity occur.
- Maintain appointments to monitor blood levels as prescribed.

     a. Gastrointestinal effects, including nausea, anorexia, and diarrhea

     b. Fatigue and lethargy

     c. Weight gain

     d. Polyuria (usually benign).

  7. Lithium toxicity is a serious side effect associated with elevated blood levels of the drug. (See *Table 15-7, Preventing lithium toxicity.*)

     a. Mild toxicity (lithium level 1.5 to 2.0 mEq/L) is characterized by apathy, diminished concentration, mild ataxia, muscle weakness, hand tremors, and muscle twitching.

     b. Moderate toxicity (lithium level 2.0 to 2.5 mEq/L) is characterized by severe diarrhea, nausea and vomiting, moderate ataxia, mild confusion, slurred speech, tinnitus, frank muscle twitching, and tremors.

     c. Severe toxicity (lithium level above 2.5 mEq/L) is characterized by nystagmus, muscle fasciculation, deep tendon hyperreflexia, decreased level of consciousness, tonic-clonic seizures, coma, and death.

  8. Treatment of lithium toxicity includes:

     a. Withholding any further doses (even if toxicity is only suspected)

     b. Obtaining an immediate serum lithium level to confirm toxicity level

     c. Monitoring vital signs and electrolyte, blood urea nitrogen, and creatinine levels

     d. I.V. therapy with normal saline

     e. Hemodialysis, if indicated for severe toxicity.

  9. **Serious side effects** include:

     a. Thyroid impairment (requires monitoring thyroid function studies every 3 to 6 months for clients on long-term lithium therapy)

     b. Renal impairment (requires monitoring renal function studies every 3 to 6 months for clients on long-term lithium therapy).

C. Anticonvulsants

  1. Mood-stabilizing anticonvulsants may be prescribed for clients with bipolar disorder. (See *Drug chart 15-3, Mood stabilizer drugs,* page 271, for a list of specific drugs.)

2. Although the mechanism of action is not well understood in treatment of bipolar disorder, it is thought to inhibit "kindling" activity in the brain (interruption of the automatic stimulating sequences of neurotransmission); it also stimulates gamma-amino butyric acid (GABA), which helps produce a calming effect.

3. **Pharmacokinetics** is as follows:
   a. The serum half-life for carbamazepine (Tegretol) is 15 to 30 hours, whereas valproic acid (Depakote) is about 8 hours; blood levels should be monitored for both these drugs.
   b. Gabapentin (Neurotin) circulates largely in a free state because of minimal binding to plasma proteins; it is not appreciably metabolized and is eliminated by the kidneys.
   c. Lamotrigine (Lamictal) is metabolized in the liver.
   d. Oxcarbazepine (Trileptal) is structurally related to carbamazepine.
   e. Topiramate (Topamax) is not extensively metabolized and is eliminated unchanged by the kidneys.

4. **Contraindications** include cardiovascular disease, hepatic impairment, hypersensitivity reactions, and blood dyscrasias.

5. **Interactions with carbamazepine** include the following:
   a. Carbamazepine levels may be increased with use of erythromycin, cimetidine, propoxyphene, isoniazid, calcium channel blockers, or SSRIs.
   b. Decreased carbamazepine levels may occur with valproic acid, phenytoin, and phenobarbital.
   c. Carbamazepine can decrease the levels of oral contraceptives, warfarin, theophylline preparations, antipsychotics, valproic acid, anticoagulants, and doxycycline.

6. **Interactions with valproic acid** are as follows:
   a. Increased valproic acid levels may occur with aspirin use.
   b. Valproic acid potentates the effect of alcohol, warfarin, and aspirin.
   c. An increased seizure risk is possible when valproic acid is used with phenytoin or clonazepam.
   d. Effects of phenobarbital, primidone, and MAOIs are increased with concurrent use of valproic acid.
   e. An increased CNS depressant effect may occur when valproic acid is combined with antihistamines, antidepressants, opioids, or sedative hypnotics.

7. **Common side effects** include (see *Table 15-1, Managing common side effects of psychotropic drugs*, pages 262 and 263):
   a. CNS effects (drowsiness, fatigue, sedation)
   b. Gastrointestinal effects (including nausea, vomiting, and indigestion, especially with valproic acid)
   c. Photosensitivity (sunburn, rash)
   d. Visual disturbances (blurred vision)
   e. Skin rash, which can be serious (may occur with lamotrigine).
   f. Renal stones (may occur with topiramate).

8. **Serious side effects** include hepatic toxicity and agranulocytosis. (See *Table 15-3, Managing serious side effects of psychotropic drugs*, page 265.)

V. ANTIANXIETY AGENTS (ANXIOLYTICS) AND SEDATIVE-HYPNOTICS

A. General information

1. Antianxiety agents include benzodiazepines (anxiolytics and sedative-hypnotics), antihistamines, and the nonbenzodiazepine anxiolytic buspirone. (See *Drug chart 15-4, Antianxiety drugs.*)
2. They are generally prescribed to treat anxiety and symptoms associated with anxiety disorders; other specific uses are discussed under the classes below.

B. Benzodiazepines (BZAs)

1. BZAs are the drug of choice for treatment of anxiety and sleep disorders; they are also used in acute alcohol withdrawal, preoperative sedation, seizure disorders, short-term treatment of acute mania, and as muscle relaxants; additionally, BZAs are used to treat agitation and hyperactivity in cognitive impairment disorders.
2. These agents are usually prescribed for adults; they must be used cautiously in children and elderly patients because of the increased risk for CNS depression; they are not recommended for use during pregnancy or lactation.
3. BZAs work by depressing subcortical levels of the CNS, particularly the limbic system and reticular formation; they also potentiate the action of GABA, thereby producing a calming effect.
4. **Pharmacokinetics** is as follows:

DRUG CHART 15-4
Antianxiety drugs

Classification	Drug
Anxiolytic benzodiazepines	alprazolam (Xanax) chlordiazepoxide (Librium) clonazepam (Klonopin) clorazepate (Tranxene) diazepam (Valium) lorazepam (Ativan) oxazepam (Serax) prazepam (Centrax)
Sedative-hypnotic benzodiazepines	flurazepam (Dalmane) temazepam (Restoril) triazolam (Halcion) zaleplon (Sonata) zolpidem (Ambien)
Antihistamines	diphenhydramine (Benadryl) hydroxyzine (Atarax, Vistaril)
Other	buspirone (BuSpar)

    a. The serum half-life for drugs in this group varies widely (5 to 30 hours for ox-azepam, 30 to 100 hours for chlorazepate).

    b. The onset of action also varies, thus leading to the use of some of these drugs as anxiolytics whereas others are primarily used as sedative-hypnotics. (See *Drug chart 15-4, Antianxiety drugs*, page 275.)

    c. BZAs produce tolerance to their effects within days, and continued use (weeks to months) may lead to dependence; abrupt cessation can precipitate withdrawal reactions.

  5. Contraindications include:

    a. Alcohol or substance abuse problems (cross-tolerant with alcohol)

    b. Hepatic or renal impairment

    c. Hypersensitivity reactions

    d. CNS depression.

  6. Interactions are as follows:

    a. Increased sedation and CNS depression may occur when these agents are combined with alcohol, barbiturates, opioids, antipsychotics, antidepressants, antihistamines, neuromuscular blocking agents, cimetidine, or disulfiram.

    b. Decreased effectiveness may occur when these agents are combined with nicotine or caffeine.

  7. Common side effects include the following (see *Table 15-1, Managing common side effects of psychotropic drugs*, pages 262 and 263):

    a. CNS effects, including sedation, fatigue, headache, and motor incoordination. (See *Table 15-8, Using benzodiazepines safely*.)

    b. Gastrointestinal effects, including nausea and dry mouth.

  8. Serious side effects include:

    a. Withdrawal syndrome, if abruptly discontinued.

    b. Respiratory depression with high doses or deliberate overdose. (See *Table 15-9, Benzodiazepine overdose*.)

    c. Paradoxical behaviors of restlessness, talkativeness, and insomnia.

C. Antihistamines

  1. These medications are used primarily to relieve allergic symptoms; however, they are also used for:

    a. Anxiety symptoms associated with a variety of mental disorders

    b. Sleep induction.

  2. Antihistamines are prescribed for adults, children, adolescents, and elderly clients; they are not recommended for use during pregnancy and lactation.

TABLE 15-8
Using benzodiazepines safely

Clients receiving benzodiazepines should be informed about the following safety precautions:
- Do not drive or operate machinery while taking the prescribed medication.
- Do not abruptly stop taking the prescribed drug because this can cause acute withdrawal symptoms.
- Do not consume alcohol or any other sedative drugs while taking the prescribed medication.

TABLE 15-9
Benzodiazepine overdose

Benzodiazepines taken alone or in therapeutic doses are relatively safe; however, if combined with alcohol or other CNS depressants, results can be fatal.

Symptoms
- Somnolence
- Confusion
- Diminished reflexes
- Hypotension
- Coma

Treatment
- Induce vomiting or gastric lavage.
- Monitor the client's vital signs and ECG readings.
- Maintain a patent airway.
- Administer the following medications as ordered:
  - levarterenol (Levophed) for hypotension
  - physostigmine (Antilirium) for acute diazepam poisoning
  - flumazenil (Mazicon), a benzodiazepine blocker, to reverse CNS depression.

3. Antihistamines produce CNS depression and sedation as a side effect of their therapeutic activity of blocking histamine; because of their relative safety, especially in elderly patients, they can be used as anxiolytics.

4. **Pharmacokinetics** is as follows:
   a. The serum half-life of these drugs is 2.4 to 7 hours; therefore, they can be used to induce sleep (sedative-hypnotic use).
   b. Unlike BZAs, these drugs are not associated with tolerance and dependence.

5. **Contraindications** include:
   a. Hypersensitivity response
   b. Hepatic disease
   c. Narrow-angle glaucoma
   d. Seizure disorders
   e. Prostatic hypertrophy.

6. **Interactions** are as follows:
   a. Additive CNS depression may occur with concurrent use of alcohol, opioids, or other sedative-hypnotics.
   b. Additive anticholinergic effects may occur with use of TCAs, guanidine, MAOIs, and other drugs causing anticholinergic responses.

7. **Common side effects** include (see *Table 15-1, Managing common side effects of psychotropic drugs*, pages 262 and 263):
   a. CNS effects (drowsiness, fatigue, dizziness)
   b. Anticholinergic effects (dry mouth, blurred vision, urinary retention, constipation).

8. **Serious side effects** include postural hypotension. (See *Table 15-3, Managing serious side effects of psychotropic drugs*, page 265.)

D. Buspirone (BuSpar)

1. This nonbenzodiazepine anxiolytic is primarily prescribed for treating generalized anxiety disorder; it also may be used for children and elderly clients with disruptive or aggressive behaviors.

2. This drug cannot be used on a p.r.n. (as needed) basis because effectiveness may not be reached for up to 2 weeks.

3. Buspirone does not act on GABA, but exerts its effects on serotonin receptors; its specific action is not well understood, but it effectively reduces anxiety.

4. Pharmacokinetics is as follows:

   a. The half-life is 2 to 7 hours.

   b. A lag time exists before buspirone exerts its antianxiety effect (it may take 10 days to 2 weeks before effectiveness occurs); clients should be encouraged to continue taking medication for this time.

   c. Tolerance and dependence are not associated with this drug.

5. **Contraindications** include hypersensitivity reactions and hepatic disease; it should not be taken during pregnancy or lactation.

6. **Interactions** include:

   a. Hypertension (can occur when used with MAOIs)

   b. Increased sedation (may occur with concurrent use of alcohol)

   c. Hepatic toxicity (risk increases when used with trazodone).

7. **Common side effects** include (see Table *15-1, Managing common side effects of psychotropic drugs*, pages 262 and 263):

   a. CNS effects, including dizziness, drowsiness, headache, fatigue, and weakness

   b. Gastrointestinal effects, including dry mouth, nausea, and diarrhea or constipation

   c. Cardiovascular effects, including palpitations and hypotension or hypertension

   d. Endocrine effects, including amenorrhea.

VI. OTHER MEDICATIONS

A. General information

1. Various types of medication may be used to treat mental health problems.

2. Some commonly prescribed classes of medications include psychostimulants, nonpsychostimulants, anticholinesterase drugs, and *N*-methyl-D-aspartate (NMDA) receptor antagonists.

3. Common uses for these medications include the treatment of attention deficit hyperactivity disorder (ADHD) and cognitive impairment associated with Alzheimer's disease.

B. Psychostimulants

1. These drugs are commonly used to treat children and adults with ADHD; they also may be used to treat narcolepsy in adults. (See *Drug chart 15-5, Drugs for treating attention deficit hyperactivity disorder.*)

   a. Psychostimulants are rarely prescribed for elderly clients.

   b. They should not be used during pregnancy or lactation.

2. Psychostimulants act directly on neuronal synapses to increase release of norepinephrine, serotonin, and dopamine.

TABLE 15-5

Drugs for treating attention deficit hyperactivity disorder

Classification	Drug
Psychostimulants	dextroamphetamine (Dexedrine) methylphenidate (Ritalin, Concerta, Adderal) pemoline (Cylert)
Nonpsychostimulants	atomoxetine (Strattera)

    a. The increased amount of norepinephrine available at the synapse accounts for the CNS excitation produced.

    b. How psychostimulants work paradoxically to decrease hyperactive and impulsive behaviors in children with ADHD is not well understood.

3. **Pharmacokinetics** is as follows:

    a. Short-acting psychostimulating medications, such as methylphenidate (Ritalin), have short half-lives and therefore require several (t.i.d.) doses throughout the day.

    b. Intermediate-acting drugs, such as methylphenidate (Concerta, Adderall) and dextroamphetamine (Dexedrine), can be administered daily or b.i.d.

    c. Long-acting preparations, such as Adderall-XR and Concerta (36 or 54 mg), are designed to be taken only once daily.

    d. Psychostimulants have a high potential for tolerance and abuse; withdrawal can occur if medications are abruptly discontinued.

4. **Contraindications** include:

    a. Substance abuse

    b. Seizure disorders

    c. Hepatic disease

    d. Cardiovascular disease

    e. Tourette syndrome and other abnormal movement disorders.

5. **Interactions** include the following:

    a. Use with MAOIs or vasopressors may cause hypertensive crisis.

    b. An additive sympathomimetic effect may occur if psychostimulants are used with other drugs that stimulate the sympathetic nervous system.

    c. Excessive use of caffeine can cause additive CNS stimulation.

    d. Antipsychotics can decrease CNS stimulation.

6. **Common side effects** include (see *Table 15-1, Managing common side effects of psychotropic drugs*, pages 262 and 263):

    a. CNS effects, including headache, insomnia, agitation, and irritability

    b. Cardiovascular effects, including hypertension and palpitations

    c. Gastrointestinal effects, including nausea, vomiting, anorexia, and diarrhea.

7. **Serious side effects** include seizures and hepatotoxicity. (See *Table 15-3, Managing serious side effects of psychotropic drugs*, page 265.)

C. Nonpsychostimulants

1. Atomoxetine (Strattera), a new nonstimulant medication developed for treating ADHD, acts to block postsynaptic norepinephrine transport in the brain, thereby improving core ADHD symptoms.
2. Because this is not a controlled substance, there is little risk of abuse.
3. The drug should not be taken with MAOIs or within 2 weeks of stopping an MAOI.
4. **Common side effects** include:
   a. GI upset
   b. Increased appetite
   c. Dizziness
   d. Fatigue
   e. Mood swings.

D. Anticholinesterase drugs

1. These agents are used to treat mild to moderate cognitive impairments associated with Alzheimer's disease and other cognitive impairment disorders. (See *Drug chart 15-6, Anticholinesterase drugs.*)
   a. Anticholinesterase drugs are prescribed for adults, especially elderly clients; they are generally not used in children.
   b. They should not be used during pregnancy or lactation.
2. They inhibit the enzyme acetylcholinesterase, which normally acts to break down acetylcholine at the synapse; therefore, increased amounts of acetylcholine are present at the synapse, and this effect is thought to lessen the memory impairment in Alzheimer's disease.
3. **Pharmacokinetics** is as follows:
   a. The serum half-life of tacrine (Cognex) is short (2 to 4 hours), requiring multiple (t.i.d.) doses daily.
   b. The serum half-life of donepezil (Aricept) is 70 hours, requiring only one dose daily.
   c. Tolerance does not develop with these drugs.
4. **Contraindications** include cardiovascular disease (especially sick sinus syndrome) and hepatic disease.
5. **Interactions** include the following:

DRUG CHART 15-6
Anticholinesterase drugs

Generic name	Trade name
donepezil	Aricept
galantamine	Reminyl
rivastigmine	Exelon
tacrine	Cognex

      a. Bleeding risk is increased when used with NSAIDs.

      b. Theophylline toxicity may occur when used concurrently with theophylline preparations.

      c. Use with cholinergic stimulants (bethanechol) potentiates the action of anticholinesterase drugs.

      d. Nicotine decreases blood levels of these drugs.

  6. **Common side effects** include the following (see *Table 15-1, Managing common side effects of psychotropic drugs*, pages 262 and 263):

      a. CNS effects, including dizziness and headache

      b. Gastrointestinal effects, including nausea, vomiting, diarrhea, and anorexia

      c. Cardiovascular effects, including bradycardia.

  7. **Serious side effects** include hepatatoxicity and gastrointestinal bleeding. (See *Table 15-3, Managing serious side effects of psychotropic drugs*, page 265.)

E. NMDA receptor antagonist

  1. Memantine (Axura) is a new *N*-methyl-D-aspartate (NMDA) receptor antagonist developed for the treatment of moderate to severe Alzheimer's disease.

  2. It acts as a neuroprotective agent by preventing release of glutamate, a neurotransmitter thought to contribute to neuronal degeneration in Alzheimer's disease.

  3. Dosing is initiated with 5 mg P.O. daily and increased weekly until a dose of 20 mg daily is reached (10 mg b.i.d.).

  4. **Common side effects** include:

      a. Constipation

      b. Cough

      c. Dizziness

      d. Headache

      e. Hypertension.

NURSING PROCESS OVERVIEW

VII. CARE OF THE CLIENT REQUIRING SOMATIC THERAPY

A. Assessment

  1. Review all data collected on the client receiving somatic therapy, including:

      a. Medical history and physical examination

      b. Laboratory and diagnostic studies, including complete blood count, blood chemistry study, thyroid profile, and liver and renal function studies

      c. Baseline ECG reading

      d. Baseline vital signs

      e. Medication and allergy history

      f. Target symptoms for the specific medication prescribed.

  2. Assess the client's and family's knowledge about the prescribed medication, including:

      a. Expected beneficial effect and when it is most likely to occur *b.* Dose frequency and instructions regarding food and fluids

  c. Minor side effects and the measures taken to counteract them

  d. Major side effects and appropriate action (stop further doses, contact health care provider)

  e. Foods, beverages, and other medications that the patient should avoid.

3. Assess the client's and family's knowledge regarding ECT therapy, including:

  a. Expected beneficial effect and when it is most likely to occur

  b. Necessity for signing informed consent

  c. Pretreatment routine, which includes:

    – Maintaining NPO status for at least 4 hours before treatment

    – Baseline vital signs

    – Removal of jewelry, glasses, contact lenses, and dentures

    – Pretreatment medications used to decrease secretions (atropine sulfate), to induce light coma (methohexital), and to prevent musculoskeletal complications from seizure activity (succinylcholine)

  d. Posttreatment routine, which includes:

    – Frequent monitoring of vital signs

    – Safety precautions (keeping bed side rails up, consuming no food or fluid until gag reflex returns)

    – Reassurance and appropriate reorientation for initial confusion following ECT.

B. Nursing diagnoses

1. Analyze all available client data, indicating any possible risk factors while the client is receiving medication or ECT therapy.

2. Establish appropriate nursing diagnosis, as needed:

  a. Anxiety

  b. Deficient knowledge (specify)

  c. Health-seeking behaviors (specify)

  d. Ineffective family therapeutic regimen management

  e. Readiness for enhanced management of therapeutic regimen

  f. Risk for injury

C. Planning and outcome identification

1. Work with the client and family in establishing realistic goals.

2. Establish desired outcome criteria for the client receiving psychotropic medications or ECT therapy.

  a. The client and family will verbalize expected benefits from treatment.

  b. The client and family will safely self-administer medications.

  c. The client and family will use appropriate measures to counteract minor side effects.

  d. The client and family will contact the health care provider if major side effects occur.

  e. The client and family will follow prescribed laboratory and other testing to monitor medications and any side effects.

D. Implementation

1. Provide the client and family with accurate information regarding medications or ECT therapy, and reinforce their understanding of all procedures and safety precautions.
2. Monitor the client for any side effects of medications.
3. Take appropriate measures to counteract any side effects the client experiences. (See *Table 15-1, Managing common side effects of psychotropic drugs*, pages 262 and 263, and *Table 15-3, Managing serious side effects of psychotropic drugs*, page 265.)
4. Monitor the client for improvement of symptoms.
5. Monitor the client's vital signs, level of consciousness, and presence of gag reflex following ECT therapy.
6. Reorient the client after ECT therapy.

E. Outcome evaluation

1. The client experiences beneficial effects from medication or ECT therapy.
2. The client safely self-administers prescribed medications.
3. The client uses appropriate measures to counteract any minor side effects.
4. The client and family contact the health care provider when any major side effects are experienced.
5. The client complies with prescribed laboratory or other testing to ensure safety while taking medications.

Study questions

1. A client who is on lithium therapy is visited by the home health nurse to have blood drawn for a routine lithium level. The nurse assesses that the client is apathetic, has difficulty responding to questions, walks with an unsteady gait, and has fine hand tremors. Which of the following would the nurse suspect the client is experiencing?
   1. An expected reaction to lithium therapy
   2. Pseudoparkinson syndrome caused by lithium therapy
   3. A medical problem unrelated to lithium therapy
   4. Toxic effects of elevated lithium levels

2. A client refuses to remain on psychotropic medications after discharge from an inpatient psychiatric unit. Which information should the community mental health nurse assess first during the initial follow-up with this client?
   1. Income level and living arrangements
   2. Involvement of family and support systems
   3. Reason for inpatient admission
   4. Reason for refusal to take medications

3. A nurse is assessing postural blood pressures for a client taking risperidone (Risperdal) for chronic schizophrenia. Which of the following results would cause the nurse to withhold the next dose of this drug?
   1. Sitting blood pressure (BP) of 124/84 mm Hg; standing BP of 104/60 mm Hg
   2. Sitting BP of 112/60 mm Hg; standing BP of 104/60 mm Hg

3. Sitting BP of 130/80 mm Hg; standing BP of 128/78 mm Hg
4. Sitting BP of 150/90 mm Hg; standing BP of 146/88 mm Hg

4. The nurse understands that the therapeutic effects of typical antipsychotic medications are associated with which neurotransmitter change?
1. Decreased dopamine level
2. Increased acetylcholine level
3. Stabilization of serotonin
4. Stimulation of GABA

5. Sertraline (Zoloft), an SSRI, is prescribed for a client with major depression. After 1 week, the client complains of no improvement and refuses to take the medication from the nurse. Which of the following would be the nurse's first response?
1. Charting the client's refusal to take this dose
2. Informing the client's doctor about noncompliance
3. Informing the client that 2 to 4 weeks is needed for a positive response
4. Reviewing the client's presenting symptoms and current complaints

6. Which information would be most important for the nurse to teach a client taking phenelzine (Nardil), an MAOI drug?
1. The need to avoid foods and beverages containing tyramine
2. The importance of maintaining regular follow-up visits
3. The drug's possible adverse effects, such as hypertension
4. The rationale for the therapeutic effect of mood elevation

7. A client who is taking the antipsychotic medication chlorpromazine (Thorazine) complains of dry mouth and constipation. Which nursing intervention would be appropriate?
1. Advise the client to chew sugarless gum and eliminate gas-forming foods.
2. Encourage the client to rinse his mouth with water and to add fiber to his diet.
3. Consult the client's doctor about changing the antipsychotic medication.
4. Question the client about his usual amount and type of daily exercise.

8. A client taking fluphenazine (Prolixin) experiences an acute dystonic reaction. Which of the following p.r.n. medications would the nurse administer to this client?
1. Acetaminophen (Tylenol), 325 mg orally
2. Diphenhydramine (Benadryl), 25 mg intramuscularly
3. Milk of magnesia, 30 ml orally
4. Thiothixene (Navane), 6 mg intramuscularly

9. While assessing a client who is taking haloperidol (Haldol), the nurse notes a temperature of 102° F (38.9° C), BP of 180/92 mm Hg, and profuse diaphoresis. Which side effect should the nurse suspect?
1. Agranulocytosis
2. Extrapyramidal reaction
3. Hepatotoxicity
4. Neuroleptic malignant syndrome

10. The nurse correctly teaches a client who is taking the benzodiazepine oxazepam (Serax) to avoid excessive intake of:
1. cheese.
2. coffee.
3. sugar.
4. shellfish.

11. Which principle should the nurse understand before planning the care of a client receiving anxiolytic medication?
1. Enhanced psychomotor coordination is expected.
2. Increased mental alertness is a common effect.
3. Medications that are CNS depressants will potentiate the sedative response.
4. Consumption of foods containing tyramine can cause hypertension.

12. To prevent the occurrence of lithium toxicity, the nurse should teach the client to maintain adequate intake of:
1. fruits and vegetables.
2. low-fat foods.
3. protein and vitamin C.
4. water and sodium.

13. Which of the following best explains why tricyclic antidepressants are used with caution in elderly patients?
1. Central nervous system effects
2. Cardiovascular system effects
3. Gastrointestinal system effects
4. Serotonin syndrome effects

14. Which of the following is the most serious side effect of the atypical antipsychotic clozapine (Clozaril)?
1. Agranulocytosis
2. Anticholinergic effects
3. Postural hypotension
4. Pseudoparkinsonism

15. A client is admitted to the emergency department after a suicide attempt involving an overdose of the tricyclic antidepressant imipramine (Tofranil). In addition to monitoring the client's vital signs and ECG reading, the nurse should prepare to provide which priority intervention?

1. Frequent stimulation
2. Electrolyte replacement
3. Patent airway
4. Quiet environment

16. The nurse should know that MAOI antidepressants can interact adversely with which drug?
1. Aspirin
2. Acetaminophen
3. Codeine
4. Norepinephrine

17. When the nurse suspects a client is experiencing either neuroleptic malignant syndrome or serotonin syndrome as a result of psychotropic medications, which action takes priority?
1. Providing adequate fluids
2. Maintaining bed rest
3. Monitoring for expected symptoms
4. Withholding further drug doses

18. The nurse is working with a client who has overdosed on a benzodiazepine. Which medication should the nurse prepare to administer?
1. carbamazepine (Tegretol)
2. diphenhydramine (Benadryl)
3. flumazenil (Mazicon)
4. physostigmine (Antilirium)

19. The nurse who is working with the family of a client who is taking tacrine (Cognex) should teach the family to be alert for early signs and symptoms of liver problems, including:
1. constipation and bloating.
2. dizziness and fatigue.
3. frequent belching and heartburn.
4. nausea and abdominal pain.

20. The nurse teaches the family of a child who is taking the psychostimulant methylphenidate (Ritalin) to manage the common side effects of nausea and anorexia. Which of the following would the nurse recommend?

1. Discourage frequent snacking of high-calorie foods.
2. Encourage the client to consume adequate calories to maintain normal weight.
3. Offer six small meals rather than three large meals.
4. Take the prescribed medication at bedtime.

21. Which nursing intervention would be the priority for a client immediately following ECT treatment?

1. Assessing vital signs and reorienting the client
2. Applying restraints to prevent injury
3. Administering previously withheld medications
4. Encouraging intake of fluids and nutritious food

22. The psychiatric nurse is teaching a group of clients about a newly prescribed SSRI antidepressant for the treatment of depression. Which of the following points should the nurse include in her teaching plan? Select all that apply.

1. These drugs act to increase the levels of a mood-elevating chemical in the brain called serotonin.
2. These drugs act quickly, so feelings of depression will decrease in a few days.
3. Clients should avoid drinking alcohol or taking antihistamine medications with these drugs.
4. Clients who have trouble falling asleep while on this medication can try taking it in the morning instead of at night.
5. Clients must remain on a special diet when taking these drugs.
6. Clients must return for weekly blood level tests to ensure the safety of these drugs.

Answer key

1. The answer is 4.

The symptoms described—apathy, difficulty concentrating, ataxia, and tremors—are those that occur because of elevated lithium levels and their effect on the CNS. These symptoms indicate the client is experiencing mild toxicity. This client's reaction is not an expected response; the goal of monitoring lithium blood levels is to prevent toxicity. Also, these are not the symptoms of pseudoparkinsonism (nor does lithium cause pseudoparkinsonism).

2. The answer is 4.

The first area for assessment would be the client's reason for refusing medication. The client may not understand the purpose for the medicine, may be experiencing distressing side effects, or may be concerned about the cost of the medicine. In any case, the nurse cannot provide appropriate intervention before assessing the client's problem with the medication. The patient's income level, living arrangements, and involvement of family and support systems are relevant issues following determination of the client's reason for refusing medication. The nurse providing follow-up care would have access to the client's medical record and should already know the reason for inpatient admission.

3. The answer is **1.**
The significant blood pressure decrease with position change is an indication of the side effect of postural hypotension. The prudent nurse would withhold the next dose and notify the doctor. The other blood pressure readings do not indicate postural hypotension.

4. The answer is **1.**
Excess dopamine is thought to be the chemical cause for psychotic thinking. The typical antipsychotics act to block dopamine receptors and therefore decrease the amount of this neurotransmitter at the synapses. The typical antipsychotics do not increase acetylcholine, stabilize serotonin, or stimulate GABA.

5. The answer is **3.**
The client may not understand that at least 2 to 4 weeks are needed before therapeutic effects of antidepressants are noticed. If the client continues to refuse medication even after the appropriate teaching, the nurse should then chart refusal and inform the doctor. The response in option 4 is irrelevant to the situation described.

6. The answer is **1.**
The most important thing the client taking an MAOI needs to understand is that foods and beverages containing tyramine must be avoided to prevent a severe hypertensive reaction. Medications containing psychostimulating drugs must also be avoided. Follow-up care is important; however, the priority teaching issue is dietary restrictions because the client could have a hypertensive reaction before any follow-up appointment if he is unaware of which foods to avoid. Option 3 is too vague. Although hypertension is possible, the client is not being informed

how to avoid this. The client may or may not want details regarding how mood elevation is achieved with an MAOI. For many clients, knowledge that their mood will elevate is sufficient; details about how this occurs are not a priority.

7. The answer is **2.**
Rinsing the mouth with water (rather than mouthwash, which is drying) will help eliminate the problem of dry mouth. Adding fiber to the diet will facilitate the passage of a normal stool and help avoid constipation. Chewing sugarless gum will help with dry mouth; however, eliminating gas-forming foods is not the treatment for constipation. Changing medications because of experiencing these common side effects is not indicated. The client should be instructed in measures to counteract the side effects. Exercise is important and it can help stimulate peristalsis; however, the problem of dry mouth is not addressed in this response.

8. The answer is **2.**
Diphenhydramine (Benadryl) is the antidote for acute dystonia. The dose needs to be given intramuscularly because a client in acute dystonia often has difficulty swallowing. The remaining medications would not treat an acute dystonic reaction and are prescribed as needed for other reasons; for example, acetaminophen would be prescribed for headache, milk of magnesia for constipation, and thiothixene for agitation.

9. The answer is **4.**
High temperatures, elevated blood pressure, diaphoresis, tachycardia, and extrapyramidal symptoms characterize neuroleptic malignant syndrome. The other reactions are all serious adverse effects of the typical antipsychotics (such as haloperidol).

10. The answer is 2.

Coffee, which contains caffeine, is psychostimulating and will counteract the intended effect of relaxation that oxazepam produces. There is no reason for the client to avoid cheese, sugar, or shellfish while taking oxazepam.

11. The answer is 3.

The nurse needs to teach the client about the serious effects of potentiation of CNS depression that can occur when taking other medicines that produce the same body reaction as the anxiolytics. Such medications would include any of the sedative-hypnotics, alcohol, and any barbiturates. Enhanced psychomotor coordination and increased mental alertness are the opposite reactions expected of anxiolytic medications; therefore, these statements do not apply. Hypertension when consuming tyramine-containing foods is a side effect of the MAOI antidepressants, not anxiolytics.

12. The answer is 4.

When sodium or water is depleted in a client taking lithium, the potential for lithium toxicity increases; the kidney will reabsorb lithium to replace depleted sodium and counteract water loss. The remaining responses are unrelated to prevention of lithium toxicity.

13. The answer is 2.

The TCAs affect norepinephrine as well as other neurotransmitters, and thus have significant cardiovascular side effects. Therefore, they are used with caution in elderly clients who may have increased risk factors for cardiac problems because of their age and other medical conditions. The remaining side effects would apply to any client taking a TCA and are not particular to an elderly person.

14. The answer is 1.

The incidence of agranulocytosis associated with clozapine therapy is 1% to 2%. Therefore, clients taking this drug must be screened weekly for the first 6 months of therapy for evidence of decreased white blood count (< 2,000 μl). Anticholinergic effects and postural hypotension can occur; however, they are not considered serious side effects. Pseudoparkinsonism is not usually associated with clozapine, and this lack of extrapyramidal side effects is one of the advantages of the atypical antipsychotics.

15. The answer is 3.

Symptoms of TCA overdose include sedation, ataxia, stupor, and, sometimes, convulsions and respiratory depression. Therefore, maintaining a patent airway is an essential component of nursing care for this client. Although the nurse would assess the client's level of consciousness and provide stimulation in order to do so, this is less essential than maintaining an airway. I.V. therapy and electrolyte replacement may be indicated, especially if the client has been treated with gastric lavage. However, this would not be as important as establishing an airway. A quiet environment may be indicated if the client has any agitation; however, airway patency precedes this measure.

16. The answer is 4.

MAOIs act to inhibit the enzyme responsible for breaking down neurotransmitters, including norepinephrine. Therefore, if medicine containing norepinephrine is taken along with the MAOI, the potential for a hypertensive crisis is increased. Norepinephrine acts peripherally to cause vasoconstriction and, therefore, increases blood pressure. The remaining medications are not contraindicated.

17. The answer is 4.

The nurse must withhold any further doses of psychotropic medications if either neuroleptic malignant syndrome or serotonin syndrome is suspected. Withholding the medications will help to avoid increasing the severity of these reactions. The remaining actions are important, but the priority is preventing symptom worsening by stopping the psychotropic drug.

18. The answer is 3.

Flumazenil (Mazicon) is the antidote for a benzodiazepine overdose; it acts to reverse the CNS depression caused by overdose. The remaining drugs will not reverse CNS depression.

19. The answer is 4.

Nausea and abdominal pain may occur if the client is developing early liver problems. Jaundice would also be an important symptom; however, it may occur later as liver dysfunction increases. Constipation, bloating, and frequent belching and heartburn may indicate gastrointestinal problems, but not liver dysfunction. Dizziness and fatigue may indicate a problem with the CNS.

20. The answer is 3.

A client (especially a child) may have increased response of nausea and lack of appetite when presented with large meals.

Offering smaller portions more frequently can help stimulate appetite. The remaining responses would not help address this problem.

21. The answer is 1.

The client will be monitored in the same manner as any postoperative client coming out of anesthesia. Applying restraints is not necessary and may cause agitation. Medications, fluids, and food will be given after the client is reoriented and his swallowing and gag reflexes return.

22. The answer is 1, 3, 4.

SSRIs will increase serotonin levels; they should not be taken with alcohol or antihistamines because this will increase the chance of CNS depression. Insomnia is a possible side effect of SSRIs, and taking the medication in the morning will help decrease the problem. Option 2 is incorrect because these drugs take 2 to 4 weeks before they are effective. No special diet is required for SSRIs (option 5); however, a tyramine-reduced diet is important for MAOIs. Weekly blood level checks (option 6) are not indicated for SSRIs.

Comprehensive Test: Questions

1. Which nursing intervention is best for facilitating communication with a psychiatric client who speaks a foreign language?
1. Rely on nonverbal communication.
2. Select symbolic pictures as aids.
3. Speak in universal phrases.
4. Use the services of an interpreter.

2. The nurse is working with a client whose culture uses the services of a special healer. The client requests this healer's services when hospitalized on a psychiatric inpatient unit. Which nursing intervention is congruent with culturally sensitive nursing care?
1. Explain to the client that this is inappropriate for a hospital setting.
2. Facilitate the client's request.
3. Explain to the client that this means an unhealthy reliance on magical healing.
4. Refer the client to the doctor.

3. A nurse and a client are talking comfortably about the client's progress as well as feelings about the therapeutic relationship. This scenario typically occurs at which phase of the therapeutic relationship?
1. Assessment
2 Orientation
3. Working
4. Termination

4. A client tells the nurse, "People think I'm no good, if you know what I mean." Which of the following responses by the nurse is most therapeutic?

1. "People don't always mean what they say about you. Perhaps you are too sensitive."
2. "I think you're a good person. So you see, at least there is one person who doesn't feel that way."
3. "I'm not sure what you mean. Tell me more about that."
4. "What is the reason people don't think you're good?"

5. The team treatment plan for a psychiatric client uses a contract approach as well as a system in which privileges are based on client participation in therapeutic activities. Which theoretical framework is being implemented?
1. Behavioral framework
2. Educational framework
3. Interpersonal framework
4. Psychodynamic framework

6. The nurse explains to a mental health care technician that a client's obsessive-compulsive behaviors are related to unconscious conflict between id impulses and the superego (or conscience). On which of the following theories does the nurse base this statement?
1. Behavioral theory
2. Cognitive theory
3. Interpersonal theory
4. Psychoanalytic theory

7. The community mental health nurse is working with a family of a client with a chronic, persistent mental illness. The family expresses concern about the client's ability to properly manage a small inheritance received

from a relative. Which legal principle should guide the nurse's response to the family's concerns?
1. ANA Code of Ethics
2. Autonomy
3. Confidentiality
4. Commitment

8. A client admitted to a psychiatric facility under an involuntary procedure has refused to take medication prescribed for psychotic symptoms. The treatment team meets to discuss this situation. Which statement made during this discussion reflects the ethical principle of beneficence?
1. "Because the client really needs the medication for self-protection, an order to give the drug as an injection should be obtained."
2. "The client has the right to refuse medications, so other treatment options should be explored."
3. "The client has been involuntarily committed and therefore does not have the right to refuse."
4. "The family should be consulted and asked to provide consent for the medication."

9. Coworkers observe that a nurse routinely responds to clients in an autocratic, controlling manner, with little consideration for their dignity and rights. After attempting to directly address the situation with the nurse in question, the coworkers plan to meet with the supervisor to express their concern about this unprofessional behavior. The plan to go to the supervisor is:
1. appropriate, because peer review is a professional activity needed to maintain quality care.
2. appropriate, because the nurse is probably looking for limits to be set on this behavior.
3. inappropriate, because it is up to the supervisor to evaluate the nurse.
4. inappropriate, because each nurse is responsible only for her own practice.

10. A client with depressive symptoms is given prescribed medications and talks with his therapist about his belief that he is worthless and unable to cope with life. Psychiatric care in this treatment plan is based on which framework?
1. Behavioral framework
2. Cognitive framework
3. Interpersonal framework
4. Psychodynamic framework

11. A nurse who explains that a client's psychotic behavior is unconsciously motivated understands that the client's disordered behavior arises from which of the following?
1. Abnormal thinking
2. Altered neurotransmitters
3. Internal needs
4. Response to stimuli

12. The nurse observes that a mother is highly anxious when caring for her infant. Which of the following theorists would state that the mother's anxiety is communicated and internalized by the infant?
1. Freud
2. Sullivan
3. Maslow
4. Erikson

13. A client with depression has been hospitalized for treatment after taking a leave of absence from work. The client's employer expects the client to return to work following inpatient treatment. The client tells the nurse, "I'm no good. I'm a failure." According to cognitive theory, these statements reflect:

1. learned behavior.
2. punitive superego and decreased self-esteem.
3. faulty thought processes that govern behavior.
4. evidence of difficult relationships in the work environment.

14. Which of the following best demonstrates how a nurse incorporates Selye's general adaptation theory in her nursing interventions?

1. By teaching clients stress-reduction techniques
2. By helping clients to develop an awareness of stressors
3. By examining a client's life events that require adaptation
4. By explaining to clients how the body responds to stress

15. The nurse observes a client pacing in the hall. Which statement by the nurse may help the client recognize his anxiety?

1. "I guess you're worried about something, aren't you?"
2. "Can I get you some medication to help calm you?"
3. "Have you been pacing for a long time?"
4. "I notice that you're pacing. How are you feeling?"

16. A client who is a Vietnam War veteran suffers from nightmares and flashbacks about his war experience. He has been diagnosed with posttraumatic stress disorder. Which of the following nursing diagnoses would be most appropriate?

1. *Fear related to intrusive images from past experiences*
2. *Ineffective coping related to failure to establish role responsibilities*
3. *Anxiety related to fear of the unknown*
4. *Chronic low self-esteem related to past experiences of inadequacy in combat*

17. A client is diagnosed with hypochondriasis. During a discussion with the nurse, the client makes all of the following statements. Which statement is most typical of a client with this diagnosis?

1. "I feel tired all the time."
2. "I think I have stomach cancer."
3. "Nobody understands my problems."
4. "I haven't been able to concentrate."

18. The nurse describes a client as anxious. Which statement about anxiety is true?

1. Anxiety is usually pathological.
2. Anxiety is directly observable.
3. Anxiety is usually harmful.
4. Anxiety is a response to a threat.

19. A client with a phobic disorder is treated by systematic desensitization. The nurse understands that this approach will do which of the following?

1. Help the client execute actions that are feared

2. Help the client develop insight into irrational fears

3. Help the client substitute one fear for another

4. Help the client decrease anxiety

20. A client with obsessive-compulsive disorder is hospitalized on an inpatient unit. Which nursing response is most therapeutic?
1. Accepting the client's obsessive-compulsive behaviors
2. Challenging the client's obsessive-compulsive behaviors
3. Preventing the client's obsessive-compulsive behaviors
4. Rejecting the client's obsessive-compulsive behaviors

21. The nurse assesses a client with generalized anxiety disorder. Which of the following characteristics are common to this disorder? Select all that apply.
1. Blank affect
2. Difficulty concentrating
3. Echolalia
4. Irritability
5. Feeling on edge
6. Suspicion

22. A 45-year-old woman with a history of depression tells a nurse in her doctor's office that she has difficulty with sexual arousal and is fearful that her husband will have an affair. Which of the following factors would the nurse identify as least significant in contributing to the client's sexual difficulty?
1. Education and work history
2. Medications used
3. Physical health status
4. Quality of spousal relationship

23. The nurse is developing a care plan for a client with borderline personality disorder who exhibits mood instability and frequent emotional outbursts. Which factor would the nurse identify as most essential for care?
1. Dealing with what is verbalized rather than underlying feelings
2. Isolating the client when intense emotions are experienced
3. Maintaining a calm, matter-of-fact response to client emotions
4. Promoting group interactions in which the client can ventilate

24. Which client outcome would best indicate successful treatment for a client with an antisocial personality disorder?
1. The client exhibits charming behavior when around authority figures.
2. The client has decreased episodes of impulsive behaviors.
3. The client makes statements of self-satisfaction.
4. The client's statements indicate no remorse for behavior.

25. The nurse is caring for a client with an autoimmune disorder at a medical clinic, where alternative medicine is used as an adjunct to traditional therapies. Which information should the nurse teach the client to help foster a sense of control over his symptoms?
1. Pathophysiology of disease process
2. Principles of good nutrition
3. Side effects of medications
4. Stress management techniques

26. The nurse assesses a young woman with anorexia nervosa and compares the client's weight with norms for age and height. Which of the following assessment findings would be expected in this client? Select all that apply.
1. Amenorrhea
2. Bradycardia
3. Diarrhea
4. Hypertension
5. Lanugo
6. Tachycardia

27. Which nursing diagnosis is most appropriate for a client with anorexia nervosa who expresses feelings of guilt about not meeting family expectations?
1. *Anxiety*
2. *Disturbed body image*
3. *Defensive coping*
4. *Powerlessness*

28. Which nursing intervention is most appropriate for a client with anorexia nervosa during initial hospitalization on a behavioral therapy unit?
1. Emphasize the importance of good nutrition to establish normal weight.
2. Ignore the client's mealtime behavior and focus instead on issues of dependence and independence.
3. Help establish a plan using privileges and restrictions based on compliance with refeeding.
4. Teach the client information about the long-term physical consequences of anorexia.

29. The nurse is providing care for a client with a somatoform disorder. Which of the following interventions should the nurse include? Select all that apply.
1. Assessing new physical symptoms
2. Encouraging independence
3. Reinforcing secondary gains
4. Focusing on emotional responses
5. Focusing on physical complaints
6. Teaching relaxation techniques

30. A nurse is evaluating therapy with the family of a client with anorexia nervosa. Which of the following would indicate that the therapy was successful?
1. The parents reinforce increased decision making by the client.
2. The parents clearly verbalize their expectations for the client.
3. The client verbalizes that family meals are now enjoyable.
4. The client tells her parents about feelings of low self-esteem.

31. The nurse is working with a client with a somatoform disorder. Which client outcome goal would the nurse most likely establish in this situation?
1. The client will recognize signs and symptoms of physical illness.
2. The client will cope with physical illness.
3. The client will take prescribed medications.
4. The client will express anxiety verbally rather than through physical symptoms.

32. Which of the following is the most distinguishing feature of a client with an antisocial personality disorder?
1. Attention to detail and order
2. Bizarre mannerisms and thoughts

3. Submissive and dependent behaviors
4. Disregard for social and legal norms

33. The nurse understands that evaluating clients with personality disorders is especially difficult because:
1. these clients are often withdrawn even after therapy and may not share results openly.
2. typically, few changes in these clients' behavior may be identified over time.
3. nurses may reject these clients because of their irritating behaviors.
4. these clients improve rapidly and wish to move on with their lives.

34. The nurse assesses a client with major depressive disorder for the physiologic effects of depression. Which of the following symptoms are common? Select all that apply.
1. Anorexia
2. Constipation
3. Increased perspiration
4. Increased thirst
5. Insomnia
6. Fatigue

35. Which method would a nurse use to determine a client's potential risk for suicide?
1. Wait for the client to bring up the subject of suicide.
2. Observe the client's behavior for cues of suicide ideation.
3. Question the client directly about suicidal thoughts.
4. Question the client about future plans.

36. A client with dysthymic disorder reports to a nurse that his life is hopeless and will never improve in the future. How can the nurse best respond using a cognitive approach?
1. Agree with the client's painful feelings.
2. Challenge the accuracy of the client's belief.
3. Deny that the situation is hopeless.
4. Present a cheerful attitude.

37. A client with a bipolar disorder exhibits manic behavior. The nursing diagnosis is *Disturbed thought processes related to difficulty concentrating, secondary to flight of ideas.* Which of the following outcome criteria would indicate improvement in the client?
1. The client verbalizes feelings directly during treatment.
2. The client verbalizes positive "self" statements.
3. The client speaks in coherent sentences.
4. The client reports feeling calmer.

38. A client with major depression has not verbalized problem areas to staff or peers since admission to a psychiatric unit. Which activity should the nurse recommend to help this client express himself?
1. Art therapy in a small group
2. Basketball game with peers on the unit
3. Reading a self-help book on depression
4. Watching a movie with the peer group

39. The home health psychiatric nurse visits a client with chronic schizophrenia who was recently discharged after a prolonged stay in a state hospital. The client lives in a boarding home, reports no family involvement, and has little social interaction. The nurse plans to refer the client to a day treatment program in order to help him with:
1. managing his hallucinations.
2. medication teaching.
3. social skills training.
4. vocational training.

40. A client with paranoid schizophrenia often directs brief, hostile verbal outbursts toward the nursing staff. Which of the following nursing actions is the most therapeutic way to address this problem?
1. Administer antipsychotic medications as needed when verbal outbursts occur.
2. Minimize the outbursts by walking away when they occur.
3. Place the client in seclusion when these episodes occur.
4. Set limits and provide a structured, predictable environment.

41. Which activity would be most appropriate for a severely withdrawn client?
1. Art activity with a staff member
2. Board game with a small group of clients
3. Team sport in the gym
4. Watching TV in the dayroom

42. A client looks frightened and states, "The unit is wired up to the FBI, and they're taking my thoughts away." Which response by the nurse would be most therapeutic?

1. "These thoughts aren't real; they're part of your illness."
2. "I don't believe this is so, but you seem scared."
3. "How long have you been thinking about this?"
4. "Let me show you that the unit is not wired."

43. A client tells a nurse, "Everyone would be better off if I wasn't alive." Which nursing diagnosis would be made based on this statement?
1. *Disturbed thought processes*
2. *Ineffective coping*
3. *Risk for self-directed violence*
4. *Impaired social interaction*

44. A client who was recently admitted to an inpatient psychiatric unit exhibits manic behavior and wears excessive make-up as well as provocative clothes. Which statement by the nurse is the most appropriate way to intervene?
1. "It's important to look appropriate on the clinical unit. Go change."
2. "Let's go back to your room and I'll help you select clothing that is better for this setting."
3. "You are dressed like you're going to a party. I think you need to change."
4. " I think you would look better in more conservative clothes."

45. A client with a *DSM-IV TR* diagnosis of schizophrenia, undifferentiated type, reports that her body is stiff and like wood. Which symptom is this client manifesting?
1. Autism
2. Ambivalence
3. Depersonalization
4. Regression

46. Which information is most essential in the initial teaching session for the family of a young adult recently diagnosed with schizophrenia?
1. Symptoms of this disease are caused by a chemical imbalance in the brain.
2. Genetic history is an important factor related to the development of schizophrenia.
3. Schizophrenia is a serious disease affecting every aspect of a person's functioning.
4. The distressing symptoms of this disorder can respond to treatment with medications.

47. A nurse is working with a client who has schizophrenia, paranoid type. Which of the following outcomes related to the client's delusional perceptions would the nurse establish?
1. The client will demonstrate realistic interpretation of daily events in the unit.
2. The client will perform daily hygiene and grooming without assistance.
3. The client will take prescribed medications without difficulty.
4. The client will participate in unit activities.

48. A nurse working in an outpatient drug and alcohol clinic interviews an 18-year-old client who was referred by her school guidance counselor. The client's history reveals that her father abandoned her at age 4, and she lives with her mother, older sister, and sister's husband, all of whom abuse alcohol and drugs. At age 16, she was raped at a party, became pregnant, and gave the child up for adoption. Her school counselor reports frequent absences, failing grades, and suspicion of drug use. Which factors in this client's life would the nurse identify as the most significant for increasing the client's vulnerability for substance abuse?
1. Abandonment by father at an early age
2. Family history of substance abuse
3. Poor school attendance and failing grades
4. Trauma of rape and subsequent pregnancy

49. A 7-year-old child has been admitted to the inpatient psychiatric unit following aggressive behavior in school and at home. He has been in three different placements in foster care since he was 2 years old. He has sporadic contact with his natural mother, who has a history of schizophrenia. He used a piece of glass to cut his fingers and stated, "I want to kill myself." A diagnosis of depressive disorder, not otherwise specified, was made on admission. The nurse understands that the most common manifestation of depression in children is:
1. acting-out behavior.
2. poor parental relationship.
3. school problems.
4. suicide attempts.

50. A client with bipolar disorder, manic type, exhibits extreme excitement, delusional thinking, and command hallucinations. Which of the following is the priority nursing diagnosis?
1. *Anxiety*
2. *Impaired social interaction*
3. *Disturbed sensory-perceptual alteration (auditory)*
4. *Risk for other-directed violence*

51. A client is admitted to an acute medical-surgical unit for treatment of multiple traumatic injuries related to a car accident. His history indicates use of both alcohol and heroin on a regular basis. Which anticipated problem would be of most concern for nursing care?

1. The client's denial of alcohol and drug abuse
2. The client's difficulty in establishing a nurse-client relationship
3. The client's demonstrating active drug-seeking behavior
4. Maintaining adequate pain control for the client

52. A client who abuses alcohol and cocaine tells a nurse that he only uses substances because of his stressful marriage and difficult job. Which defense mechanisms is this client using?

1. Displacement
2. Projection
3. Rationalization
4. Sublimation

53. A client has developed tolerance to CNS depressants. Which of the following is the correct interpretation of tolerance?

1. Concurrent abuse of two different substances
2. Continued use of a substance despite absence of life problems
3. Need to increase the dose to obtain the desired effect
4. Occurrence of physiologic symptoms when the drug is discontinued

54. The nurse assesses a client in a substance abuse unit for symptoms of alcohol withdrawal. Which of the following symptoms are common? Select all that apply.

1. Agitation
2. Bradycardia
3. Increased blood pressure
4. Decreased blood pressure
5. Drowsiness
6. Tachycardia

55. The nurse is planning care for a family in which violence commonly occurs. Which statement about nonvictim members of violent families is correct?

1. These family members do not require intervention because they are not involved.
2. These family members often experience more trauma than do actual victims.
3. These family members should be encouraged to seek alternative living arrangements.
4. These family members commonly experience fear and guilt from their exposure to violence.

56. An 11-year-old child diagnosed with conduct disorder is admitted to the psychiatric unit for treatment. Which of the following behaviors would the nurse assess?

1. Restlessness, short attention span, hyperactivity
2. Physical aggressiveness, low stress tolerance, disregard for the rights of others
3. Deterioration in social functioning, excessive anxiety and worry, bizarre behavior
4. Sadness, poor appetite and sleeplessness, loss of interest in activities

57. A mental health treatment team recommends family systems therapy for a family with a history of violence toward both adults and children in the family. The nurse understands that this treatment method is recommended for the primary purpose of:
1. allowing family members to verbalize feelings.
2. establishing responsible self-functioning of family members.
3. identifying the perpetrators of violence in the family.
4. treating child victims of abusive behaviors.

58. A pregnant woman has abused heroin for the past 3 years. She is unemployed and obtains money by prostitution and stealing. Which intervention should be the nurse's first priority in this situation?
1. Counsel the client about her lifestyle and needed changes.
2. Reflect on personal attitudes about heroin addiction and prostitution before initiating actions.
3. Help the client to identify the legal implications of stealing, the health risks associated with prostitution, and the effects of drugs on her fetus.
4. Review literature on substance abuse and dependence and its impact on the health of pregnant women before initiating therapy.

59. The nurse understands that if a client continues to be dependent on heroin throughout her pregnancy, her baby will be at high risk for:
1. mental retardation.
2. heroin dependence.
3. addiction in adulthood.
4. psychological disturbances.

60. The emergency department nurse is assigned to provide care for a victim of a sexual assault. When following legal and agency guidelines, which intervention is most important?
1. Determine the assailant's identity.
2. Preserve the client's privacy.
3. Identify the extent of injury.
4. Ensure an unbroken chain of evidence.

61. Which factor is least important in the decision regarding whether a victim of family violence can safely remain in the home?
1. The availability of appropriate community shelters
2. The nonabusing caretaker's ability to intervene on the client's behalf
3. The client's possible response to relocation
4. The family's socioeconomic status

62. A family member of a client with schizophrenia questions the nurse about the cause of this disorder. Which response by the nurse is most accurate?
1. The disorder is thought to result from disturbed family relations and communication problems.
2. The disorder is thought to result from brain alterations in the frontal lobe.
3. The disorder is thought to result from a combination of biologic, genetic, and psychosocial factors.
4. The disorder is thought to result from altered dopamine transmission in the brain.

63. A psychiatric nurse generalist works with a support group of individuals who have experienced the death of a spouse. The primary purpose of this group would be to:
1. Focus on problems in group living and encourage coping strategies
2. Help members improve interaction and plan enjoyable activities
3. Provide empathy for members and reinforce existing strengths
4. Provide educational information and encourage self-management

64. While providing group therapy for clients on an inpatient unit, the nurse should take which action when a conflict among members develops?
1. Discuss the situation privately with the individual clients involved in the conflict.
2. Encourage an open discussion among group members.
3. Ignore the situation unless it becomes a group problem.
4. Provide specific information on how to resolve the conflict.

65. The nurse would expect a client with early Alzheimer's disease to have problems with:
1. balancing a checkbook.
2. self-care measures.
3. relating to family members.
4. remembering his own name.

66. The nurse understands that delirium is a cognitive impairment disorder characterized by which factors? Select all that apply.
1. Acute onset of disease
2. Gradual onset of disease
3. Subtle initial symptoms, such as difficulty planning meals
4. Dramatic initial symptoms, such as acute confusion
5. Motor changes from agitation to somnolence
6. Pacing and wandering, especially at night

67. A client with a history of multiple suicide attempts is admitted to the inpatient unit with a diagnosis of major depression, recurrent, with psychotic features. The doctor orders all of the following medications. Which medication should help decrease the client's irrational thinking?
1. lorazepam (Ativan) 1 mg P.O., q6h, p.r.n.
2. clonazepam (Klonopin) 0.5 mg P.O. daily at 5 p.m.
3. sertraline (Zoloft) 50 mg P.O. daily at bedtime
4. olanzapine (Zyprexa) 5 mg P.O. b.i.d.

68. Which nursing intervention is most appropriate for a client with Alzheimer's disease who has frequent episodes of emotional lability?
1. Attempt humor to alter the client's mood.
2. Explore reasons for the client's altered mood.
3. Reduce environmental stimuli to redirect the client's attention.
4. Use logic to point out reality aspects.

69. Which neurotransmitter has been implicated in the development of Alzheimer's disease?
1. Acetylcholine
2. Dopamine
3. Epinephrine
4. Serotonin

70. The daughter of a client with Alzheimer's disease reports feeling chronic fatigue and mild depression. Further assessment reveals that this daughter has been responsible for feeding, cleaning, and doing laundry for her parent while maintaining a full-time job and caring for two teenagers. Which nursing diagnosis would the nurse establish for the client's daughter?
1. *Interrupted family coping*
2. *Disabled family coping*
3. *Caregiver role strain*
4. *Social isolation*

71. Which factors are most essential for the nurse to assess when providing crisis intervention for a client?
1. The client's communication and coping skills
2. The client's anxiety level and ability to express feelings
3. The client's perception of the triggering event and availability of situational supports
4. The client's use of reality testing and level of depression

72. A seriously ill client dies much sooner than expected. Family members are called and told about the death when they arrive. At this time, the nurse can expect family members to:
1. demonstrate shock and disbelief.
2. exhibit helplessness and withdrawal.
3. share fond memories about their deceased loved one.
4. state how much they miss their family member.

73. The nurse considers a client's response to crisis intervention successful if the client:
1. changes coping skills and behavioral patterns.
2. develops insight into reasons why the crisis occurred.
3. learns to relate better to others.
4. returns to his previous level of functioning.

74. Two nurses are co-leading group therapy for seven clients in the psychiatric unit. The leaders observe that the group members are anxious and look to the leaders for answers. Which phase of development is this group in?
1. Conflict resolution phase
2. Initiation phase
3. Working phase
4. Termination phase

75. A nurse is leading a therapeutic social skills group and tells the members, "This is our group and the purpose of meeting is to learn different ways of talking to people. It's important that we practice listening. Our group is designed to help with talking and listening." These statements by the nurse are:
1. nontherapeutic because group spontaneity will be restricted.
2. therapeutic because group cohesiveness will be enhanced.
3. nontherapeutic because group norms are not addressed.
4. therapeutic because group conflict will be prevented.

76. The nurse leading group therapy documents that the group is in the working phase of treatment based on which evaluative data?
1. They begin to comment on their behaviors.
2. They ask the nurse for advice regarding their problems.
3. They talk about someone outside the group.
4. They focus on their past relationships.

77. Group members have worked very hard, and the nurse reminds them that termination is approaching. Termination is considered successful if group members:
1. decide to continue.
2. evaluate group progress.
3. focus on positive experiences.
4. stop attending prior to termination.

78. When providing family therapy, the nurse validates that the family practices good communication skills based on which data?
1. Evidence that children accept and adopt the parental value system
2. Family members' expression of agreement on issues and problems
3. Open and clear discussion of issues and feelings among members
4. Parental statement that they have no problems communicating with children

79. A nurse is caring for an adolescent hospitalized for depression. The parents ask the nurse to encourage the adolescent to attend college. The nurse can intervene most therapeutically by:
1. encouraging family members to discuss their individual feelings about this issue.
2. explaining to the parents that the adolescent can make her own decision about college.
3. talking to the adolescent about the advantages of higher education.
4. refusing to get involved in this issue, which is unrelated to the client's treatment.

80. A client hospitalized with a diagnosis of schizophrenia recently started taking oral trifluoperazine (Stelazine), 2 mg three times daily. The client complains of progressively stiff, painful, and tense neck muscles. Given this data, the nurse suspects that the client is experiencing:
1. increased tension related to the illness.
2. an acute dystonic reaction.
3. symptoms of pseudoparkinsonism.
4. neuroleptic malignant syndrome.

81. The nurse is teaching a group of clients about the mood-stabilizing medication lithium carbonate. Which medications should she instruct the clients to avoid because of the increased risk of lithium toxicity?
1. Antacids
2. Antibiotics
3. Diuretics
4. Hypoglycemic agents

82. A client has been taking haloperidol (Haldol), 5 mg three times daily, to treat schizophrenia. The nurse routinely assesses for extrapyramidal side effects, which include all of the following except:
1. dry mouth and urine retention.
2. eyes rolling upward uncontrollably.
3. excessive motor restlessness.
4. tremors and shuffling gait.

83. When providing family therapy, the nurse analyzes the functioning of healthy family systems. Which situations would not increase stress on a healthy family system?
1. An adolescent's going away to college
2. The birth of a child
3. The death of a grandparent
4. Parental disagreement

84. A client with generalized anxiety disorder has been taking diazepam (Valium), 5 mg three times daily, for the past 2 weeks. At the outpatient clinic, the nurse assesses the client's knowledge about this drug. Which of the following statements indicates the need for further client instruction?
1. "I know this drug can be addicting."
2. "I understand that when I no longer need this drug, I'll gradually have to stop taking it."
3. "I won't drink alcohol while I'm taking this drug."
4. "I will take this drug only when I'm feeling upset."

85. Prior to administering chlorpromazine (Thorazine) to an agitated client, the nurse should:
1. assess skin color and sclera.
2. assess the radial pulse.
3. take the client's blood pressure.
4. ask the client to void.

86. The nurse evaluates the effectiveness of the neuroleptic drug olanzapine (Zyprexa) by noting which expected client outcome?
1. The client has increased motivation and improved social interaction.
2. The client has a decreased level of anxiety and normal sleep patterns.
3. The client has increased withdrawal and decreased interest in activities.
4. The client has decreased excitement and fewer episodes of panic.

87. A client taking the monoamine oxidase inhibitor (MAOI) antidepressant isocarboxazid (Marplan) is instructed by the nurse to avoid which foods and beverages?
1. Aged cheese and red wine
2. Milk and green, leafy vegetables
3. Carbonated beverages and tomato products
4. Lean red meats and fruit juices

88. A client who has been taking paroxetine (Paxil) for depression for the past 7 days reports no improvement in her mood and asks if the drug should be discontinued. The nurse responds correctly that the client should continue taking the medication based on which data?
    1. The drug's onset of action is 24 to 48 hours.
    2. The drug's onset of action is 2 to 3 weeks.
    3. The drug's effect may be diminished in major depression.
    4. The drug's effect may not always be readily observed by the client.

89. The nurse understands that electroconvulsive therapy is primarily used in psychiatric care for the treatment of:
    1. anxiety disorders.
    2. depression.
    3. mania.
    4. schizophrenia.

90. The nurse administering a typical antipsychotic medication, such as fluphenazine (Prolixin), by the oral route would know that this drug should be given:
    1. at least 2 hours after eating.
    2. at mealtimes or with milk.
    3. with plenty of water.
    4. without regard to meals.

91. Which atypical antipsychotic drug requires weekly testing of white blood cell counts for the first 6 months of treatment?
    1. clozapine (Clozaril)
    2. pimozide (Orap)
    3. olanzapine (Zyprexa)
    4. sertindole (Serdolect)

92. The nurse would expect an elderly client to have which of the following tests prior to initiation of therapy with tricyclic antidepressants?
    1. Electroencephalogram
    2. Baseline electrocardiogram
    3. Liver function studies
    4. Serum electrolyte studies

93. A client taking the MAOI phenelzine (Nardil) tells the nurse that he routinely takes all of the medications listed below. Which medication would cause the nurse to express concern and therefore initiate further teaching?
    1. acetaminophen (Tylenol)
    2. diphenhydramine (Benadryl)
    3. furosemide (Lasix)
    4. isosorbide dinitrate (Isordil)

94. Bupropion (Zyban) has been prescribed for a client as an aid in smoking cessation. Which medical problem would contraindicate the use of this drug?
    1. Angina pectoris
    2. Food allergies
    3. Rheumatoid arthritis
    4. Seizure disorder

95. The nurse is administering a psychotropic drug to an elderly client who has a history of benign prostatic hypertrophy. It is most important for the nurse to teach this client to:
    1. add fiber to his diet.
    2. exercise on a regular basis.
    3. report incomplete bladder emptying.
    4. take the prescribed dose at bedtime.

96. A client is admitted with major depressive disorder, not otherwise specified, following the recent divorce from his wife. He complains of sleep disturbance, poor energy level, and feeling helpless and hopeless. The nursing diagnosis is *Ineffective coping related to response to loss, secondary to recent divorce.* Which client outcome is most appropriate for this diagnosis?

1. The client will contact his wife and request a reconciliation.
2. The client will identify three strategies to use to handle his feelings related to the divorce.
3. The client will list the stressors that contributed to the marital problems.
4. The client will verbalize thoughts and feelings of hopelessness.

97. Which intervention is the priority when a nurse suspects a client is experiencing either neuroleptic malignant syndrome or serotonin syndrome?

1. Ensuring the client receives adequate fluids
2. Maintaining the client on bed rest
3. Monitoring the client frequently
4. Withholding further drug doses

98. The nurse correctly teaches a client taking the benzodiazepine oxazepam (Serax) to avoid excessive intake of:

1. cheese.
2. coffee.
3. sugar.
4. shellfish.

99. The nurse provides a referral to Alcoholics Anonymous to a client who describes a 20-year history of alcohol abuse. The primary function of this group is to:

1. encourage the use of a 12-step program.
2. help members maintain sobriety.
3. provide fellowship among members.
4. teach positive coping mechanisms.

100. Which client outcome is most appropriately achieved in a community-approach setting in psychiatric nursing?

1. The client performs activities of daily living and learns about crafts.
2. The client is able to prevent aggressive behavior and monitors his use of medications.
3. The client demonstrates self-reliance and social adaptation.
4. The client experiences anxiety relief and learns about his symptoms.

101. A client with panic disorder experiences an acute attack while the nurse is completing an admission assessment. List the following interventions according to their level of priority.

1. Remain with the client.
2. Encourage physical activity.
3. Encourage slow, deep breathing.
4. Reduce external stimuli.
5. Teach coping measures.

102. The doctor has prescribed haloperidol (Haldol) 2.5 mg. I.M. for an agitated client. The medication is labeled *haloperidol 10 mg/2 ml.* The nurse prepares the correct dose by drawing up how many milliliters in the syringe?

_____

Comprehensive Test: Answers

1. The answer is 4.

An interpreter will enable the nurse to better assess the client's problems and concerns. Nonverbal communication is important; however, for the nurse to fully determine the client's problems and concerns, the assistance of an interpreter is essential. The use of symbolic pictures and universal phrases may assist the nurse in understanding the basic needs of the client; however, these are insufficient to assess the client with a psychiatric problem.

2. The answer is 2.

The client's request is congruent with his cultural beliefs and should be honored. The nurse can help by acting as the client's advocate. Commenting on the appropriateness of a special healer in the hospital setting is a value judgment on the nurse's part; it would be inappropriate for the nurse to say this to the client. Reflecting that the client is seeking magical healing is an interpretative response based on the nurse's belief system and does not reflect the client's culture. A nurse who provides culturally sensitive nursing care would facilitate the request rather than referring this to the doctor. The client has the right to practice religious and cultural beliefs.

3. The answer is 4.

Termination is an important phase in the therapeutic relationship. The nurse and the client reassess the client's progress, evaluate goal attainment, and explore how the therapeutic relationship was experienced. It is also important to deal with feelings about termination during this phase. Assessment is an ongoing part of

the therapeutic relationship and occurs in all phases. The therapeutic relationship is also characterized by establishing trust (orientation phase) and planning outcomes and interventions to assist the client to meet goals (working phase).

4. The answer is 3.

When a client makes vague, global statements, the therapeutic approach is to seek clarification. Seeking clarification helps the client become more aware of thoughts, feelings, and ideas. In the responses of options 1 and 2, the nurse is making assumptions about the meaning of the client's statement and replying in such a way that further exploration of this client's concern is cut off. In option 4, the nurse is challenging the client to explain behaviors while reinforcing the notion that the client's belief is correct.

5. The answer is 1.

The behavioral framework is based on the premise that maladaptive behaviors are learned and can be changed by altering the environment that reinforces these behaviors. Techniques such as establishing a behavioral contract can be a form of operant conditioning in which the individual agrees to modify behavior according to specific rewards. Although the client learns to change behaviors, there is no established educational framework in psychiatric nursing. Neither an interpersonal framework nor a psychodynamic framework uses a reward system for change.

6. The answer is 4.

Psychoanalytic theory is based on Freud's beliefs regarding the importance of unconscious motivation for behavior and the role of the id and superego in opposition to each other. Behavioral, cognitive, and interpersonal theories do not emphasize unconscious conflicts as the basis for symptomatic behavior.

7. The answer is 2.
The client has the basic right to make decisions in areas affecting his life; this is the principle of autonomy. Managing funds is an example of one area in which the client exercises the right of autonomy. Unless a court declares the client incompetent, the family is legally unable to exert control in this area. Although the ANA Code of Ethics guides nursing practice, it does not address the legality of clients' rights. Confidentiality refers to the client's right to control disclosure of information related to health status and treatment. Commitment is the legal process governing psychiatric admission.

8. The answer is 2.
The principle of beneficence requires the nurse to act in ways that benefit the client. Offering other treatment options demonstrates the nurse's commitment to respect and honor client choices. Options 1 and 3 reflect a lack of understanding on the nurse's part of the legal issues of psychiatric nursing regarding the client's rights and the commitment process. Finally, the family cannot provide consent because, despite involuntary commitment, the client is still considered competent until judged otherwise by a court.

9. The answer is 1.
The ANA's Standards of Psychiatric and Mental Health Practice call for peer review as a mechanism for maintaining quality care. In the situation described, it would be better if a formal peer review system were in place to evaluate the nurse's performance. However, the colleagues are correct in expressing their concerns to the supervisor. The remaining answer choices do not address the nurses' responsibilities for upholding professional standards of practice.

10. The answer is 2.
Cognitive therapy focuses on the client's misperceptions about self, others, and the world that impact functioning and contribute to symptoms. Using medications to alter neurotransmitter activity is a psychobiologic approach to treatment. The other answer choices are frameworks for care, but they are not applicable to this situation

11. The answer is 3.
The concept that behavior is motivated and has meaning comes from the psychodynamic framework. According to this perspective, behavior arises from internal wishes or needs. Much of what motivates behavior comes from the unconscious. The remaining responses do not address the internal forces thought to motivate behavior.

12. The answer is 2.
Sullivan believed that a child develops a sense of self from the appraisal received from significant others. According to Sullivan, the infant will internalize the mother's increased anxiety levels. The other theorists do not place emphasis on the relationship process.

13. The answer is 3.
The client is demonstrating faulty thought processes that are negative and that govern his behavior in his work situation—issues that are typically examined using a cognitive theory approach. Issues involving learned behavior are best explored through behavior theory, not cognitive

theory. Issues involving ego development are the focus of psychoanalytic theory. Option 4 is incorrect because there is no evidence in this situation that the client has conflictual relationships in the work environment.

14. The answer is 4.

According to Selye's general adaptation theory, the body responds to stress in three stages: the first stage is the alarm reaction, the second is resistance, and the third is exhaustion if the stress continues. The best way to incorporate this information into a nursing intervention is to explain how the body responds to stress. The other answer choices reflect specific actions the nurse would implement with clients in a stress management program.

15. The answer is 4.

By acknowledging the observed behavior and asking the client to express his feelings, the nurse can best assist the client to become aware of his anxiety. In option 1, the nurse is offering an interpretation that may or may not be accurate; the nurse is also asking a question that may be answered by a "yes" or "no" response, which is not therapeutic. In option 2, the nurse is intervening before accurately assessing the problem. Option 3, which also encourages a "yes" or "no" response, avoids focusing on the client's anxiety, which is the reason for his pacing.

16. The answer is 1.

Flashbacks and nightmares from past experiences are common in those suffering from posttraumatic stress disorder. Clients with this disorder respond with intense fear to these "relived" events. Insufficient data is available to establish the nursing diagnoses in options 2 and 4. Option 3 is incorrect because the client with posttraumatic stress disorder has a known

fear that is directly related to the traumatic events precipitating his disorder.

17. The answer is 2.

The fear of having a serious disease is the essential feature of a person with hypochondriasis. The statement in option 1 is more typical of someone with a somatoform disorder. The statements in options 3 and 4 could apply to many psychiatric disorders.

18. The answer is 4.

Anxiety is a response to a threat arising from internal or external stimuli. The remaining answer choices are incorrect.

19. The answer is 1.

Systematic desensitization is a behavioral therapy technique that helps clients with irrational fears and avoidance behavior to face the thing they fear, without experiencing anxiety. There is no attempt to promote insight with this procedure, and the client will not be taught to substitute one fear for another. Although the client's anxiety may decrease with successful confrontation of irrational fears, the purpose of the procedure is specifically related to performing activities that typically are avoided as part of the phobic response.

20. The answer is 1.

A client with obsessive-compulsive behavior uses this behavior to decrease anxiety. Accepting this behavior as the client's attempt to feel secure is therapeutic. When a specific treatment plan is developed, other nursing responses may also be acceptable. The remaining answer choices will increase the client's anxiety and therefore are inappropriate.

21. The answer is 2, 4, 5.

Difficulty concentrating or focusing and feeling irritable and on edge are all symptoms of generalized anxiety disorder. Blank affect and echolalia are characteristic symptoms of someone with a schizophrenic disorder. Suspicion is a common symptom of a paranoid disorder.

22. The answer is 1.
Education and work history would have the least significance in relation to the client's sexual problem. Age, health status, physical attributes, and relationship issues have great influence on sexual expression.

23. The answer is 3.
In this situation, the nurse should maintain a calm, matter-of-fact response to avoid increasing the client's anxiety, which typically is elevated during emotional outbursts. This response will also help defuse the client's anger. Ignoring the client's underlying feelings would not help the client gain control of outbursts. Isolating a client with borderline personality disorder will further increase anxiety because those with borderline personality disorder usually fear being alone. Promoting group interaction would be inappropriate because such clients tend to be narcissistic and might monopolize the group; also the increased stimuli of a group setting could elevate the client's anxiety.

24. The answer is 2.
A client with antisocial personality disorder typically has frequent episodes of acting impulsively with poor ability to delay self-gratification. Therefore, decreased frequency of impulsive behaviors would be evidence of improvement. Charming behavior when around authority figures and statements indicating no remorse are examples of symptoms typical of someone with this disorder and would not indicate successful treatment. Self-satisfaction would be viewed as a positive

change if the client expresses low self-esteem; however, this is not characteristic of a client with antisocial personality disorder.

25. The answer is 4.
In autoimmune disorders, stress and the response to stress can exacerbate symptoms. Stress management techniques can help the client reduce the psychological response to stress, which in turn will help reduce the physiologic stress response. This will afford the client an increased sense of control over his symptoms. The nurse can address the remaining answer choices in her teaching about the client's disease and treatment; however, knowledge alone will not help the client to manage his stress effectively enough to control symptoms.

26. The answer is 1, 2, 5.
In anorexia nervosa, amenorrhea results from loss of estrogen stores in fat tissue. Decreased heart rate (bradycardia) results from the decreased metabolic rate and loss of heart muscle tissue that occurs with starvation. Lanugo, the downy body hair characteristic of anorexic clients, results from loss of subcutaneous tissue. Diarrhea, hypertension, and tachycardia are not expected with this disorder.

27. The answer is 4.
The client with anorexia typically feels powerless, with a sense of having little control over any aspect of life besides eating behavior. Often, parental expectations and standards are quite high and lead to the client's sense of guilt over not measuring up.

28. The answer is 3.
Inpatient treatment of a client with anorexia usually focuses initially on establishing a plan for refeeding to combat the effects

of self-induced starvation. Refeeding is accomplished through behavioral therapy, which uses a system of rewards and reinforcements to assist in establishing weight restoration. Emphasizing nutrition and teaching the client about the long-term physical consequences of anorexia may be appropriate at a later time in the treatment program. The nurse needs to assess the client's mealtime behavior continually to evaluate treatment effectiveness.

29. The answer is 1, 2, 4, 6.
New physical symptoms should be assessed because organic causes of illness are possible and must be ruled out in somatoform disorder. The nurse should encourage independent behavior to help increase the client's self-esteem and sense of control. Focusing on the client's underlying emotional responses or feelings rather than on his chronic physical symptoms is one of the goals of therapy. Teaching relaxation techniques will help decrease the client's anxiety, thereby reducing his need to displace his feelings onto physical symptoms.

30. The answer is 1.
One of the core issues concerning the family of a client with anorexia is control. The family's acceptance of the client's ability to make independent decisions is key to successful family intervention. Although the remaining options may occur during the process of therapy, they would not necessarily indicate a successful outcome; the central family issues of dependence and independence are not addressed in these responses.

31. The answer is 4.
The client with a somatoform disorder displaces anxiety onto physical symptoms. The ability to express anxiety verbally indicates a positive change toward improved

health. The remaining responses do not indicate any positive change toward increased coping with anxiety.

32. The answer is 4.
Disregard for established rules of society is the most common characteristic of a client with an antisocial personality disorder. Attention to detail and order is characteristic of someone with obsessive-compulsive disorder. Bizarre mannerisms and thoughts are characteristic of a client with schizoid or schizotypal disorder. Submissive and dependent behaviors are characteristic of someone with a dependent personality.

33. The answer is 2.
Behavioral changes are often subtle in persons with personality disorders. Withdrawn behavior is not typical, and improvement does not occur rapidly with these clients. The nurse may allow personal feelings to overrule professional judgment; however, this problem would probably affect the entire nurse-client relationship, not just the evaluation phase.

34. The answer is 1, 2, 5, 6.
A client with major depression typically experiences loss of appetite and constipation related to decreased food and fluid intake and lack of activity. The client may have difficulty sleeping and usually feels tired and fatigued as a result of disturbed sleep patterns. Increased perspiration and thirst are not commonly associated with depression.

35. The answer is 3.
Directly questioning a client about suicide is important to determine suicide risk. The client may not bring up this subject for several reasons, including guilt regarding suicide, wishing not to be discovered, and his lack of trust in staff. Behavioral cues are

important, but direct questioning is essential to determine suicide risk. Indirect questions convey to the client that the nurse is not comfortable with the subject of suicide and, therefore, the client may be reluctant to discuss the topic.

36. The answer is 2.

Use of cognitive techniques allows the nurse to help the client recognize that his negative beliefs may be distortions and that, by changing his thinking, he can adopt more positive beliefs that are realistic and hopeful. Agreeing with the client's feelings and presenting a cheerful attitude are not consistent with a cognitive approach and would not be helpful in this situation. Denying the client's feelings is belittling and may convey that the nurse does not understand the depth of the client's distress.

37. The answer is 3.

A client exhibiting flight of ideas typically has a continuous speech flow and jumps from one topic to another. Speaking in coherent sentences is an indicator that the client's concentration has improved and his thoughts are no longer racing. The remaining options do not relate directly to the stated nursing diagnosis.

38. The answer is 1.

Art therapy provides a nonthreatening vehicle for the expression of feelings, and use of a small group will help the client become comfortable with peers in a group setting. Basketball is a competitive game that requires energy; the client with major depression is not likely to participate in this activity. Recommending that the client read a self-help book may increase, not decrease, his isolation. Watching a movie with a peer group does not guarantee that interaction will occur; therefore, the client may remain isolated.

39. The answer is 3.

Day treatment programs provide clients with chronic, persistent mental illness training in social skills, such as meeting and greeting people, asking questions or directions, placing an order in a restaurant, and taking turns in a group setting or activity. Although management of hallucinations and medication teaching may also be part of the program offered in day treatment, the nurse is referring the client in this situation because of his need for socialization skills. Vocational training generally takes place in a rehabilitation facility; the client described in this situation would not be a candidate for this service.

40. The answer is 4.

Setting firm, nonpunitive limits and providing a structured environment are the best approaches to handling a verbally hostile client. Administering antipsychotic medication and the use of seclusion are too severe, considering that the outbursts are brief and there is no escalation to physical violence. Walking away when the outbursts occur would not be as useful in setting clear limits on inappropriate behavior.

41. The answer is 1.

The best approach with a withdrawn client is to initiate brief, nondemanding activities on a one-to-one basis. This approach gives the nurse an opportunity to establish a trusting relationship with the client. A board game with a group of clients or playing a team sport in the gym may overwhelm a severely withdrawn client. Watching TV is a solitary activity that will reinforce the client's withdrawal from others.

42. The answer is 2.

The best approach to delusional ideas is to avoid arguing with them while simultaneously acknowledging reality. It is also important to respond to the underlying message or the predominant feeling of the client. In this case, the client is frightened, so the nurse addresses this by saying she believes that the client is safe here. Option 1 would be premature; when the client has some improvement, it may be possible to discuss delusions as part of the illness. Options 3 and 4 place too much emphasis on the delusions and, therefore, they are inappropriate.

43. The answer is 3.

The nurse should take any statements indicating suicidal thoughts seriously and further assess for other risk factors. The remaining diagnoses fail to address the seriousness of the client's statement.

44. The answer is 2.

This response allows the nurse to handle the issue of inappropriate dress in a way that preserves the client's dignity and provides an opportunity for her to select more appropriate clothes. Option 1 is incorrect because this does not directly address the client's distorted thinking (she may choose another inappropriate outfit). Option 3 would embarrass the client and, again, does not provide any specific direction for more appropriate clothing. Option 4 is too vague (the client may not understand what the nurse means by "more conservative clothes").

45. The answer is 3.

Depersonalization is a feeling of strangeness or unreality about one's own body or body parts. Autism is a focus inward; the individual may create a fantasy world. Ambivalence is having strong opposing emotions about a person or situation. Regression is a defense mechanism whereby the individual returns to an earlier, more comfortable form of behavior.

46. The answer is 4.

This statement provides accurate information and an element of hope for the family of a schizophrenic client. Although the remaining statements are true, they do not provide the empathic response the family needs after just learning about the diagnosis. These facts can become part of the ongoing teaching.

47. The answer is 1.

A client with schizophrenia, paranoid type, has distorted perceptions and views people, institutions, and aspects of the environment as plotting against him. The desired outcome for someone with delusional perceptions would be to have a realistic interpretation of daily events. The client with a distorted perception of the environment would not necessarily have impairments affecting hygiene and grooming skills. Although taking medications and participating in unit activities may be appropriate outcomes for nursing intervention, these responses are not related to client perceptions.

48. The answer is 2.

In this situation, the client's family history presents the most significant stressor affecting her vulnerability for substance abuse. Genetic theory and cognitive-behavioral theory have both established this factor as highly significant. Abandonment by the father and the trauma of the rape and subsequent pregnancy are stressors that may significantly affect the client's normal growth and development, possibly increasing her susceptibility to either depressive illness or posttraumatic stress disorder. The client's poor school attendance and failing grades are symptomatic of significant problem areas, not the cause of the substance abuse.

49. The answer is 1.
In children, depression is often manifested by acting-out behaviors (in contrast to an adult in which behavior is often withdrawal from interaction with others). Excessive sadness, hopelessness, and helplessness may also be seen in a child with depression. A poor parental relationship is a factor that would increase the child's vulnerability to depressive illness. School problems may be associated with multiple psychiatric problems in children and are not specific to depression. Although suicide attempt is a sign of depressive illness, it is not commonly seen in a young child. The fact that this child has demonstrated this would warrant his hospitalization in order to provide a safe environment and decrease the risk of suicide.

50. The answer is 4.
A client with these symptoms would have poor impulse control and would therefore be prone to acting-out behavior that may be harmful to either himself or others. All of the remaining nursing diagnoses may apply to the client with mania; however, the priority diagnosis would be risk for violence.

51. The answer is 4.
A client who has a history of substance abuse will have cross-tolerance to the medications used for analgesia. In this situation, in which the client has traumatic injuries, pain control will be a priority concern for nursing care. The client history already has documented use of an abusive substance; the client's denial of this would be a defense mechanism and would not be of priority concern. Difficulty

establishing a nurse-client relationship may or may not occur with this client; it would not be of priority concern. Drug-seeking behaviors would be anticipated; however, this client has multiple traumatic injuries, and therefore pain control would be a priority concern.

52. The answer is 3.
Rationalization is the defense mechanism that involves offering excuses for maladaptive behavior. The client is defending his substance abuse by providing reasons related to life stressors. This is a common defense mechanism used by clients with substance abuse problems. None of the remaining defense mechanisms involves making excuses for behaviors.

53. The answer is 3.
Tolerance is the need for increased amounts of a substance to obtain the desired effect. It is one of the characteristics of substance dependence. Concurrent abuse of two different substances is polydrug use. Continued use of a substance in the absence of life problems would be the criterion for substance dependence. Occurrence of physiologic symptoms when the drug is discontinued is the phenomenon of withdrawal.

54. The answer is 1, 3, 6.
Alcohol withdrawal is characterized by central nervous system stimulation, including agitation and increased pulse and blood pressure. Drowsiness, bradycardia, and decreased blood pressure do not occur in alcohol withdrawal.

55. The answer is 4.
These nonvictim family members have been witnesses to violent acts and are part of a dysfunctional family system. They require help in coping with their emotional responses, which may include fear and

guilt. Available data do not support the assumption that nonvictims are more traumatized. Encouraging nonvictim family members to seek alternative living arrangements encourages family alienation and is not indicated.

56. The answer is 2.

Physical aggressiveness, low stress tolerance, and a disregard for the rights of others are common behaviors in clients with conduct disorders. Restlessness, short attention span, and hyperactivity are typical behaviors in a client with attention deficit hyperactivity disorder. Deterioration in social functioning, excessive anxiety and worry, and bizarre behaviors are typical in schizophrenic disorders. Sadness, poor appetite, sleeplessness, and loss of interest in activities are behaviors commonly seen in depressive disorders.

57. The answer is 2.

Family systems therapy aims to promote responsible self-functioning in families in which there are blurred generational boundaries and evidence of undifferentiated family ego mass. Family members may be encouraged to verbalize their feelings; however, this is not the primary purpose of treatment. Identifying perpetrators of violence is part of the assessment process; it is not the primary purpose of therapy. The child victims of abuse will be helped by the adult members who are developing more responsible self-functioning.

58. The answer is 2.

The nurse's attitudes can affect the treatment of the client. Negative attitudes can be indirectly communicated and can damage the client's self-esteem. Neither counseling the client about her lifestyle and needed changes nor identifying the legal implications, health risks, and drug effects on her fetus would be the first intervention; these interventions should be done only when the nurse can demonstrate respect and a nonjudgmental attitude. Reviewing literature on substance abuse and its impact on pregnant women is incorrect as the first intervention, although it may prove helpful for the nurse who lacks information about female addicts.

59. The answer is 2.

Babies born to heroin-dependent women are also heroin-dependent and need to go through withdrawal. There is no evidence to support any of the remaining answer choices.

60. The answer is 4.

Establishing an unbroken chain of evidence is essential in order to ensure that the prosecution of the perpetrator can occur. The nurse will also need to preserve the client's privacy and identify the extent of injury. However, it is essential that the nurse follow legal and agency guidelines for preserving evidence. Identifying the assailant is the job of law enforcement, not the nurse.

61. The answer is 4.

Socioeconomic status is not a reliable predictor of abuse in the home, so it would be the least important consideration in deciding issues of safety for the victim of family violence. The availability of appropriate community shelters and the ability of the nonabusing caretaker to intervene on the client's behalf are important factors when making safety decisions. The client's response to possible relocation (if the client is a competent adult) would be the most important factor to consider; feelings of empowerment and being treated as a competent person can help a client feel less like a victim.

62. The answer is 3.

As with many psychiatric disorders, a combination of factors (including biological, genetic, and psychosocial factors) contributes to the cause of schizophrenia. Disturbed family relations and communication problems are not considered true based on research findings. Options 2 and 4 have been implicated in the cause; however, they are not the only causative factors involved.

63. The answer is 3.

A support group functions to provide empathy for members who have experienced similar problems and also focuses on reinforcing existing strengths. Option 1 would be appropriate for a community living group, such as an inpatient unit. Option 2 would be more appropriate for a socialization group. Option 4 would be appropriate for an educational group.

64. The answer is 2.

Open and honest discussion of conflict will promote healthy interaction and the ability of members to tolerate differences and negotiate solutions. Discussing the situation privately with the individual clients involved and providing specific information on how to resolve the conflict are not appropriate interventions because the nurse is solving the problem rather than encouraging the group process to handle and resolve the conflict. If the nurse ignores the existence of conflict in a group, the group loses an opportunity to learn how to resolve differences.

65. The answer is 1.

In the early stage of Alzheimer's disease, complex tasks (such as balancing a checkbook) would be the first cognitive deficit to occur. The loss of self-care ability, problems with relating to family members, and difficulty remembering one's own name are all areas of cognitive decline that occur later in the disease process.

66. The answer is 1, 4, 5.

Delirium occurs rapidly, usually related to an acute physiologic cause; it is characterized by sudden onset of acute confusion as well as motor changes ranging from agitation to somnolence. Dementia is a cognitive impairment disorder, characterized by gradual onset and subtle initial symptoms. Pacing and wandering at night are part of the sundowning effect of dementia.

67. The answer is 4.

Olanzapine is an atypical antipsychotic (neuroleptic) that is used to decrease psychiatric or irrational thinking. Lorazepam is a benzodiazepine (antianxiety agent) ordered for anxiety on an as-needed basis. Clonazepam is also a benzodiazepine ordered to decrease anxiety. Sertraline is an antidepressant used to decrease depressive symptoms.

68. The answer is 3.

The client with Alzheimer's disease can have frequent episodes of labile mood, which can best be handled by decreasing a stimulating environment and redirecting the client's attention. An overstimulating environment may cause the labile mood, which will be difficult for the client to understand. The client with Alzheimer's disease loses the cognitive ability to respond to either humor or logic. The client lacks any insight into his or her own behavior and therefore will be unaware of any causative factors.

69. The answer is 1.

A relative deficiency of acetylcholine is associated with this disorder. The drugs used in the early stages of Alzheimer's disease will act to increase available acetylcholine in the brain. The remaining neurotransmitters have not been implicated in Alzheimer's disease.

70. The answer is 3.

The client's daughter has the characteristic signs of a caretaker who is becoming overwhelmed with her role. Such signs may include feelings of stress in the relationship with the care receiver, depression, and possibly anger. Although the family's processes may be interrupted and its usual coping mechanisms disabled, the symptoms described in this situation reflect caregiver role strain. There is no evidence that the caregiver is socially isolated in this situation.

71. The answer is 3.

The most important factors to determine in this situation are the client's perception of the crisis event and the availability of support (including family and friends) to provide basic needs. Although the nurse should assess the other factors, they are not as essential as determining why the client considers this a crisis and whether he can meet his present needs.

72. The answer is 1.

The first stage of grieving consists of shock and disbelief. In this phase, the family is faced with the realization that their loved one is dead. Exhibiting helplessness and withdrawal are more typical of the second phase of grief. Sharing fond memories about the deceased and stating how much they miss their family member typically occur after grief is resolved.

73. The answer is 4.

Crisis intervention is based on the idea that a crisis is a disturbance in homeostasis (steady state). The goal is to help the client return to a previous level of equilibrium in functioning. The remaining answer choices are not considered the primary outcome of crisis intervention, although they may occur as a side benefit.

74. The answer is 2.

Increased anxiety and uncertainty characterize the initiation phase in group therapy. Group members are more self-reliant during the working and termination phases.

75. The answer is 2.

The use of the pronouns "our" and "we" enhances the sense of the group as a viable unit. The nurse is also clarifying the purpose of the group, which will not restrict spontaneity. Her statements address group norms. The purpose of group therapy is not to prevent conflict, but to work on resolving problem areas.

76. The answer is 1.

As the group progresses into the working phase, group members assume more responsibility for the group. The leader becomes more of a facilitator. Comments about behavior in a group are indicators that the group is active and involved. The remaining answer choices would indicate the group progress has not advanced to the working phase.

77. The answer is 2.

During the termination phase, group members need to evaluate the progress of the group and themselves. Deciding to continue the group denies the termination process; not attending any more sessions avoids the issue entirely. Focusing on positive experiences would fail to deal with all the issues of termination (both negative and positive experiences should be reviewed).

78. The answer is 3.
In good family communication, family members openly encourage clear, direct discussions of issues and feelings. Members recognize that their feelings and thoughts are important and valued, which fosters their ability to initiate discussion. Evidence that the children accept and adopt the parental value system does not necessarily indicate good communication. Children may adopt the parental value system in a family where communication is maladaptive. Agreement among family members may indicate good communication; however, members may be enmeshed, in which case individuals are not free to express differences. Parents may feel that they communicate to their children; however, good communication requires feedback. The nurse must further assess whether children can communicate freely with the parents.

79. The answer is 1.
When working with families, the nurse needs to remain neutral and avoid taking sides. Encouraging each family member to discuss this issue will promote communication among members and allow for clarification of individual feelings. The answers in options 2 and 3 indicate that the nurse has chosen to agree with either the adolescent or the parents on this issue. Option 4 is not therapeutic and dismisses an opportunity to encourage family communication.

80. The answer is 2.
These are classic symptoms of dystonia. The specificity of symptoms is more definitive of dystonia than of tension.

Parkinsonian symptoms include akinesia or generalized rigidity, drooling, and pill-rolling movements. Neuroleptic malignant syndrome, a rare condition, is characterized by high fever, muscle rigidity, hypertension, and diaphoresis.

81. The answer is 3.
The use of diuretics would cause sodium and water excretion, which would increase the risk of lithium toxicity. Clients taking lithium carbonate should be taught to increase their fluid intake and to maintain normal intake of sodium. Concurrent use of any of the remaining medications will not increase the risk of lithium toxicity.

82. The answer is 1.
Dry mouth and urinary retention are anticholinergic side effects that can occur with use of neuroleptic medications, not extrapyramidal effects. All of the remaining symptoms are extrapyramidal side effects that would be assessed routinely while a client is taking haloperidol.

83. The answer is 4.
In a functional family, parents typically do not agree on all issues and problems. Open discussion of thoughts and feelings is healthy, and parental disagreement should not cause system stress. The remaining answer choices are life transitions that are expected to increase family stress.

84. The answer is 4.
This statement is incorrect and would cause the nurse to question the client's ability to take the medication as prescribed. Further teaching is needed. The remaining statements are correct and indicate that the client has a good understanding of the medication's use and effects.

85. The answer is 3.

Because chlorpromazine (Thorazine) can cause a significant hypotensive effect (and possible client injury), the nurse must assess the client's blood pressure (lying, sitting, and standing) before administering this drug. If the client had taken the drug previously, the nurse would also need to assess the skin color and sclera for signs of jaundice, a possible drug side effect; however, based on the information given here, there is no evidence that the client has received chlorpromazine before. Although the drug can cause urine retention, asking the client to void will not alter this anticholinergic effect.

86. The answer is 1.

This atypical antipsychotic is especially effective for both the negative and positive symptoms of schizophrenia. Therefore, an expected outcome would be increased motivation and improved social interaction. This medication is not used to decrease anxiety levels or to normalize sleep. Increased withdrawal and decreased interest in activities would indicate a worsening of the negative symptoms of schizophrenia and would not be the expected outcome of this drug. This medication is not used for either excitation or panic responses.

87. The answer is 1.

Aged cheese and red wines contain the substance tyramine which, when taken with an MAOI, can precipitate a hypertensive crisis. The other foods and beverages do not contain significant amounts of tyramine and, therefore, are not restricted.

88. The answer is 2.

The onset of action of the SSRI antidepressant paroxetine occurs around 3 to 4 weeks after drug therapy begins. Therefore, a client will seldom notice improvement before this time. Continuing to take the drug is important for this client.

89. The answer is 2.

Electroconvulsive therapy is used primarily in the treatment of depression, generally when a client has not responded to antidepressant medications. Electroconvulsive therapy is not used for anxiety disorders, mania, or schizophrenia.

90. The answer is 1.

Oral absorption of the typical antipsychotic medications is significantly affected by food and stomach acidity level. Therefore, these agents should be taken at least 2 hours after eating and not used concurrently with antacids or histamine$_2$-blocking agents.

91. The answer is 1.

Because clozapine may cause agranulocytosis, the FDA mandates white blood cell count testing as described. The remaining atypical agents are not associated with agranulocytosis; therefore, weekly white blood cell count testing is not required.

92. The answer is 2.

Tricyclic antidepressants are associated with an increased risk of cardiovascular effects, especially in elderly clients; therefore, a baseline electrocardiogram is expected. The remaining studies are not routinely done prior to antidepressant therapy in elderly clients.

93. The answer is 2.

Over-the-counter medications used for allergies and cold symptoms are contraindicated because they will increase the sympathomimetic effects of MAOIs, possibly causing a hypertensive crisis.

None of the remaining medications will increase the sympathomimetic response and, therefore, are not contraindicated.

94. The answer is 4.
Bupropion increases the risk of seizures; therefore, a client with a history of seizure disorder would not be able to take this drug. None of the remaining medical problems would constitute a problem for a client taking bupropion.

95. The answer is 3.
Urinary retention is a common anticholinergic side effect of psychotic medications, and the client with benign prostatic hypertrophy would have increased risk for this problem. Adding fiber to one's diet and exercising regularly are measures to counteract another anticholinergic effect, constipation. Depending on the specific medication and how it is prescribed, taking the medication at night may or may not be important. However, it would have nothing to do with urinary retention in this client.

96. The answer is 2.
At this point, the client is not coping effectively; with intervention, he should be able to identify strategies that will improve his coping ability. Contacting the wife and requesting reconciliation would not be an expected outcome because it does not address the reality of the client's problem, which is adjusting to the divorce. Listing stressors that contributed to the marital problems and verbalizing thoughts and feelings of hopelessness would be appropriate as initial steps in gathering data related to the client's problem.

97. The answer is 4.
Both neuroleptic malignant syndrome and serotonin syndrome are life-threatening complications of psychotropic medications. Neuroleptic malignant syndrome may occur with neuroleptic medications, whereas serotonin syndrome may occur with antidepressant medications. In either case, any further doses of medication would be contraindicated. All of the remaining measures may be used, but the priority is avoiding further doses of the offending medications.

98. The answer is 2.
Coffee contains caffeine, which has a stimulating effect on the central nervous system that will counteract the effect of the antianxiety medication oxazepam. None of the remaining foods is contraindicated.

99. The answer is 2.
The primary purpose of Alcoholics Anonymous is to help members achieve and maintain sobriety. Although each of the remaining answer choices may be an outcome of attendance at Alcoholics Anonymous, the primary purpose is directed toward sobriety of members.

100. The answer is 3.
A therapeutic community is designed to help individuals assume responsibility for themselves, to learn how to respect and communicate with others, and to interact in a positive manner. The remaining answer choices may be outcomes of psychiatric treatment, but the use of a therapeutic community approach is concerned with promotion of self-reliance and cooperative adaptation to being with others.

101. The answer is 14325.

The nurse should remain with the client to provide support and promote safety. Reducing external stimuli, including dimming lights and avoiding crowded areas, will help decrease anxiety. Encouraging the client to use slow, deep breathing will help promote the body's relaxation response, thereby interrupting stimulation from the autonomic nervous system. Encouraging physical activity will help him to release energy resulting from the heightened anxiety state; this should be done only after the client has brought his breathing under control. Teaching coping measures will help the client learn to handle anxiety; however, this can only be accomplished when the client's panic has dissipated and he is better able to focus.

102. The answer is 0.5.

Set up the problem as follows:

$$\frac{2.5 \text{ mg}}{10 \text{ mg}} = \frac{X \text{ ml}}{2 \text{ ml}}$$

$$X = 0.5 \text{ ml}$$

Selected References

Aguilera, D.C. *Crisis Intervention: Theory and Methodology,* 8th ed. St. Louis: Mosby-Year Book, Inc., 1998.

American Nurses Association. *Scope and Standards of Psychiatric-Mental Health Practice.* Washington, D.C.: American Nurses Publishing, 2000.

American Pharmaceutical Association. *Medication Management Considerations in Schizophrenia.* Washington, D.C.: American Pharmaceutical Association, 2002.

American Psychiatric Association. *Diagnostic and Statistical Manual of Mental Disorders,* 4th ed., Text Revision. Washington, D.C.: American Psychiatric Association, 2000.

Andrews, M.M., and Boyle, J.S. *Transcultural Concepts in Nursing Care,* 4th ed. Philadelphia: Lippincott Williams & Wilkins, 2002.

Baier, M., and Murray, R.L.E. "A Descriptive Study of Insight into Illness Reported by Persons with Schizophrenia," *Journal of Psychosocial Nursing and Mental Health Services* 37(1): 14–21, 1999.

Bailey, K.P. "Psychopharmacology Grand Rounds: Aripiprazole," *Journal of Psychosocial Nursing and Mental Health Services* 41(2): 4-18, 2003.

Bain, L.J. "Defining the Basis of Manic Depression," *NARSAD Research Newsletter* 10(4): 14, 1998.

"Battling Back from Childhood Sexual Abuse—And Surviving the Journey," *Journal of Psychosocial Nursing and Mental Health Services* 36(12): 13–17, 1998.

Berlinger, J. "Why Don't You Just Leave Him?" *Nursing98* 28(4): 34–39, 1998.

Bisson, J.I. and Kitchiner, N.J. "Early Psychosocial and Pharmacological Interventions after Traumatic Events," *Journal of Psychosocial Nursing and Mental Health Services* 41(10): 42-51, 2003.

Bonnel, W.B. "Not Gone and Not Forgotten: A Spouse's Experience of Late-Stage Alzheimer's Disease," *Journal of Psychosocial Nursing and Mental Health Services* 34(8): 23–27, 1996.

Bowen, M. *Family Therapy in Clinical Practice.* New York: Jason Aronson, 1978.

Bradley, K.A., et al. "Alcohol Screening Questionnaires in Women: A Critical Review," *JAMA* 280(2): 166–171, 1998.

Brightman, H. "Manic and Depressive Recurrences: Search for Mechanisms and Treatments," *NARSAD Research Newsletter* 10(2): 14, 1998.

Brown, A., and Lempa, M. "Update on Potential Causes and New Treatments for Anxiety Disorders," *NARSAD Research Newsletter Fall/Winter:* 13-18, 1996.

Brown, A., and Weaver R. "How Related Are Autism and Childhood Schizophrenia?" *NARSAD Research Newsletter Fall* (10): 13–19, 1998.

Brown, S.W., et al. "Process-Oriented Critical Pathways in Inpatient Psychiatry: Our First Year," *Journal of Psychosocial Nursing and Mental Health Services* 36(6): 31–36, June 1998.

Burgess, A.W. *Psychiatric Nursing: Promoting Mental Health.* Stamford, Conn.: Appleton & Lange, 1997.

Burgess, A.W. "Connections," *Alzheimer's Disease Education and Referral Center* 7(2), 1998.

Burkhardt, M.A., and Nathaniel, A.K. *Ethics and Issues in Contemporary Nursing.* Albany, N.Y.: Delmar Pubs., 2002.

Chez, N. "Helping the Victim of Domestic Violence," *American Journal of Nursing* 94(7): 32–37, 1994.

Deglin, J.W., and Hazard-Vallerand, A.H. *Davis's Drug Guide for Nurses,* 9th ed. Philadelphia: F.A. Davis Co., 2004.

Evans, B., et al. "Complementary Therapies and HIV Infection," *American Journal of Nursing* 99(2): 42–45, Feb. 1999.

Fine, J.I., and Rouse-Bane, S. "Using Validation Techniques to Improve Communication with Cognitively Impaired Older Adults," *Journal of Gerontological Nursing* 21(6): 39–45, 1995.

Finfgeld, D.L. "Use of Brief Interventions to Treat Individuals with Drinking Problems," *Journal of Psychosocial Nursing and Mental Health Services* 37(4): 23–30, 1999.

Fontaine, K.L., and Fletcher, J.S. *Mental Health Nursing,* 5th ed. Upper Saddle River, N.J.: Prentice-Hall, 2003.

Fortinash, K.M., and Holoday-Worret, P.A., eds. *Psychiatric-Mental Health Nursing,* 3rd ed. St. Louis: Mosby-Year Book, Inc., 2004.

Frisch, N., et al. *Psychiatric Mental Health Nursing,* 2nd ed. Albany, N.Y.: Delmar Pubs., 2002.

Giger, J.N., and Davidhizer, R.E. *Transcultural Nursing: Assessment and Intervention,* 4th ed. St. Louis: Mosby-Year Book, Inc., 2002.

Glod, C.A. *Contemporary Psychiatric-Mental Health Nursing: The Brain–Behavior Connection.* Philadelphia: F.A. Davis, 1998.

Goodman, M.B., and Ahmann, E. "Child Abuse," *Pediatric Nursing* 1(1): 69-72, 2001.

Greenwald, J., and Blackman, A. "Herbal Healing," *Time* 152(21): 58, Nov. 1998.

Haggerty, B.M. "Advances in Understanding Major Depressive Disorder," *Journal of Psychosocial Nursing and Mental Health Services* 33(11): 27–34, 1995.

Health Care Financing Administration. *Hospital Conditions of Participation: Patients' Rights: Interim Final Rule.* Washington, D.C.: HCFA, 1999.

Hobbs, H., et al. "The Alumni Program: Redefining Continuity of Care in Psychiatry," *Journal of Psychosocial Nursing and Mental Health Nursing* 37(1): 23–29, 1999.

Hockenberry, M.J. *Wong's Essentials of Pediatric Nursing,* 7th ed. St. Louis: Mosby-Year Book, Inc., 2005.

Johnson, B.S. "The 5 R's of Becoming a Psychiatric Nurse Practitioner: Rationale, Readying, Roles, Rules, and Reality," *Journal of Psychosocial Nursing and Mental Health Services* 38(9): 20–24, 1998.

Jones, J.E. "Chronic Anxiety and the Adrenocortical Response and Differentiation," *Family Systems: Journal of Natural Systems Thinking in Psychiatry and the Sciences,* 1(2): 30–38, 1994.

Keltner, N.L., et al. *Psychiatric Nursing,* 4th ed. St. Louis: Mosby-Year Book, Inc., 2003.

Keltner, N.L., et al. *Psychobiological Foundation of Psychiatric Care.* St. Louis: Mosby-Year Book, 1998.

Kerr, M. "A Systems Model for Disease," *Theory and Practice.* Washington, D.C.: Georgetown Family Center, 1997.

Keys, S.G., et al. "Transforming School Counseling to Serve Mental Health Needs of At-Risk Youth," *Journal of Counseling and Development,* 76(4): 381–87, 1998.

Kneisl, C.R., et al., eds. *Contemporary Psychiatric-Mental Health Nursing.* Upper Saddle River, N.J.: Prentice-Hall, 2004.

Leonard, B. "Quality Nursing Care Celebrates Diversity," *Online Journal of Issues in Nursing* 6(2), May 2001.

Lesseig, D.Z. "Pharmacotherapy for Long-Term Care Residents with Dementia-Associated Behavioral Disturbance," *Journal of Psychosocial Nursing and Mental Health Services* 36(2): 27–31, 1998.

Lisofsky, T. "New Treatment for Opioid Dependence," *General Community Pharmacy Newsletter.* Wilkes-Barre: Wyoming Valley Health Care System, 2003.

Mayfield, D.G., et al. "The CAGE Questionnaire: Validation of a New Alcoholism Screening Instrument," *American Journal of Psychiatry* 131(10): 1112-23, 1974.

Mendlewicz, J. "Genetic Vulnerability," *NARSAD Research Newsletter,* 10(4), 11–13, 1998.

Minuchin, S. *Families and Family Therapy.* Cambridge, Mass.: Harvard University Press, 1974.

Mohr, W.K. "Cross-Ethnic Variations in Care of Psychiatric Patients: A Review of Contributing Factors and Practice Considerations," *Journal of Psychosocial Nursing and Mental Health Services* 36(5): 16–21, 1998.

Mohr, W.K. *Johnson's Psychiatric-Mental Health Nursing,* 5th ed. Philadelphia: Lippincott Williams & Wilkins, 2002.

Mohr, W.K. "Updating What We Know About Depression in Adolescents," *Journal of Psychosocial Nursing and Mental Health Services* 36(9): 12–19, 1998.

Morse, J.M. "Exploring Empathy: A Conceptual Fit for Nursing Practice?" *Image: Journal of Nursing Scholarship* 24(4): 273-80, Winter 1992.

Myers, S. *ADHD Management, 2001 Update for Pediatric Practitioner.* Unpublished paper, 2001.

Mynatt, S. "A Model of Contributing Risk Factors to Chemical Dependency in Nurses," *Journal of Psychosocial Nursing and Mental Health Services* 34(7): 13–22, 1996.

NARSAD (National Alliance for Research on Schizophrenia and Depression) *NARSAD Research Newsletter,* 9(34), 1997.

NARSAD. *NARSAD Research Newsletter,* 10(2), 1998.

NARSAD. *NARSAD Research Newsletter,* 10(4), 1998.

National Institute on Drug Abuse (NIDA). *NIDA Infofax: Nationwide Trends.* Bethesda, Md.: National Institutes of Health, 2004.

Nemeroff, C.B. "Neurobiology of Depression," *Scientific American* 298(6): 42-47, 1998.

Newman, C.F. "Cognitive Therapy with Depressed and Suicidal Adolescents," *Healing Magazine,* 4(1): 24–27, 1999.

Nugent, E. "Try to Remember: Reminiscence As a Nursing Intervention," *Journal of Psychosocial Nursing and Mental Health Services,* 3(11): 7–11, 1995.

Poliafico, F.J. "Abstinence Is Not the Only Answer," *RN* 62(1): 58–60, Jan. 1999.

Ratey, J.J. *A User's Guide to the Brain: Perception, Attention, and the Four Theaters of the Brain.* New York: Pantheon Books, 2001.

Richman, D. "To Restrain or Not to Restrain?" *RN* 61(7): 55–58, 1998.

Satir, V. *Conjoint Family Therapy.* Palo Alto, Calif.: Science and Behavior Books, 1964.

Shea, C., et al. "Breaking Through the Barriers to Domestic Violence Intervention," *American Journal of Nursing* 97(6): 26–33, 1997.

Spencer, V.E. "Combined Therapy in OCD," *Journal of Psychosocial Nursing and Mental Health Services* 34(7): 37–40, 1996.

Townsend, M. *Essentials of Psychiatric/Mental Health Nursing,* 3rd ed. Philadelphia: F.A. Davis, 2005.

Wakefield, M., and Pallister, R. "New Hope for a Disabling Condition: Cognitive-Behavioral Approaches to Panic Disorder," *Journal of Psychosocial Nursing and Mental Health Services* 35(3): 12–20, 1997.

Wilson, J.H., and Hobbs, H. "The Family Educator: A Professional Resource for Families," *Journal of Psychosocial Nursing and Mental Health Services* 37(6): 22–27, 1999.

Wolfe, S. "Look for Signs of Abuse," *RN* 61(8): 48–54, 1998.

Yalom, I.D. *The Theory and Practice of Group Psychotherapy,* 4th ed. New York: Basic Books, 1994.

Zanarini, M.C., et al. "Reported Pathological Childhood Experiences Associated with Development of Borderline Personality Disorders," *American Journal of Psychiatry* 154(8): 1101-06, 1997.

Zook, R. "Take Action Before Anger Builds," *RN* 59(4): 46–50, 1996.

INDEX

i refers to an illustration; t refers to a table.

i refers to an illustration; t refers to a table.

i refers to an illustration; t refers to a table.

i refers to an illustration; t refers to a table.

i refers to an illustration; t refers to a table.

i refers to an illustration; t refers to a table.

About the CD-ROM

Lippincott's Review Series CD-ROMs provide a convenient way to assess readiness for academic tests and licensure exams. More than 200 carefully selected multiple-choice and alternate-formate questions are provided for study and simulated testing.

Minimum system requirements

- Windows 98
- Pentium 166
- 128 MB RAM
- 8 MB of free hard-disk space
- SVGA monitor with high color (16-bit)
- CD-ROM drive

Installation

Place the CD in your CD-ROM drive. After a few moments, the install process will automatically begin. *Note:* If the install process doesn't automatically begin, click the Start button and select Run. At the command line, type *D:\setup.exe*. (Note: The letter D represents the CD-ROM drive. If your drive is designated by a different letter, use your drive letter instead.) Click OK. Follow the installation instructions.

Technical support

For technical support, call toll-free 1-800-638-3030, Monday through Friday, 8:30 a.m. to 5 p.m. Eastern Time. You may also write to Lippincott Williams & Wilkins Technical Support, 351 W. Camden Street, Baltimore, MD 21201-2436, or e-mail us at techsupp@lww.com.